Clinical Practice of Medical Mycology in Asia

Arunaloke Chakrabarti
Editor

Clinical Practice of Medical Mycology in Asia

Springer

Editor
Arunaloke Chakrabarti
Department of Medical Microbiology
Postgraduate Institute of Medical Education and Research (PGIMER)
Chandigarh
India

ISBN 978-981-13-9461-4 ISBN 978-981-13-9459-1 (eBook)
https://doi.org/10.1007/978-981-13-9459-1

This Springer imprint is published by the registered company Springer Nature Singapore Pte Ltd.
The registered company address is: 152 Beach Road, #21-01/04 Gateway East, Singapore 189721, Singapore

Distinctive Features of the Book

- The book will cover **fungal infections specific to Asian countries**
- The **unique epidemiology** of fungal infections in Asian countries will be covered
- **Diagnosis and management** of fungal infections **in resource-limited environment** will be stressed
- Chapters will be comprehensive in such way that **busy clinicians can go through** it quickly
- The book will **NOT be exhaustive** on each disease, but will provide knowledge of salient features required while managing fungal diseases in Asian countries
- Each chapter will be **summarized in a box** for quick recollection; **more tables rather than description**

Contents

Editors and Contributors

About the Editor

Arunaloke Chakrabarti graduated from Calcutta Medical College, Calcutta University, India, and completed his MD at the Postgraduate Institute of Medical Education and Research, Chandigarh, India, where he is currently a Professor and Head of the Department of Medical Microbiology. He has a keen interest in the epidemiology of fungal sinusitis, sporotrichosis, mucormycosis, and hospital-acquired fungal infections, and he has published over 300 papers in the field. He is Co-Chair of Asian Fungal Working Group and Chair of Fungal Infections Study Forum. He is a Section Editor/Associate Editor/Deputy Editor of five international journals. He is currently the President of the International Society for Human and Animal Mycology.

Contributors

O. C. Abraham Department of Medicine and Infectious Diseases, Christian Medical College, Vellore, Tamil Nadu, India

Ritesh Agarwal Department of Pulmonary Medicine, Post Graduate Institute of Medical Education and Research (PGIMER), Chandigarh, India

Suhail Ahmad Department of Microbiology, Faculty of Medicine, Kuwait University, Safat, Kuwait

Sanjay Bhattacharya Department of Microbiology, Tata Medical Center, Kolkata, India

Arunaloke Chakrabarti Department of Medical Microbiology, Postgraduate Institute of Medical Education and Research (PGIMER), Chandigarh, India

Pranatharthi H. Chandrasekar Division of Infectious Diseases, Department of Medicine, Wayne State University, School of Medicine, Detroit, MI, USA

Karmanos Cancer Center, Detroit, MI, USA

Yee-Chun Chen Division of Infectious Diseases, Department of Internal Medicine, National Taiwan University Hospital, Taipei, Taiwan

Department of Medicine, National Taiwan University, College of Medicine, Taipei, Taiwan

National Institute of Infectious Diseases and Vaccinology, National Health Research Institutes, Miaoli County, Taiwan

Ariya Chindamporn Mycology Unit, Department of Microbiology, Faculty of Medicine, Chulalongkorn University, Bangkok, Thailand

Anup Ghosh Department of Medical Microbiology, Postgraduate Institute of Medical Education and Research (PGIMER), Chandigarh, India

Harsimran Kaur Department of Medical Microbiology, Postgraduate Institute of Medical Education and Research (PGIMER), Chandigarh, India

Ziauddin Khan Department of Microbiology, Faculty of Medicine, Kuwait University, Safat, Kuwait

Pankaj Malhotra Department of Internal Medicine, Postgraduate Institute of Medical Education and Research (PGIMER), Chandigarh, India

Valliappan Muthu Department of Pulmonary Medicine, Post Graduate Institute of Medical Education and Research (PGIMER), Chandigarh, India

Suganthini Krishnan Natesan John D. Dingell VA Medical Center, Detroit, MI, USA

Division of Infectious Diseases, Department of Medicine, Wayne State University, School of Medicine, Detroit, MI, USA

Atul K. Patel Infectious Diseases Clinic, "VEDANTA" Institute of Medical Sciences, Ahmedabad, India

Shivaprakash M. Rudramurthy Department of Medical Microbiology, Postgraduate Institute of Medical Education and Research (PGIMER), Chandigarh, India

Dipika Shaw Department of Medical Microbiology, PGIMER, Chandigarh, India

Tanu Singhal Kokilaben Dhirubhai Ambani Hospital and Medical Research Institute, Mumbai, India

Department of Paediatrics, Kokilaben Hospital, Mumbai, India

Rajeev Soman Department of Medicine and Division of Infectious Diseases, P.D. Hinduja Hospital and Medical Research Centre, Mumbai, India

Jupiter Hospital, Pune, India

Ayesha Sunavala Department of Medicine, Division of Infectious Diseases, PD Hinduja Hospital, Mumbai, India

Subramanian Swaminathan Gleneagles Global Hospitals, Chennai, India
Gleneagles Global Hospitals, Bengaluru, India

Ban-Hock Tan Department of Infectious Diseases, Singapore General Hospital, Singapore, Singapore

Subhash Todi Director Critical Care, AMRI Hospitals, Kolkata, India

Navaporn Worasilchai Mycology Unit, Department of Microbiology, Faculty of Medicine, Chulalongkorn University, Bangkok, Thailand

1 Introduction

Arunaloke Chakrabarti

Of nearly 1.5 million fungi in the environment, nearly 400–500 species are now known to cause human disease. The spectrum of fungi causing human infection is ever increasing with the rise of susceptible population at risk for invasive mycoses. This has happened largely due to climate change, healthcare related factors, and adaptation of fungi in human host. For all benefits to mankind, modern medicine has developed this expanding population with low immunity and anatomical barrier break. The traditional group of patients who are known to be at risk of acquiring fungal infections include the patients with hematological malignancies undergoing chemotherapy, transplant recipients, patients with AIDS, severe burns, prematurity, and autoimmune diseases. During the last decade, the range of susceptible patients has increased. New risk factors like admission in ICU, chronic liver and renal diseases, diabetes, and post H1N1 influenza are added to this list. Even the so-called immunocompetent hosts are occasionally found to acquire invasive fungal infections (IFIs) due to direct introduction of fungi through indwelling devices, trauma or due to exposure of large inoculums of fungal spores in respiratory tract. Fungal spore count in the environment of the hospital and community is very high in majority of the Asian countries [1]. The exact burden of IFIs in Asian countries is still not known, as the disease is largely unrecognized, not notified, and difficult to diagnose. The limitation of diagnostic mycology laboratories in those countries is another challenge [2]. The awareness of IFIs among clinicians is also limited to few tertiary care centers only. It is estimated that over 800 millions people globally suffer from IFIs and annual death due to IFIs (1,660,000) is comparable to malaria (445,000) or to tuberculosis (1,700,000) [3].

While discussing IFIs in Asia, one should remember that more than half of world's population lives in this region. The population is a large economically deprived section who do not get proper healthcare facilities and a small portion of

A. Chakrabarti (✉)
Department of Medical Microbiology, Postgraduate Institute of Medical Education and Research (PGIMER), Chandigarh, India

A. Chakrabarti (ed.), *Clinical Practice of Medical Mycology in Asia*,
https://doi.org/10.1007/978-981-13-9459-1_1

privileged section who get modern management including transplants and advanced medical interventions. Both extremes of population develop IFIs for different reasons. A large number of untrained health professionals, misuse of steroids and broad-spectrum antibiotics, intravenous drug abuse, and compromised hospital care practices in this region add to the risk of IFIs. Many countries of this region are in tropical zone where fungi thrive easily and disperse large number of spores in the air. Construction activities in the hospital without protective covering from the patient care area, climate change, and natural disasters have contributed further in the epidemiology of IFIs [4, 5].

IFIs can be broadly classified into endemic and opportunistic mycoses. The prevalent endemic mycoses in Asian countries include histoplasmosis, talaromycosis (penicilliosis), and sporotrichosis. Blastomycosis and emergomycosis are occasionally reported [6, 7]. Few cases of coccidioidomycosis have been reported as imported mycoses. Only one case of imported paracoccidioidomycosis has been recognized in Japan [8]. Among opportunistic mycoses, invasive candidiasis is the commonest disease followed by aspergillosis and mucormycosis. In certain center, cryptococcosis has been reported at high rate. Other opportunistic fungal infections like fusariosis and scedosporiosis are occasionally reported. The rarity of non-*Aspergillus* molds may be due to limited facilities for identification of these infections [9, 10].

Though the importance of fungal infections is increasingly recognized in Asian countries, the understanding of the magnitude of problem and its socio-economic impact remains largely unknown. The available limited data predict high incidence of IFIs in Asian countries. Invasive candidiasis has been recorded at 4–15 times higher frequency compared to developed countries. The disease may have different epidemiology in Asian countries. In an Indian study covering intensive care units, candidemia was reported as early infection in young patients with less morbidity [11]. The incidence of mucormycosis has been estimated at nearly 70 times the generally accepted rates in western countries. Endemic disease, talaromycosis is restricted only in south-east Asian countries. Allergic fungal rhinosinusitis is highly prevalent in certain geographical locations. Many new fungi have emerged in Asian countries causing human infections and are linked with unique presentation of IFIs. Recent emergence of multi-drug resistant *C. auris* infection globally was first reported from Japan. Subsequently reported from South Korea, India, Pakistan, Kuwait, Oman, Singapore, Thailand, and China. *C. auris* infected patients possibly exist in all Asian countries, but failed to be recognized or identified due to difficulty in identification of the fungus by conventional procedures [12, 13]. Infection due to *Apophysomyces variabilis* is highly prevalent in India; *Mucor irregularis* has been reported to cause cutaneous mucormycosis mainly in South-East China and few places of India; *Ramichloridium mackenziei* and *Veronea botryosa* are known to cause phaeohyphomycosis only in Asian Countries. High prevalence of cerebral abscess due to *Cladophialophora bantiana* has been recorded in India. All these unique features stress the need of systematic epidemiological studies of IFIs in Asia [9, 14].

Despite the development of many new antifungal agents in last two decades, the mortality of IFIs has not come down significantly. This is largely due to delay in diagnosis of IFIs. By the time antifungal drugs are prescribed, the IFIs are widely disseminated and fail to respond to therapy. Early diagnosis is the need of the hour. The diagnosis of IFIs still relies largely on conventional techniques including direct microscopy and culture. The limitations of conventional techniques are poor sensitivity and long turnaround time. Proper sample collection from deep tissue is also a challenge, as the patients are mostly thrombocytopenic and/or neutropenic. High resolution CT scan has improved the suspicion of IFIs, but HRCT is not available in all tertiary care centers. Moreover, by the time lesion is macroscopic and visible on CT scan, the prognosis of the disease becomes poor for obvious reasons. Alternative procedures like galactomannan, beta-glucan, mannan detection, and DNA detection by polymerase chain reaction have been attempted in diagnosis of IFIs. The results are encouraging, as it improved the sensitivity of diagnostic tests and IFIs could be diagnosed early. But the techniques are either not validated or not available in most of the centers of Asian countries. In a recent survey of seven Asian countries, it was noted that biomarker tests are largely not available in Thailand, Philippines, and Indonesia [2]. Therefore, diagnosis of IFIs remains a challenge in this region and clinicians rely more on empiric than on targeted therapy [15].

To treat the IFIs, three groups of antifungal agents—polyene, azoles, and echinocandins—are available. Though conventional polyene-amphotericin B deoxycholate is considered as the pan-antifungal agent, its use in developed countries has seriously been curtailed due to its toxicity. The lipid preparations of amphotericin B are commonly used to treat IFIs. However, in Asian countries amphotericin B deoxycholate is widely used due to its low cost. Among azoles, voriconazole and posaconazole have broad spectrum of activity compared to fluconazole and itraconazole. In Asian countries, fluconazole and to certain extent itraconazole are widely used due to the same reason of resource limitation. The new triazole, isavuconazole is still not available. 5-fluorocytosine is also not available in majority of the countries. All three echinocandins—caspofungin, anidulafungin, and micafungin—are available in major part of Asian market and have cidal activity against *Candida*, but its use is limited to the patients who can afford it. For optimal use of antifungal agents, antifungal stewardship program is also essential in Asian region [16].

In conclusion, the devastating IFIs in Asia has drawn the attention of clinicians, medical mycologists, and epidemiologists to work together to face the challenge and improve the patient management. Different chapters of the book have highlighted the unique epidemiology, challenges in diagnosis and possible management guidelines in greater details. In each chapter, the major issues are highlighted in a box.

Important Features of Invasive Fungal Infections (IFIs) in Asia

- Incidence—Within available limited data, IFIs are 3–15 times more common in Asian countries than western world. Possible reasons of high incidence:
  - Many countries in Asia are located in tropics where fungi thrive easily due to congenial weather.

- Over-capacity patient load in public sector hospitals leads to compromise in healthcare.
- Solid organ and bone marrow transplant centers are increasing in all countries, but majority patients cannot afford to buy medicines post-transplant.
- Systemic steroid and antibiotics are available over the counters and misused by so-called "quacks" (untrained health professional).
- Sub-optimal infection control practices.
- Very large number of diabetics with poor compliance to therapy—may be the reason of high incidence of mucormycosis.

• Diseases
  - Endemic mycoses.

    Histoplasmosis and talaromycosis cases have increased in patients with HIV infections.

    Talaromycosis is only endemic in South-east Asia.

    Sporotrichosis—high incidence in certain geographical areas.
  - Opportunistic mycoses

    Candidiasis—*C. tropicalis* is commonest agent in majority of the countries especially in tropical region; outbreak due to unusual *Candida* species has been reported; *Candida auris* infection is prevalent in Asian countries; *Candida* pancreatitis is an emerging problem.

    Aspergillosis—High number of cases is related to high fungal spore count in the environment (hospital and community); fungal rhinosinusitis is prevalent in certain areas; *Aspergillus* endophthalmitis is an important challenge especially in rural population; *A. flavus* rather than *A. fumigatus is* common in rhinosinusitis, endophthalmitis, and central nervous system infections.

    Mucormycosis—very high incidence in India and China; associated more with uncontrolled diabetes; isolated renal mucormycosis is a new clinical entity in China and India; *Apophysomyces variabilis* is an emerging mucoraceous fungus in India; new rare pathogens are reported to cause mucormycosis—*Rhizopus homothallicus, Rhizomucor variabilis, Saksenaea vasiformis, Thamnostylum lucknowense.*

    Cryptococcosis—the incidence is still very high in HIV positive population despite introduction of antiretroviral therapy in all countries; the reason of high incidence may be poor affordability for antiretroviral drug or poor compliance; *C. grubii* and *C. gattii* are reported from majority countries, but the frequency of *C. gattii* infection is very limited; both varieties are isolated from environment of Asian countries.

• Diagnosis—challenges
  - Awareness about fungal infections is still limited.
  - Very few competent diagnostic mycology laboratories.
  - Existing laboratories rely on conventional techniques.
  - Galactomannan and beta-glucan are available in limited laboratories.
  - Delay in diagnosis leads to higher mortality in IFIs.

- Therapy
  - Common antifungal agents are now available in majority of the countries in Asia, but the antifungal use remains restricted to amphotericin B deoxycholate, fluconazole, and itraconazole in majority of cases due to poor affordability.
  - Attributable mortality in IFIs is high—reason may be multifactorial: delay in seeking medical attention, delay in diagnosis, compromise in use of antifungal agents, confounding factors, etc.
  - Empiric therapy is common occurrence due to insensitivity of available diagnostic procedures.
  - Comparatively higher resistance to antifungal drugs among prevailing fungi.
  - No country-specific management guideline for IFIs is available.

References

1. Rudramurthy SM, Singh G, Hallur V, Verma S, Chakrabarti A. High fungal spore burden with predominance of Aspergillus in hospital air of a tertiary care hospital in Chandigarh. Indian J Med Microbiol. 2016;34:529–32.
2. Chindamporn A, Chakrabarti A, Li R, Sun PL, Tan BH, Chua M, Wahyuningsih R, Patel A, Liu Z, Chen YC, Chayakulkeeree M. Survey of laboratory practices for diagnosis of fungal infection in seven Asian countries: An Asia Fungal Working Group (AFWG) initiative. Med Mycol. 2018;56:416–25.
3. Brown GD, Denning DW, Levitz SM. Tackling human fungal infections. Science. 2012;336:647.
4. Chakrabarti A, Chatterjee SS, Shivaprakash MR. Overview of opportunistic fungal infections in India. Jpn J Med Mycol. 2008;49:165–72.
5. Chakrabarti A, Singh R. The emerging epidemiology of mould infections in developing countries. Curr Opin Infect Dis. 2011;24:521–6.
6. Chakrabarti A, Slavin MA. Endemic fungal infections in Asia-Pacific region. Med Mycol. 2011;49:337–44.
7. Malik R, Capoor MR, Vanidassane I, Gogna A, Singh A, Sen B, Rudramurthy SM, Honnavar P, Gupta S, Chakrabarti A. Disseminated Emmonsia pasteuriana infection in India: a case report and a review. Mycoses. 2016;59:127–32.
8. Onda H, Komine M, Murata S, Ohtsuki M. Letter: imported paracoccidioidomycosis in Japan. Dermatol Online J. 2011;17:11.
9. Slavin MA, Chakrabarti A. Opportunistic fungal infections in the Asia-Pacific region. Med Mycol. 2012;50:18–25.
10. Arunaloke C, Sekhar CS, Ashim D, Shivaprakash MR. Invasive aspergillosis in developing countries. Med Mycol. 2011;49 (Suppl. I:S35–47.
11. Chakrabarti A, Sood P, Rudramurthy SM, Chen S, Kaur H, Capoor M, Chhina D, Rao R, Eshwara VK, Xess I, Kindo AJ, Umabala P, Savio J, Patel A, Ray U, Mohan S, Iyer R, Chander J, Arora A, Sardana R, Roy I, Appalaraju B, Sharma A, Shetty A, Khanna N, Marak R, Biswas S, Das S, Harish BN, Joshi S, Mendiratta D. Incidence, characteristics and outcome of ICU acquired candidemia in India. Intensive Care Med. 2015;41:285–95.
12. de Cássia Orlandi Sardi J, Silva DR, Soares Mendes-Giannini MJ, Rosalen PL. Candida auris: epidemiology, risk factors, virulence, resistance, and therapeutic options. Microb Pathog. 2018;125:116–21.

13. Jeffery-Smith A, Taori SK, Schelenz S, Jeffery K, Johnson EM, Borman A, Candida auris Incident Management Team, Manuel R, Brown CS. Candida auris: a review of the literature. Clin Microbiol Rev. 2017;31. pii:e00029–17.
14. Chakrabarti A, Shivaprakash MR, Curfs-Breuker I, Baghela A, Klaassen CH, Meis JF. Apophysomyces elegans: epidemiology, AFLP typing, and in vitro antifungal susceptibility pattern. J Clin Microbiol. 2010;48:4580–5.
15. Perfect JR. Fungal diagnosis: how do we do it and can we do better? Curr Med Res Opin. 2013 Apr;29(Suppl 4):3–11.
16. Wattal C, Chakrabarti A, Oberoi JK, Donnelly JP, Barnes RA, Sherwal BL, Goel N, Saxena S, Varghese GM, Soman R, Loomba P, Tarai B, Singhal S, Mehta N, Ramasubramanian V, Choudhary D, Mehta Y, Ghosh S, Muralidhar S, Kaur R. Issues in antifungal stewardship: an opportunity that should not be lost. J Antimicrob Chemother. 2017;72:969–74.

Part I

Epidemiology in Asia

Epidemiology of Superficial Fungal Infections in Asia

2

Shivaprakash M. Rudramurthy and Dipika Shaw

2.1 Introduction

Superficial fungal infections are the large group of infections of the skin and mucous membrane due to fungi. Most common superficial fungal infections include dermatophytosis (tinea or ringworm), pityriasis versicolor, oral thrush, and vulvovaginal candidiasis. Keratitis, which is the inflammation of the cornea caused due to fungi, is also considered under superficial fungal infections. In addition, seborrheic dermatitis/dandruff, the sub-acute or chronic superficial inflammatory skin conditions associated *Malassezia* may also be included under this group of infections. Rare superficial fungal infections are tinea nigra, white piedra, and black piedra.

Superficial fungal infections are common fungal infections that have worldwide distribution. The prevalence of these infections varies across different geographical regions and is more prevalent in the regions with hot and humid climate including the tropical regions of Asia. Though the clinical presentation of the disease is generally similar, there are certain differences in distribution of individual fungal species across different geographic regions. Due to the extensive distribution of the diseases under this group of infections, the current chapter will only discuss cutaneous fungal infections/disease and fungal keratitis.

2.2 Epidemiology of Dermatophytosis in Asia

Dermatophytes are the oldest group of fungi implicated with superficial infections affecting 20–25% of general population throughout the world [1, 2]. Infections due to dermatophytes are known since its first description in 1830s from the clinical samples of tinea by Robert Remark, a Polish physician. Infection mainly spread through direct contact with infected humans, animals, and soil [1, 3]. Dermatophytes belong to group

S. M. Rudramurthy (✉) · D. Shaw
Department of Medical Microbiology, Postgraduate Institute of Medical Education and Research (PGIMER), Chandigarh, India

A. Chakrabarti (ed.), *Clinical Practice of Medical Mycology in Asia*,
https://doi.org/10.1007/978-981-13-9459-1_2

of keratinophilic fungi. They damage the keratinous tissue of skin, hair, and nail, thus causing tinea or ringworm infection (dermatophytosis) [4]. Tinea infection can be classified according to the site involved such as tinea corporis (body), tinea cruris (groin), tinea barbae (beard), tinea faciei (face), tinea incognito (steroid modified), tinea unguium (nail), and tinea capitis (hair) [5, 6]. The fungi under the broad group called "Dermatophytes" belong to three closely related genera: *Epidermophyton, Trichophyton,* and *Microsporum.* On the basis of natural habitat, they are classified as geophilic (dermatophytes that are naturally present in the soil), zoophilic (animals), and anthropophilic (humans) [1]. Diagnosis can be easily achieved based on the clinical presentation and direct microscopic examination of the skin scrapings using potassium hydroxide-calcofluor wet mount preparation (Fig. 2.1a). Over the past several years upsurge in the frequency of dermatophytosis cases has been noted. Management of dermatophytosis is becoming challenging due to increase in the number of cases of treatment failure, relapses (re-occurrence of the dermatophyte infection within few weeks, after completion of treatment), and chronicity (persistent dermatophytosis that runs a chronic course with episodes of remission and exacerbation) [7–10]. Dermatophytes can thrive in hot and humid climatic conditions and occur mainly in tropics and subtropical countries. They also can cause an epidemic outbreak in area of overcrowding and poor hygienic conditions [11–13].

Trichophyton species are the major causative agents with prevalence rate of 70–90% of onychomycosis cases and 53.1–86% with other tinea infection [14, 15]. The epidemiology of dermatophytosis is widely studied and has been shown that it varies with time and geographic area [16]. Before 1980s, *M. audouinii* and *T. schoenleinii* were recognized as main etiological agents for tinea capitis in British island, Europe and America [17]. *T. rubrum* rarely caused scalp infection but was commonly associated with other form of tinea worldwide. *T. mentagrophytes* and *E. floccosum* (Fig. 2.1b–d) were also frequently involved in skin and nail infections [16]. Various epidemiological surveys conducted from the Asian countries revealed *T. violaceum* (India) and *M. ferrugineum* (China and Japan) as the predominant causative agent of tinea capitis [18, 19]. Compared to worldwide data, a smaller number of tinea capitis cases have been reported in Asian countries [17]. Post 1980s, worldwide, the commonest species causing tinea infection other than tinea capitis was *T. rubrum* followed by *T. mentagrophytes* [13]. Whereas, the common causative agent of tinea capitis shifted to *M. canis* in Europe and Asia and *T. tonsurans* (Fig. 2.1e, f) in Americas and United Kingdom [16].

2.3 Epidemiology of Dermatophytes in India

The epidemiology of dermatophytosis has been significantly changed in India especially in terms of increasing number of cases of chronic, relapse, or recurrent infection even after completing full course of treatment, wide distributions of lesions, and resistance to the major classes of antifungal drugs (allylamines and azoles) [10, 20]. Depending on clinical settings, 15–20% of patients visiting dermatology outpatient departments (OPD) and clinics present with chronic or recurrent

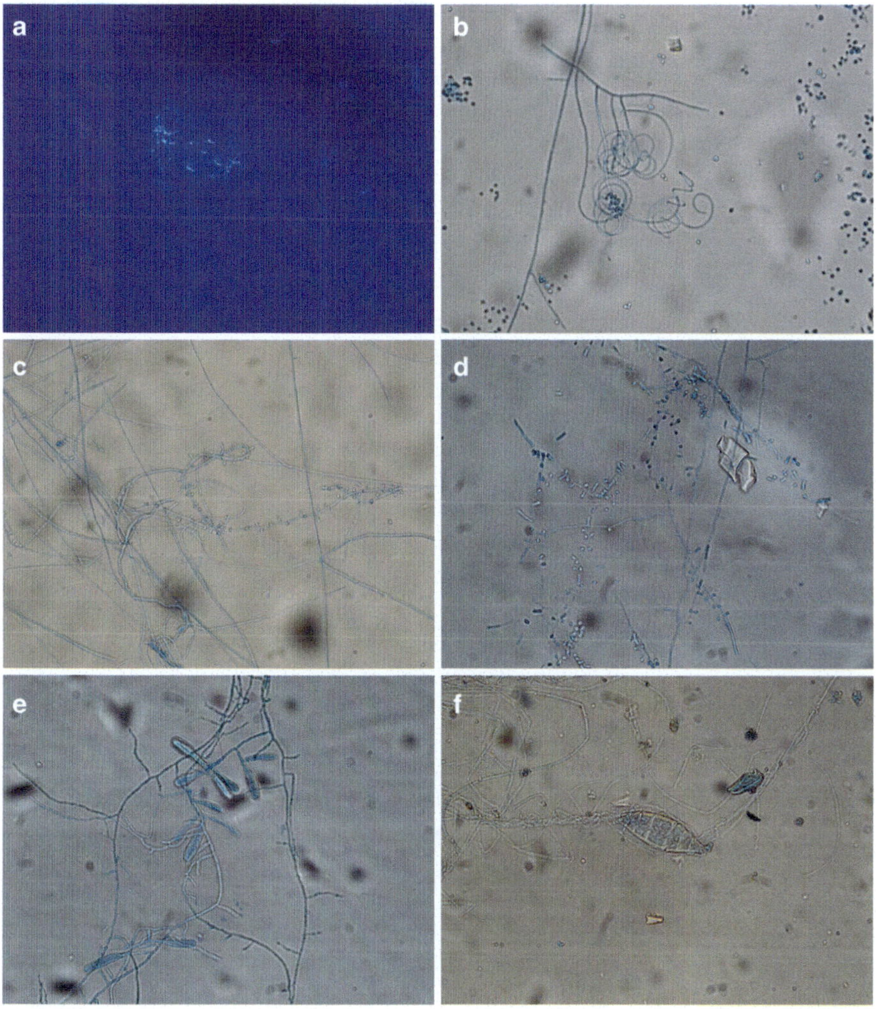

Fig. 2.1 (**a**) Direct microscopy of skin scrapings under calcofluor- pottasium hydroxide wet-mount examination, (**b**) *Trichophyton mentagrophytes complex,* (**c**) *Trichophyton rubrum*, (**d**) *Trichophyton tonsurans*, (**e**) *Epidermophyton floccosum*, (**f**) *Microsporum canis*

dermatophytosis. Though the reasons for this phenomenon are not clear, it has been related to several factors such as the use of irrational combination of creams containing corticosteroids, inadequate treatment regimen, discontinuation of medication, difficulties in eliminating predisposing factors, and re-infection due to inadequate source control [21]. In addition, resistance to the major class of antifungals has also been attributed to some extent [22].

Earlier, majority of patients usually presented with classical tinea lesion that includes erythematous papule or plaque that spreads centrifugally resulting in annular ring lesion with scales and well-defined margins. Of late, majority of patients present with widespread atypical lesions such as loss of active erythematous edges, lesions spreading with irregular margins mimicking other dermatological conditions such as eczema, erythema multiforme, seborrheic dermatitis, lupus erythematosus, dermatitis herpetiformis, rosacea, eczematous dermatitis, psoriasis, impetigo, and polymorphous light eruption. These atypical lesions have been attributed to rampant usage of topical cream with irrational fixed-dose combination (FDC) containing high-potency steroid- antifungal- antibiotic for varying time period (Fig. 2.2a–e) [23]. Such clinical presentations of tinea rarely reported in literature

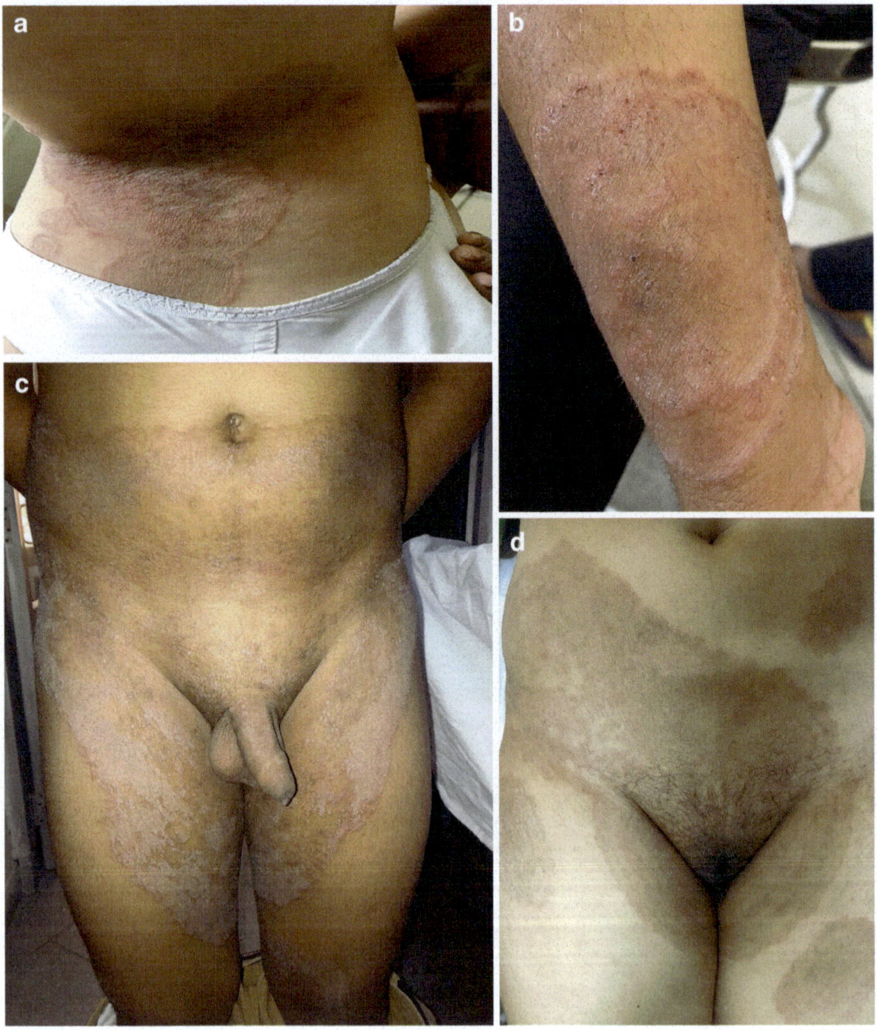

Fig. 2.2 (**a**) Tinea corporis with typical presentation, (**b**) Tinea corporis ring within ring presentation, (**c**, **d**) Tinea cruris with atypical presentation, (**e**) Tinea faciei with atypical presentation, (**f**) Seborrheic dermatitis, (**g**) Pityriasis versicolor

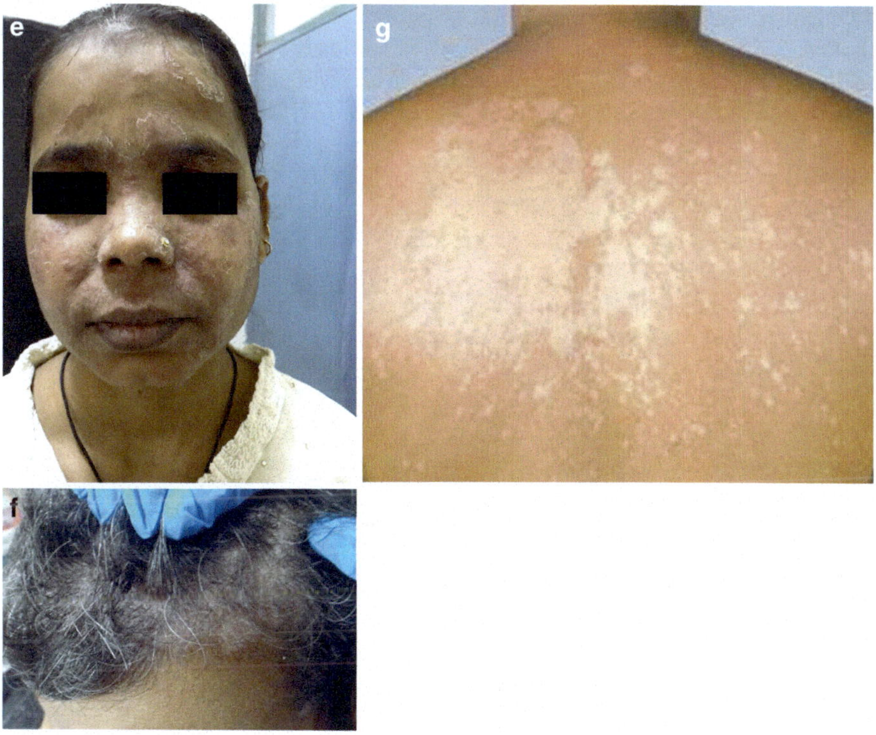

Fig. 2.2 (continued)

are now being routinely seen in India [23, 24]. Recently, Nenoff et al. reported 81.3% of dermatophytosis cases with steroid modified dermatophytosis due to the use of fixed-dose combinations (FDC) creams available over the counter without prescription [24]. Though corticosteroids may alleviate itching and redness, it does not eliminate the fungus from the skin surfaces, rather lead to apparent remission with atypical appearance [25, 26]. The current prevalence rate of dermatophytosis in India ranges between 36.6 and 78.4% [27] with a higher prevalence (27–36%) among the younger age group and in males [28–31]. This may be attributed to the involvement of younger age group in various outdoor activities and recreational activities increasing the chances of contracting dermatophyte infection [32]. Close contact with infected person and domestic pets is one of the major risk factors for dermatophytosis [33]. The prevalence of dermatophytosis in school children is reported around 4% affecting boys more than girls [34].

Increase in resistance to common antifungal has been attributed to some extent in those isolates. Recently, Rudramurthy et al. showed that 17% of the *T. interdigitale* isolates and 14.3% of *T. rubrum* isolates had high MICs for terbinafine, the most effective systemic anti-dermatophytic agent [21]. Fluconazole resistance was noted in 35% isolates. Resistance to drug could be due to several mechanisms like modification in the target site, increased drug efflux mechanism, and decrease in the uptake of drug [22]. In India, Rudramurthy et al. first time reported the mutation in squalene epoxidase gene responsible for allylamine resistance in *T. interdigitale* and *T. rubrum* isolated from relapse/recurrent cases. A T1189C mutation was observed in *T. interdigitale* and *T. rubrum* isolates that exhibited high MICs to allylamines [21]. Later another study from India reported similar findings [35].

The distribution of dermatophytes in India varies across different geographical areas, wherein either *T. rubrum* [11, 29, 36, 37], or *T. interdigitale/T. mentagrophytes* [9, 21, 32, 38, 39] is reported as the most predominant etiologic agent, except in studies by Pathan et al. in which *T. violaceum* was predominant [40] and Kaur et al. where *T. tonsurans* (59.7%) was reported as emerging dermatophyte from Northern India [41].

Tinea corporis (30–50%) remains as the most common clinical presentation followed by tinea cruris (16–29%), tinea pedis (7–16%), tinea capitis (2–15%), tinea manuum (9–13%), and tinea faciei (2.5%) [14, 21, 32, 38, 42, 43]. Majority of the patients presents with single-site involvement, whereas multiple-site involvement with coexistence of tinea corporis and tinea cruris (9.2%) are also seen. (Table 2.1) Grover et al. screened 214 pediatric cases suspected with tinea capitis and found that noninflammatory type as more common variety (56.5%) in 8–10 years of age group. Majority of cases showed the growth of *T. violaceum* (64.4%) [44].

2.4 Epidemiology of Dermatophytes in China

In China, a retrospective study was conducted over the period of 10 years (2004–2014) to determine the epidemiological profile from both inpatients and outpatients in Guangzhou (Southern China). Of the 3365 patients enrolled in the study, only 697 cultures were positive for fungal growth. Among the total number of positive cultures, 83.46% showed growth of dermatophytes. *T. rubrum* and *T. mentagrophytes* were found to be the most common species isolated from tinea infection [45]. In another study, it was shown that the causative agent of tinea capitis shifted towards *M. canis* compared to the previous data (1956–1985), wherein *T. violaceum* (28.8%) followed by *T. schoenleinii* (44.7%) and *M. ferrugineum* (20.7%) were the common causative agents [16, 46]. Tao- Xiang et al. conducted a study during 2002–2003 in the northwestern part of China and found that most prevalent species to cause dermatophytosis were *T. rubrum* (43.9%) and *T. mentagrophytes* (29.4%) from cases with tinea pedis (38.7%), tinea unguium (27.8%), and tinea manuum (13.5%) [47] (Table 2.2). An outbreak in 30% of dairy workers due to *T. verrucosum* was reported in 2006 [48]. Screening of 5204 school children for tinea capitis revealed only 189 cases with *T. violaceum* (41.24%) as the common agent affecting more of male children in the age group of 6–12 years [49].

Zhan et al. analyzed the distribution of dermatophytes in tinea capitis cases in mainland China since 1956. In the 1950s and 1960s, several provinces in eastern and northwest China were hyper-endemic for favus, with *T. schoenleinii* followed by *M. ferrugineum* as the most common pathogens. In 1965, in Jiangxi region the prevalence of favus reached 3410 per 100,000 population. Due to the free treatment

Table 2.1 Epidemiology of dermatophytosis in India

Sl no	YOP	Study period	No of cases	Sample	Clinical presentation										
					Tu/ony	Tco	Tc	Tcap	Tp	Tf	Tma	Tg	Tb	Tco + Tc	Mul
1	2018	2015–2016	38	S,N,H	5.26	18.42	42.1	2.63	7.89	2.63	5.26			15.78	
2	2018	2015	150	S		17.3	18								64.6
3	2018	2014-2015	195	S,H		30.2	28.2	1	7.1	2.5				9.2	
4	2018	2015-2016	152	N	100										
5	2017	2014-2015	129	N	100										
6	2017	2011-2014	243	N	100										
7	2017	2014-2015	124	S,N,H	8.8	29	37.9	8	11.2	2.41	1.6				
8	2017	2015	192	S,N,H	15.6	54.4	14.58	3.12	10.4	0.5	0.5				
9	2016	2014	150	H				100							
10	2016		130	S,N,H	13.84	50.76	19.23	7.69	5.38				3.07		
11	2016	2013	162	S,N,H	21.6	40.7	4.3	7.4	10.5	2.5	13				
12	2015	2012-2013	351	S,N,H											
13	2015		110	S,H		40	9.09	8.19	4.55	6.36	5.45		0.91	25.45	
14	2015	2011-2012	297	S,N,H	6	78	10		0.7	1.8	2.5				
15	2015		105	S,N,H	15.24	44.76	18.09	7.62	3.81	3.81	1.9			5.71	
16	2014	2011-2012	300	S,N,H	37.3	13.7	13	11	3.7	3	2		1.7		
17	2014	2008-2009	100	S,N,H	15	21	17	5	8	3	5		3		23
18	2014	2013	321	S,N	6.9	44.2	29.9		11.5		4.7		2.8		
19	2014	2005-2006	149	S,N,H	8.1	44.3	38.2		2.7	1.3	3.3		2.1		
20	2014	2012	202	S,N,H	23.26	30.19	17.32	3.9	16.83	3.4	3.9	0.4	0.4		
21	2014		100	N	100										
22	2014		90	S,N,H	2	46	19		4						
23	2013		160	S,N,H	11	4	5	30	2	1	2			5	
24	2013	2011-2012	150	N	100										
25	2013		83	S,N,H	7.1	35.2	8.4	25.3	17		4.2		2.8		

(continued)

Table 2.1 (continued)

Sl no	YOP	Study period	No of cases	Sample	Clinical presentation										
					Tu/ony	Tco	Tc	Tcap	Tp	Tf	Tma	Tg	Tb	Tco + Tc	Mul
26	2012		120	N	100										
27	2012	2008-2009	140	S,H		77.8	11.1	5.6	2.2	1.1					
28	2011	2008-2009	165	S,N,H	11	45	3	34	2		5				
29	2010	2003-2004	198	S,H		56.57	5.56	11.11	6.06	1.01	9.09		1.51		
30	2009	2 year	34	N	100										

DM	C/S	Etiological agent														Condition	References
		Ti	Tm	Tr	Tvi	Tve	Ts	Tt	Tspp	Ma	Mn	Mg	*Mf*	Mc	Ef		
86.84	81.57		19.35	58.06	12.9					6.45				3.22		HIV patients population	[120]
98.7	60	11.1	40	32.2	1		1	3.3				4.4		2.2		Recurrent dermatophytosis cases	[39]
100	68.2	66.1		26.3				3				3		1.5		Clinically suspected cases	[21]
60.52	44.7		20	35												Clinically suspected cases	[121]
65.89	58.91		47.05	38.23				3.61							2.94	Clinically suspected cases	[122]
46.1	53.5		11.5	16.9	0.8	1.5	0.8	7.7							2.3	Clinically suspected cases	[54]
74.19	53.2	56.06		7.5	4.5	1.5		25.7				4.5				Clinically suspected cases	[123]
55.21	63.54		19.6	3.2			16.3	8.1							1.6	Clinically suspected cases	[124]
76.67	84			13.48	10.32	4.76	6.35	61.11								Children upto 14 years age included	[57]

75.38	53.8		22.85	38.57	4.28					21.42		11.43			1.43	Clinically suspected cases	[125]
51.8	56.7		48.2	32.1	3.6	1.8	1.8	10.7				1.8				Clinically suspected cases	[38]
53.5	61.2		2.1	4.6	1	3.2	2.1			0.5						Clinically suspected cases	[126]
58.18	56.35		22.58	58.06	6.45		3.22	3.22							6.45	Clinically suspected cases	[127]
50.5	75.6		14.5	79								3.2		3.2		Clinically suspected cases	[4]
70.48	70.48		43.24	51.35											2		[29]
84.67	30			34.2	11.3	0.4		8.3		6.2				1.7		Clinically suspected cases	[128]
80	68		19.11	66.17	7.35	2.94		1.47				1.47			1.47	Clinically suspected cases	[129]
	59.5		27.2	38.2	2.1			12.6				9.9		4.2	5.8	Clinically suspected cases	[42]
65.7	26.8		20	67.5			2.5			2.5				2.5	5	Clinically suspected cases	[130]
100	36.6															Clinically suspected cases without antifungal therapy	[32]
100	100	61		34		5										Clinically suspected cases	[131]
	78.8		19.7	73.2								2.8			4.2	Clinically suspected cases	[132]

(continued)

Table 2.1 (continued)

62.5	37.5		5	8.3	21.6			10		10	6.6				5	Clinically suspected cases	[40]
56	40		26.66	35												Clinically suspected cases	[133]
	85.5		12.6	42.25	9.8		7	5.6	5.6	1.4		9.8				Clinically suspected cases from cancer hospital	[134]
55	59.26		14.81	33.33				7.41							3.7	Clinically suspected cases	[135]
53.8	64.3		16.6	75.5	1.1							3.3		1.1		Clinically suspected cases	[43]
89.6	83		25	5		10.5	7	20		5			9.5		3	Clinically suspected cases	[136]
			21.3	36	4	2.7	1.3								1.3	Clinically suspected cases	[137]
94.12	82.35		22.22	11.11		11.11		44.44		11.11						Clinically suspected cases	[138]

YOP year of publication, *S,N,H* skin scrapping, hair, nail clipping, *Tu/Ony* tinea unguium/onychomycosis, *Tco* tinea corporis, *Tc* tinea cruris, *Tcap* tinea capitis, *Tp* tinea pedis, *Tf* tinea faciei, *Tma* tinea manuum, *Tg* tinea gladiatorum, *Tb* tinea barbae, *Tco* + *Tc* tinea corporis and tinea cruris, *Com* mixed infection, *DM* direct microscopy, *C/S* culture positive, *Ti Trichophyton interdigitale*, *Tm T. mentagrophytes*, *Tr T. rubrum*, *Tvi T. violaceum*, *Tve T. verrucosum*, *Ts T. schoenleinii*, *Tt T. tonsurans*, *Tspp Trichophyton species*, *Ma Microsporum audouinii*, *Mn M. nanum*, *Mg M. gypseum*, *Mf M. ferrugineum*, *Mc M. canis*, *Ef Epidermophyton floccosum*

Table 2.2 Epidemiology of dermatophytosis in China

Sl no	Study period	Year	No. of cases	Clinical Sample								C/S	Etiological agent										
					Tu/ony	Tco	Tc	Tcap	Tp	Tf	Tma		Tm	Tr	Tvio	Ts	Tcere	Tt	Mg	*Mf*	Mc	Ef	References
1	2004-2014	2016	3385	SHN	28.5	8.75	10.33	15.6	15	3.16	2.87	84.36	13.35	56.24	30.01			0.28	1.01		10.19	0.28	[45]
2	1986	2011	9096										20	47	7	2				2	5	2	[139]
	1996	2011	19,009										12	40							2	1	
	2006	2011	33,022										7	30							3		
3	1993-2008	2010	867	H				100				82.4	2.5	3.8	19		0.31	9.8	1.8		62.4		[140]

YOP year of publication, *S,N,H* skin scrapping, hair, nail clipping, *Tu/Ony* tinea unguium/onychomycosis, *Tco* tinea corporis, *Tc* tinea cruris, *Tcap* tinea capitis, *Tp* tinea pedis, *Tf* tinea faciei, *Tma* tinea manuum, *C/S* culture positive, *Tm Trichophyton mentagrophytes*, *Tr T. rubrum*, *Tvio T. violaceum*, *Ts T. schoenleinii*, *Tcere T. cerebriform*, *Tt T. tonsurans*, *Mg Microsporum gypseum*, *Mf M. ferrugineum*, *Mc M. canis*, *Ef Epidermophyton floccosum*

provided to all the patients, the incidence of tinea capitis came down to 7.2/100,000 population by 2000. In the late 1980s, *T mentagrophytes* and *T. violaceum* became predominant and *M. canis* begun to increase gradually and presently is the major agent of tinea capitis in the areas of high economic growth of China. In some areas, 80% of infection are due to zoophilic species *M. canis,* suggesting animal contact as the main source of infection [49]. The prevalence of asymptomatic carriers of dermatophytes was 0.1–49% [50]. In addition to the animal contact, the asymptomatic carrier can also be responsible for the spread of infection.

2.5 Epidemiology of Dermatophytes in Iran

Recently, many cases (9485) with clinically suspected cutaneous fungal infection were investigated for dermatophytosis. A total of 1502 patients were infected with dermatophytes. Large number of patients presented with tinea corporis (35.2%) followed by tinea cruris (17%). *T. interdigitale* (49.36%) was the main etiological agent responsible for dermatophytosis followed by *T. rubrum* (18.98%), *E. floccosum* (13.29%), *M. canis* (9.17%), *A. benhamiae* (5.38%), and *T. tonsurans* (3.79%) [51]. In a study conducted from northeast part of Iran of 1100 suspected onychomycosis cases, fungi could be isolated in 625 (56.8%) cases. *T. mentagrophytes* (17.7%) and *T. rubrum* (1.7%) were the common dermatophytes implicated [52]. Southwest part of Iran noticed a high occurrence of infection with *T. interdigitale* (58.7%) that was not noted before and *A. benhamiae* emerged as a new agent of dermatophytosis. Tinea corporis (32%) was the common clinical presentation followed by tinea cruris (21.9%), tinea capitis (12%), tinea manuum (11.2%), tinea pedis (10.3%), tinea unguium (6.9%), tinea faciei (5.16%), and tinea barbae (0.35%) [13] (Table 2.3).

Table 2.3 Epidemiology of dermatophytosis in Iran

Sl. no	YOP	No of cases	Clinical sample	Clinical presentation								DM	C/S	Etiological agent														References
				Tu/ony	Tco	Tc	Tcap	Tp	Tf	Tma	Tb			Ti	Tm	Tr	Tvi	Tve	Ts	Tt	Mg	Mc	Mp	Mco	Mv	Ef	Ab	
1	2018	170	N	100										4.7		2.9				0.5								[141]
2	2018	405	SHN	4.6	22.7	20.5	10.2	31.8	4.6	5.7		21.7	[3 (3.4%) (C/S)] [(21.7%) (Molecular)]	36.4		27.3				11.4	2.3	4.5				17	1.1	[142]
3	2018	257	SH	70	69.2	15.4		3.8		11.5		66.9	68.9	52.9		29.4				17.6								[143]
4	2018	180	N	65.5								65.5	66.9		43	49.3		1.27		3.8						2.53		[144]
5	2016	169					100					71.6	100	8	12	24	32	4		4		16						[145]
6	2015	9485	SHN	6.9	35.2	17	12.8	11.3		11	5.8	15.8	15.8	49.36		18.9				3.7		9.17				13.2	5.3	[51]
7	2015	13,469	SHN	4	24	7	52.7	8.9	0.4	2.8		11.5		17.6	2.5	4.1	12	40.6	4	1.5	1.8	2.8		0.1		13		[146]
8	2015	139										18.7	18.7		38.5	23	15.4	11.5				7.7				3.8		[147]
9	2013	560	SHN	0.6	33.1	10.2	32.5	5.4		17.5	0.6	29.6	29.6		21.6	1.4	27.7	1.4	12.8				0.7		11.4	21.6		[148]
10	2012	3976	SHN	3.3	28.9	2.1	8.8	8.4	13.8	34.7		15.2			28			9.3			0.3	2.2						[149]
11	2011	110											100	3.8	1.9	5.8		1.9		82.7						3.8		[53]
12	2011	6325			32.1	14.3	5.4	8.9	26.8	12.5			0.9		28.6	12.5	3.6	33.9	1.8			8.9				10.7		[150]
13	2010	308											40.2	16.9	4	24.2		1.6								3.2		[62]

YOP year of publication, *S,N,H* skin scrapping, hair, nail clipping, *Tu/Ony* tinea unguium/onychomycosis, *Tco* tinea corporis, *Tc* tinea cruris, *Tcap* tinea capitis, *Tp* tinea pedis, *Tf* tinea faciei, *Tma* tinea manuum, *Tb* tinea barbae, *DM* direct microscopy, *C/S* culture positive, *Ti Trichophyton interdigitale*, *Tm T. mentagrophytes*, *Tr T. rubrum*, *Tvi T. violaceum*, *Tve T. verrucosum*, *Ts T. schoenleinii*, *Tt T. tonsurans*, *Mg Microsporum gypseum*, *Mc M. canis*, *Mco M. cookie*, *Mv M. vanbreuseghemii*, *Ef Epidermophyton floccosum*, *Ab Arthroderma benhamiae*

Another interesting feature noted in Iran is the outbreak of tinea gladiatorum in wrestlers. Of 612 cases of outbreak, *T. tonsurans* was isolated from >90% and was found to be more frequent in individuals between the ages of 10 and 20 years of age (72.7%). Direct human to human contact was identified as a source that leads to transmission of infection leading to outbreak [50]. Later, survey showed that 33% of the wrestling mats were heavily contaminated with *T. tonsurans* indicating possibility of both man–man and mat–man transmission [53].

Antifungal susceptibility profile of the dermatophytes isolated from Iran varied to that reported from India. Overall terbinafine resistance was noted in 5% of the tested isolates but none of their *T. interdigitale* isolates were resistant to this drug. Two isolates also showed Leu393 Phe substitution. Out of 99 dermatophyte isolates, only 5 isolates [*T. rubrum* ($n = 2$); *T. tonsurans* ($n = 2$), and *E. floccosum* ($n = 1$)] showed reduced susceptibility to terbinafine. Griseofulvin was susceptible to all the *T. interdigitale* isolates [54].

2.6 Epidemiology of Dermatophytes in Other Asian Countries

In 1995, the prevalence of tinea was examined in Japanese self-defense force (SDF) population. Among the SDF population, tinea pedis (93.2%) was most usual form of tinea infection, whereas tinea corporis was rare [55]. Noguchi et al. in 2014 reported *T. rubrum* (43.7%) as a common cause of tinea faciei in Japan [56]. In 2017, Yamada et al. reported that 1% of their isolates had reduced susceptibility to terbinafine. Squalene epoxidase gene sequencing of those resistant isolates showed single amino acid substitution in *Trichophyton rubrum* at Leu393, Phe397, Phe415, and His440 [57]. Increased prevalence of tinea corporis has also been noted from Nepal and Kuwait with *T. mentagrophytes* as a predominant causative agent [5, 58] (Table 2.4).

2.7 Onychomycosis Due to Non-dermatophytic Molds

Onychomycosis is a common superficial fungal infection of nails and caused by dermatophytes, non-dermatophyte molds (NDM), and yeasts. It needs special consideration as it is difficult to treat due to the chronicity of infection [59, 60]. Incidence of onychomycosis is frequently increasing due to several risk factors such as advanced age diabetes and poor peripheral circulation, compromised immune status of hosts, sports participation, wearing occlusive footwear, and genetic susceptibility due to defect in immune system [28, 61]. The prevalence rate of onychomycosis varies by age, predisposing factor, social class, occupation, climate, living environment, and frequency of travel [28]. In Asian and middle eastern countries, dermatophytes account for 40–48% of cases, 43–46% are due to yeasts, and 8–11% are caused by non-dermatophyte molds [59]. The most common non-dermatophyte molds responsible for onychomycosis are *Aspergillus* spp., *Fusarium* spp., and

Table 2.4 Epidemiology of dermatophytosis in other Asian countries

Sl no	Country	YOP	Study period	No of cases	Sample	Clinical presentation											
						Tu/ony	Tco	Tc	Tcap	Tp	Tf	Tma	Tfav	Tg	Tb	Tv	Com
1	Singapore	2018	2005-2014	229													
2	Vietnam	2017	2015-2016	160	SHN												
3	Malaysia	2017	2011-2015	1,357	N	100											
4	Kazakhstan	2017	2014	195	SH		27.17	13.3	43.07								16.41
5	Nepal	2016	2014	200	SN	17.5	25	17		13							
6	Yemen	2015		112	SHN	17.9	21.4	4.5	22.3	17	2.7	11.6	1.8		0.9		
7	Saudi Arabia	2015	2005-2006	640	SHN	7.7	14.8	6.9	28.6	21.1						11.6	
8	Saudi Arabia	2014	2012-2013	170	N	100											
9	Japan	2014	2008-2014	80							100						
10	Jordan	2011	2004-2009	39	N				100								100
11	Turkey	2011	2005-2006	372	SHN	50.6	4.5		0.18	37.4		1.8			0.36		55.3
12	Kuwait	2009	2000-2005	2,730	SHN	35	22	8	10	8		1		16			
13	Turkey	2009	2000-2007	9,150	SHN	40	8	11	1	28		9				3	

DM	C/S	Etiological agent																	Condition	References
		Ti	Tm	Tr	Tvi	Tve	Ts	Tc	Tt	Tsou	Tspp	Ma	Mn	Mg	*Mf*	Mi	Mc	Ef		
			26.2	40.6	0.4	0.9			4.4	0.4	24.9							2.2	Retrospective study	[151]
		12.5		66.9	0.9				9.6							8.1	2.2		Clinically suspected cases	[152]
	7.4		15.8	27.7					34.6										Retrospective study	[153]
97.9				42.6	0.5			10.3							1	20.4			Clinically suspected cases	[154]

DM	C/S	Etiological agent																Condition	References
		Ti	Tm	Tr	Tvi	Tve	Ts	Tc	Tt	Tsou	Tspp	Ma	Mn	Mg	*Mf*	Mi	Mc	Ef		
44.5	55.5		39.6	11.7					5.4								5.4	2.7	Clinically suspected cases	[5]
	46.4		9.6	15.3	19.2	11.4	3.8	1.9				7.7					25	5.8	Clinically suspected cases	[155]
	51.5	7.2	14.8	11.8					36					14	4.2		25.7		Clinically suspected cases	[156]
45.3	45.3			11.6		5.3													Clinically suspected cases	[60]
		3.8	43.7	2.5	2.5					23.8			2.5			21.3			Clinically suspected cases	[56]
64.1	76.9				46.6	10	6.6		10								26.6		Microscopic positive cases	[157]
	26.8	3.3	87.25						0.67	1.34									Clinically suspected cases	[158]
39	23		39	10	2.4	0.4		6.2								16			Clinically suspected cases	[58]
		7	47						2								7		Clinically suspected cases	[159]

YOP year of publication, *S,N,H* skin scrapping, hair, nail clipping, *Tu/Ony* tinea unguium/onychomycosis, *Tco* tinea corporis, *Tc* tinea cruris, *Tcap* tinea capitis, *Tp* tinea pedis, *Tf* tinea faciei, *Tma* tinea manuum, *Tfav* tinea favosa, *Tg* tinea gladiatorum, *Tb* tinea barbae, *Tv* tinea versicolor, *Com* mixed infection, *DM* direct microscopy, *C/S* culture positive, *Ti Trichophyton interdigitale*, *Tm T. mentagrophytes*, *Tr T. rubrum*, *Tvi T. violaceum*, *Tve T. verrucosum*, *Ts T. schoenleinii*, *Tc T. concentricum*, *Tt T. tonsurans*, *Tsou T. soudanense*, *Tspp Trichophyton species*, *Ma Microsporum audouinii*, *Mn M. nanum*, *Mg M. gypseum*, *Mf M. ferrugineum*, *Mi M. incurvatum*, *Mc M. canis*, *Ef Epidermophyton floccosum*

Scopulariopsis spp. Among yeasts, the predominant causative agent is *C. albicans,* followed by *C. tropicalis*, *C. glabrata,* and other non-albicans *Candida* [62].

2.8 Superficial Diseases Caused by *Malassezia* Species

Malassezia species are often found as commensals on human skin. It has also been associated with many skin disorders such as pityriasis versicolor (PV), seborrheic dermatitis/dandruff (SD/D), pityrosporum folliculitis (PF), psoriasis (PS), and atopic dermatitis (AD). The current literature supports strong association of *Malassezia* with PV, SD/D, and PF. Association of *Malassezia* with atopic dermatitis and psoriasis is not strong and hence would not be discussed further.

2.8.1 *Malassezia* and Seborrheic Dermatitis/Dandruff

Seborrheic dermatitis, a common dermatoses estimated to affect around 3–10% of the general population and up to 50% of the adult male population. When the disease presents with mild flakes on the scalp, it is generally referred as dandruff and when it presents with large visible flakes on the scalp with severe inflammation it is referred as seborrheic dermatitis (Fig. 2.2f). SD/D is a multifactorial disease caused due to increased colonization by *Malassezia* species, along with individual's predispositions and host interactions with *Malassezia*, rather than the mere presence of *Malassezia*. Predisposing factors include immune-compromised patients (HIV/AIDS patients, organ transplant recipients, and patients with lymphoma) and neurological disorders (psychiatric disorders, facial palsy, spinal cord injury, mood depression). Increased incidence in the adult male indicates that androgen may have a role in predisposition [63].

Malassezia is lipophilic yeast and the lipase enzymes secreted by them hydrolyzes human sebum triglycerides and releases unsaturated fatty acids causing inflammation and clinical features of SD/D. Several factors such as breach in the epidermal layer and individual's susceptibility to the disease have also been described [63]. *Malassezia* species associated with SD/D depends upon the geographical region and the sampling methods used in the study. In skin fungal microbiota study, *Malassezia* species were identified directly from the clinical samples of Japanese patients using molecular technique. The study showed higher presence of *M. restricta* at lesional sites and *M. globosa* at non-lesional sites [64]. Nakabayashi et al. used the culture-based technique and reported significantly high rates of *M. furfur* (35%) and *M. globosa* (22%) from lesion area of SD/D patients [65]. The level of *Malassezia* colonization at lesional sites was approximately three-fold higher than at non-lesional sites with *M. restricta* as significantly more common species than *M. globosa* [66]. In HIV patients, the incidence of SD/D from Thailand, Malaysia, and Korea were 46%, 19.2%, and 17.1%, respectively [67–69]. In India, *M. restricta* and *M. globosa* are the most prevalent species among dandruff patients of northern India, whereas *M. furfur,*

M. restricta, and *M. globosa* were predominantly isolated in southern Indian population [70]. Honnavar et al. reported significantly higher association of *M. restricta* in SD/D patients compared to normal individuals [71]. They also identified a novel species, *M. arunalokei* from patients with mild and moderately severe SD/D cases [71].

2.8.2 Pityriasis Versicolor (PV)

Worldwide, pityriasis versicolor or tinea versicolor is one of the most common pigmentary disorders [72, 73]. PV is characterized by hypopigmented or hyperpigmented round or oval macules with fine scales. Though PV is reported from young children and older individuals, it is generally seen in teenagers and young adult possibly due to increased activity of sebaceous gland and sebum secretion, which acts as lipid source for *Malassezia* to proliferate [74]. Majority of the patients usually present with multiple hypopigmentation (Fig. 2.2g). *Malassezia* species is considered as the causative agent responsible for the clinical manifestation of PV. Several factors that predispose an individual to PV include malnutrition, use of oral contraceptives, corticosteroids, immunosuppressants, certain disease conditions (HIV, visceral leishmaniasis), mood disorders, climatic condition, and the use of cosmetics. The incidence of PV is more in tropical region compared to temperate region [73]. In tropical countries of Asia, the incidence may go up as high as 50% [75]. The species of *Malassezia* implicated with PV varies with the region. From Japan, the *M. globosa* (55%) was the major species isolated from the skin lesions. Their results suggest that *M. globosa*, a normal commensal of skin, may become pathogenic and produces PV lesion when the environment becomes conducive [65]. A study from Iran showed that involvement of species depends on the site affected; *M. globosa* was most frequent in groin region, whereas *M. pachydermatis* on face and *M. furfur* on trunk [76]. When the survey for PV was conducted in the students population, they did not find any significant association between the fatty skin and distribution of *Malassezia* species [77]. In China, recurrence of PV was more in cases having positive family history of PV compared to the negative family history [78]. A report from Indonesia recorded increased isolation of *M. furfur* with patients presenting with hypopigmentation (64.3%) and hyperpigmentation (19.4%) [79] Among northeast Indian population, the *Malassezia* species isolated from lesional vs non-lesional sites of PV cases were *M. furfur* (72.8% vs. 66.1%), *M. globosa* (14.9% vs. 4.4%), *M. obtusa* (4.8% vs. 0.0%), *M. sympodialis* (3.4% vs. 14.7%), *M. restricta* (2.7% vs. 19.1%), *M. slooffiae.* (0.7% vs. 0.0%), and *M. japonica* (0.7% vs. 0.0%) [80]. Other studies from northeast India also showed the predominance of *M. furfur* in the PV cases [81, 82]. In central India, *M. globosa* (57.5%) was the most common species, followed by *M. sympodialis* (17.2%), *M. furfur* (6.9%), *M. obtusa* (6.9%), and *M. restricta* (3.4%) [83], whereas from the southern India, *M. sympodialis* (58.33%) was most frequent, followed by *M. globosa* (39.58%) and *M. restricta* (2.08%) [84] (Table 2.5).

Table 2.5 Epidemiology of *Malassezia* infection in Asia

C	DOS	No. of cases	Sample	Diagnosis	DM (%)	C/S (%)	Etiological agent (%)													Ref
							MF	MS	MG	MP	MG + MSy	MG + MF	M Sy	MJ	MO	MR	MN	MIX	U	
India	2 years	262	S	PV			77		12				2.7			2.7				[82]
India	1 years	120	DS	D	120	70	36	2.3	38				3.5			55				[70]
India	8 months	65	S	PV	89	93.1		18	51					31	3.7					[160]
India		100	S	PV	90	87	7		58				25		7	3				[83]
India	2 years	271	S	PV	72.3															[161]
India		427	S	PV	100	58.5	29		54		4.8	4.4						16	3.2	[162]
China		246	L	SD	100				51							48				[163]
Indonesia		96	S	PV	100		42	7.7	13				27		7.7	2.2			7.1	[79]
Iran		189	S	PV	22.2	22.2	11		30				19			38				[77]
Iran	11 months	713	S	PV	9.5	80.9	23	7.28	36	29					3.6					[76]
Iran		100	L	SD	100	77	32		55				1.3	1.3		9.1				[164]
Iran	1 years	166	S	PV	60.2	69.8	29	5.3	44	10			9.3		8.1	10.3				[165]
Iran		94	S	PV			25	4	53											[166]
Israel		75	S	PV	100	97.3			97							1.3				[167]
Turkey	2 years 6 months	146	S	PV	36.4	74.7	0.9		65					7.4	17	1.8	3.7			[168]
Turkey	1 years 3 months	97	S	PV	100	45	36	15												[169]

C Country, *DOS* Duration of study, *S* Skin scrapping, *L* lesional skin, *DS* Dandruff sample *PV* Pityriasis versicolor, *SD* Seborrheic dermatitis, *D* Dandruff cases, *DM* Direct microscopy, *C/S* Culture positive, *MF Malassezia furfur*, *MS M. slooffiae*, *MG M. globosa*, *MP M. pachydermatis*, *MG + MSy M. globosa + M. sympodialis*, *MG + MF M. globosa + M. furfur*, *MSy M. sympodialis*, *MJ M. japonica*, *MO M. obtuse*, *MR M. restricta*, *MN M. nana*, *U* Unidentified species, *Ref* References, *MIX* Mixed organism isolated

2.8.3 Pityrosporum Folliculitis

Pityrosporum/*Malassezia* folliculitis (PF/MF) is a common inflammatory or fungal acneiform eruption caused by overgrowth of yeast naturally present on the skin surface. This infection is often misdiagnosed as acne vulgaris. PF/MF is a chronic form of infection and distributed worldwide, especially in the hot tropical climatic region [85]. The main predisposing factors for PF include hot and humid environment, use of topical and systemic steroids, and immunosuppression [85]. This condition is mainly observed in the adult population. In Japan, of the 32 cases PF/MF cases diagnosed, *M. globosa* was the predominant species isolated from the lesions [86]. Similarly, in another study from Turkey, *M. globosa* (69.4%) was predominant species followed by *M. sympodialis, M. restricta,* and *M. furfur* [87].

2.9 Tinea Nigra

Tinea nigra is a rare superficial fungal infection and first identified by Horta in 1921. The causative agent for tinea nigra is *Hortaea werneckii* (*Phaeoannellomyces werneckii, Exophiala werneckii, Cladosporium werneckii*) [88]. *Hortaea werneckii* is a halophilic fungus and can utilize decomposed lipids in the stratum corneum [73]. Due to halophilic nature of this agent, this disease is being increasingly associated with the beach recreational activities. Tinea nigra mainly affects the children and young adult population and is predominant in female [88]. Though this infection occurs on any of the body part with sweat glands, palms and soles are commonly affected areas. Hyperhidrosis may be the major risk factor for tinea nigra [73]. Of the 7 case reports available from India, 5 cases are from southern India and one case each from the north and eastern India [89, 90]. Of the 40 cases of tinea nigra reported from Japan, 80% presented with the lesion on palms [91]. In 2008, 3 cases of tinea nigra were reported among school children in Taiwan [92] (Table 2.6).

2.10 Piedra

Piedra is a superficial fungal infection of the hair shaft. Clinically two types of piedra; white piedra and black piedra has been described.

White piedra usually affects the hair shaft (pubic hair, axillary hair, mustaches, scalp, eyebrows, and eyelashes) by forming soft nodules. The etiological agent for white piedra is *Trichosporon* spp. (*T. cutaneum, T. asahii, T. mucoides, T. ovoides, T. asteroides,* and *T. inkin*). In India, Kamlam et al. reported white piedra as a rare superficial fungal infection with the prevalence rate of 0.1%. All the four cases of white piedra reported by them were caused by *Trichosporon beigelii*. A higher incidence seen in women may be due to hairdressing fashion and social custom such as wearing a turban or burka [93, 94]. Cases of white piedra have also been reported from other Asian countries like Saudi Arabia and Kuwait [95, 96] (Table 2.6).

Table 2.6 Epidemiology of piedra and tinea nigra infection in Asia

			Diagnosis				Organism isolated								
References	Country	No. of cases	WP	BP	Mixed	TN	Ts	Tb	Tc	Tm	Ta	Ph	Ts + Ph	Tb + Ph	Pw
[98]	India	3	1	1	1		1					1	1		
[170]	India	4	3	1				4				1			
[95]	Saudi Arabia	6	6						6						
[99]	Saudi Arabia	1			1									1	
[171]	Yemen	8	8						4	2	2				
[92]	Taiwan	3				3									3

WP White piedra, *BP* Black piedra, *MP* Mixed piedra, *Ts Trichosporon* spp., *Tb T. beigelii*, *Tc T. cutaneum*, *Tm T. mucoides*, *Ta T asahii*, *Ph Piedraia hortae*, *Pw Phaeoannellomyces werneckii*, *TN* Tinea nigra

Black piedra is the rare and asymptomatic infection of the hair in which hard nodules are formed along the hair shaft. *Piedraia hortae,* the causative agent of black piedra is present in soil, stagnant water, and crops [88]. Like white piedra this infection is also observed in the regions of hot and humid climate. Few cases of black piedra have been reported from India, Malaysia, and Saudi Arabia [97–99].

2.11 Fungal Keratitis

Fungal keratitis is the inflammation or infection of the cornea, which can be either superficial (involve outer layer) or deep (involve the deeper layer). Fungal keratitis is one of the important causes of the vision loss or blindness. The incidence of fungal keratitis has been significantly increased in Asian countries and contributes to nearly half of the world's fungal keratitis cases [100]. The predisposing factors for development of keratitis include trauma to eye due to vegetative material or ophthalmic surgeries, insect fall, use of contaminated ophthalmic solutions, use of contact lens, steroids application, traditional eye remedies, and other host factors (diabetes mellitus, immunocompromised status, and ocular disorders—dry eye, bullous keratopathy, and lagophthalmos) [101]. Unlike in western countries, wherein FK is more associated with use of contact lens wearer, in Asian countries this disease is seen mainly in farmers (52.3%) and laborers (22.9%) who are prone for trauma of the eye as protective eyewear is rarely used by them [100, 102]. Bharathi et al. from India reported corneal trauma (92.15%) as predominant predisposing factor for FK; trauma inflicted by vegetable matter was highest (61.28%) [103]. Among all the trauma agents causing FK in central China, agricultural material was common (16.86%) [104]. Fungal keratitis occurs more frequently during monsoon season and in the young male individuals [101]. Trauma to the eye is the main (60.5%) predisposing factor of FK in India [102]. Generally, any agent that is prevalent in the air, soil, vegetative matter, or water can cause FK [105]. Among all the etiological agents, filamentous fungi is the major cause of fungal keratitis throughout the world.

Fungal agents that predominantly causes keratitis vary among different regions. In India, the studies clearly show difference in etiological agents with geogrpahical regions. Ghosh et al. from North India showed that *Aspergillus* spp. as the commonest ($n = 187$, 47.6%) agent followed by melanized fungi ($n = 86$, 21.9%) and *Fusarium* spp. ($n = 64$, 16%) [106]. In contrast, Bharathi et al. from Southern India reported *Fusarium* spp. (42.82%) as a predominant etiological agent of fungal keratitis [103]. Among *Aspergillus* spp., the most common species to cause infection is *Aspergillus flavus* in India and Nepal, whereas in China and Bangladesh *Aspergillus fumigatus* is commonest [106–108]. Among *Fusarium* spp., *F. solani* is the predominant species in India, China, and Bangladesh [103, 109, 110]. In China, from culture-proven cases of keratitis 123 different species were identified belonging to 51 fungal genera. Among them, *Fusarium* spp. (56.93%) was the most common followed by *Aspergillus* spp. (15.26%) and *Alternaria* spp. (7.32%) [104].

Recently, keratitis due to *Pythium* species is increasingly being implicated from Asian countries particularly from Thailand and India. The prevalence of Pythium keratitis in southern India is 5.9% [111]. The aquatic environment is considered as an important risk factor for Pythium keratitis [112], but recently it has been shown that non-aquatic environment also has the same potential to cause this infection [111]. Use of contact lens as a risk of acquiring Pythium keratitis has been reported from Thailand [113]. The previous history of exposure to water or involvement of agricultural work may give a clue to the clinician to suspect Pythium etiology. In Thailand, an outbreak of Pythium keratitis was reported during the rainy season [112].

Microsporidia, recently being classified as fungi under Ascomycota, is emerging as an opportunistic pathogen particularly causing FK. The prevalence of Microsporidial keratitis from southern India was around 0.4% [114]. Microsporidial keratitis is a rare disease and infects both immune-compromised and immune-competent individual. In those using contact lens or immune-compromised individuals, infection presents as kerato-conjunctivitis, whereas in immune-competent individual stromal involvement is common [115]. Most of the cases of Microsporidial keratitis were seen during the monsoon season [116] and this agent has been detected in stagnant water [115]. *Colletotrichum* spp. has been noted as an emerging agent of ophthalmic infection [117–119]. *Colletotrichum* is ubiquitous fungi and is reported to cause the anthracnose of many crops in India and Thailand. Case series of fungal keratitis due to *C. truncatum* has been mainly reported from India [117].

References

1. Weitzman I, Summerbell RC. The dermatophytes. Clin Microbiol Rev. 1995;8:240–59.
2. Havlickova B, Czaika VA, Friedrich M. Epidemiological trends in skin mycoses worldwide. Mycoses. 2008;51:2–15.
3. Ajello L. Natural history of the dermatophytes and related fungi. Mycopathol Mycol Appl. 1974;53:93–110.
4. Ganeshkumar P, Sr M, Hemamalini M, Madhavan R, Lakshmanan A. Epidemiological and clinical pattern of dermatomycoses in rural India. Indian J Med Microbiol. 2015;33:134–6.
5. Khadka S, Sherchand JB, Pokharel DB, Pokhrel BM, Mishra SK, Dhital S, Rijal B. Clinicomycological characterization of superficial mycoses from a tertiary care hospital in Nepal. Dermatol Res Pract. 2016;2016:1–7.
6. Hayette M-PP, Sacheli R. Dermatophytosis, trends in epidemiology and diagnostic approach. Curr Fungal Infect Rep. 2015;9:164–79.
7. Majid I, Sheikh G, Kanth F, Hakak R. Relapse after oral terbinafine therapy in dermatophytosis: a clinical and mycological study. Indian J Dermatol. 2016;61:529–33.
8. Ahmed S, Jeelani S, Lanker A, Qayoom S, Sameem F. Relapse of cutaneous fungal infection in healthy individuals—a rising concern. Br J Med Med Res. 2016;11:1–8.
9. Sahoo AK, Mahajan R. Management of tinea corporis, tinea cruris, and tinea pedis: a comprehensive review. Indian Dermatol Online J. 2016;7:77–86.
10. Dogra S, Uprety S. The menace of chronic and recurrent dermatophytosis in India: is the problem deeper than we perceive? Indian Dermatol Online J. 2016;7:73–6.
11. Venkatesan G, Singh AJAR, Murugesan AG, Janaki C, Shankar SG. *Trichophyton rubrum* – the predominant etiological agent in human dermatophytoses in Chennai. India African J Microbiol Res. 2007;52:9–12.

12. Chakrabarti A, Sharma SC, Talwar P. Isolation of dermatophytes from clinically normal sites in patients with tinea cruris. Mycopathologia. 1992;120:139–41.
13. Rezaei-Matehkolaei A, Rafiei A, Makimura K, Gräser Y, Gharghani M, Sadeghi-Nejad B. Epidemiological aspects of dermatophytosis in Khuzestan, southwestern Iran, an update. Mycopathologia. 2016;181:547–53.
14. Balakumar S, Rajan S, Thirunalasundari T, Jeeva S. Epidemiology of dermatophytosis in and around Tiruchirapalli, Tamilnadu, India. Asian Pacific J Trop Dis. 2012;2:286–9.
15. Garg A, Venkatesh V, Singh M, Pathak KP, Kaushal GP, Agrawal SK. Onychomycosis in central India: a clinicoetiologic correlation. Int J Dermatol. 2004;43:498–502.
16. Zhan P, Liu W. The changing face of dermatophytic infections worldwide. Mycopathologia. 2017;182:77–86.
17. Philpot CM. Geographical distribution of the dermatophytes: a review. J Hyg (Lond). 1978;80:301–13.
18. Desai SC. Epidemic and clinical features of *T. rubrum* infections in the tropics. Int J Dermatol. 1966;5:222–4.
19. Khan KA, Anwar AA. Study of 73 cases of tinea capitis and tinea favosa in adults and adolescents. J Invest Dermatol. 1968;51:474–7.
20. Bishnoi A, Vinay K, Dogra S. Emergence of recalcitrant dermatophytosis in India. Lancet Infect Dis. 2018;18:250–1.
21. Rudramurthy SM, Shankarnarayan SA, Dogra S, Shaw D, Mushtaq K, Paul RA, Narang T, Chakrabarti A. Mutation in the Squalene Epoxidase Gene of *Trichophyton interdigitale* and *Trichophyton rubrum* Associated with Allylamine Resistance. Antimicrob Agents Chemother. 2018;62:1–9.
22. Martinez-Rossi NM, Peres NTA, Rossi A. Antifungal resistance mechanisms in dermatophytes. Mycopathologia. 2008;166:369–83.
23. Dogra S, Narang T. Emerging atypical and unusual presentations of dermatophytosis in India. Clin Dermatology Rev. 2017;1:12–8.
24. Nenoff P, Verma SB, Vasani R, Burmester A, Hipler U-C, Wittig F, Krüger C, Nenoff K, Wiegand C, Saraswat A, Madhu R, Panda S, Das A, Kura M, Jain A, Koch D, Gräser Y, Uhrlaß S. The current Indian epidemic of superficial dermatophytosis due to *Trichophyton mentagrophytes*-A molecular study. Mycoses. 2019;62:336–56.
25. Verma S. Steroid modified tinea. BMJ. 2017;356:j973.
26. Verma S, Madhu R. The Great Indian epidemic of superficial dermatophytosis: an appraisal. Indian J Dermatol. 2017;62:227–36.
27. Naglot A, Shrimali DD, Nath BK, Gogoi HK, Veer V, Chander J, Tewari R, Centre C. Recent trends of dermatophytosis in northeast india (assam) and interpretation with published studies. IntJCurrMicrobiolAppSci. 2015;4:111–20.
28. Kashyap B, Bhalla P, Kaur R. A five-year survey of onychomycosis in New Delhi, India: Epidemiological and laboratory aspects. Indian J Dermatol. 2009;52:39–42.
29. Lavanya V, Solabannavar SS. Prevalence and socio-economic correlation of dermatophytes isolated from clinical samples in a tertiary care centre in South India. Asian J AdvBasicSci. 2015;4:1–4.
30. Singal A, Rawat S, Bhattacharya SN, Mohanty S, Baruah MC. Clinico-myocological profile of tinea capitis in North India and response to griseofulvin. J Dermatol. 2001;28:22–6.
31. Sachin K, Seema B. Clinico-mycological profiles of dermatophytosis in Jaipur, India. African J Microbiol Res. 2016;10:1477–82.
32. Bhatia VK, Sharma PC. Epidemiological studies on Dermatophytosis in human patients in Himachal Pradesh, India. Springerplus. 2014;3:134–40.
33. Mattei AS, Beber MA, Madrid IM, Souza Mattei A. Dermatophytosis in small animals. SOJ Microbiol Infect Dis. 2014;2:1–6.
34. Upendra Y, Sendur S, Keswani N, Pallava A. Prevalence of dermatoses among the tribal children studying in residential schools of South Chhattisgarh, India. Indian J Paediatr Dermatology. 2018;19:15–20.

35. Singh A, Masih A, Khurana A, Singh P, Kumar GM, Hagen F, Jacques FM, Chowdhary A. High terbinafine resistance in *Trichophyton interdigitale* isolates in Delhi, India harbouring mutations in the squalene epoxidase gene. Mycoses. 2018;61:477–84.
36. Kannan P, Janaki C, Selvi GS. Prevalence of dermatophytes and other fungal agents isolated from clinical samples. Indian J Med Microbiol. 2006;24:212–5.
37. Peerapur BV, Inamdar AC, Pushpa PV, Srikant B. Clinicomycological study of dermatophytosis in Bijapur. Indian J Med Microbiol. 2004;22:273–4.
38. Kaur I, Thakur K, Sood A, Mahajan VK, Gupta PK. Clinico-mycological profile of clinically diagnosed cases of dertmatophytosis in North India- a prospective cross sectional study. IJHSR. 2016;6:54–60.
39. Pathania S, Rudramurthy SM, Narang T, Saikia UN, Dogra S. A prospective study of the epidemiological and clinical patterns of recurrent dermatophytosis at a tertiary care hospital in India. Indian J Dermatol Venereol Leprol. 2018;84:678–84.
40. Pathan N, Sharma R, Vyas L, Vyas A. A clinicomycological study of cutaneous mycoses in Sawai Man Singh Hospital of Jaipur, North India. Ann Med Health Sci Res. 2013;3:593–7.
41. Kaur I, Chaudhary A, Singh H. Clinico-microbiological aspects of tinea corporis in North India: emergence of Trichophyton tonsurans. Int J Res Dermatology. 2019;5:144–9.
42. Maulingkar SV, Pinto MJW, Rodrigues S. A clinico-mycological study of dermatophytoses in Goa, India. Mycopathologia. 2014;178:297–301.
43. Sharma M, Sharma R. Profile of dermatophytic and other fungal infections in Jaipur. Indian J Microbiol. 2012;52:270–4.
44. Grover C, Arora P, Manchanda V. Tinea capitis in the pediatric population: A study from North India. Indian J Dermatol Venereol Leprol. 2010;76:527–32.
45. Cai W, Lu C, Li X, Zhang J, Zhan P, Xi L, Sun J, Yu X. Epidemiology of superficial fungal infections in Guangdong, Southern China: a retrospective study from 2004 to 2014. Mycopathologia. 2016;181:387–95.
46. Zhan P, Li D, Wang C, Sun J, Geng C, Xiong Z, Seyedmousavi S, Liu W, de Hoog GS. Epidemiological changes in tinea capitis over the sixty years of economic growth in China. Med Mycol. 2015;53:691–8.
47. Tao-Xiang N, Zhi-Cheng L, Sao-Mao W, Wen-Zhu L. Analysis of dermatomycoses in Lanzhou District of Northwestern China. Mycopathologia. 2005;160:281–4.
48. Ming PX, Ti YLX, Bulmer GS. Outbreak of *Trichophyton verrucosum* in China transmitted from cows to humans. Mycopathologia. 2006;161:225–8.
49. Deng S, Bulmer GS, Summerbell RC, De Hoog GS, Hui Y, Gräser Y. Changes in frequency of agents of tinea capitis in school children fromWestern China suggest slow migration rates in dermatophytes. Med Mycol. 2008;46:421–7.
50. Bassiri-Jahromi S, Khaksar A. Outbreak of tinea gladiatorum in wrestlers in Tehran (Iran). Indian J Dermatol. 2008;53:132–6.
51. Saham A, Mohammad H, Zomorodian K, Pakshir K, Badali H, Abdollah R, Ravandeh Mostafa SS. Molecular characterization and in vitro antifungal susceptibility of 316 clinical isolates of dermatophytes in Iran. Mycopathologia. 2016;181:89–95.
52. Afshar P, Khodavaisy S, Kalhori S, Ghasemi M, Razavyoon T. Onychomycosis in North-East of Iran. Iran J Microbiol. 2014;6:98–103.
53. Aghamirian MR, Ghiasian SA. A clinico-epidemiological study on tinea gladiatorum in Iranian wrestlers and mat contamination by dermatophytes. Mycoses. 2011;54: 248–53.
54. Banik A, Durairaj E, Lyngdoh W, Khyriem AB, Sabhapandit D. Clinico-aetiologic profile of Onychomycoses in a tertiary care centre in northeast India. Trop Dr. 2018;48:136–42.
55. Noguchi H, Hiruma M, Kawada A, Ishibashi A, Kono S. Tinea pedis in members of the Japanese Self-defence Forces: relationships of its prevalence and its severity with length of military service and width of interdigital spaces. Mycoses. 1995;38:494–9.
56. Noguchi H, Jinnin M, Miyata K, Hiruma M, Ihn H. Clinical features of 80 cases of tinea faciei treated at a rural clinic in Japan. Drug Discov Ther. 2014;8:245–8.

57. Bhat YJ, Zeerak S, Kanth F, Yaseen A, Hassan I, Hakak R. Clinicoepidemiological and mycological study of tinea capitis in the pediatric population of Kashmir valley: a study from a tertiary care centre. Indian Dermatol Online J. 2017;8:100–3.
58. Yehia MA, El-Ammawi TS, Al-Mazidi KM, El-Ela MAA, Al-Ajmi HS. The spectrum of fungal infections with a special reference to dermatophytoses in the Capital area of Kuwait during 2000-2005: A retrospective analysis. Mycopathologia. 2010;169:241–6.
59. Gupta AK, Mays RR, Versteeg SG, Piraccini BM, Takwale A, Shemer A, Babaev M, Grover C, Di Chiacchio NG, Taborda PRO, Taborda VBA, Shear NH, Piguet V, Tosti A. Global perspectives for the management of onychomycosis. Int J Dermatol. 2018:1–12.
60. Shahzad M, Alzolibani AA, Al Robaee AA, Bin Saif GA, Babikir IHK, Abdel-Magied EM, Elsayed AE. Onychomycosis in Qassim region of Saudi Arabia: A clinicoaetiologic correlation. J Clin Diagnostic Res. 2014;8:1–4.
61. Gupta AK, Konnikov N, MacDonald P, Rich P, Rodger NW, Edmonds MW, McManus R, Summerbell RC. Prevalence and epidemiology of toenail onychomycosis in diabetic subjects: a multicentre survey. Br J Dermatol. 1998;139:665–71.
62. Aghamirian MR, Ghiasian SA. Onychomycosis in Iran: epidemiology, causative agents and clinical features. Japanese J Med Mycol. 2010;51:23–9.
63. Borda LJ, Wikramanayake TC. Seborrheic dermatitis and dandruff: a comprehensive review. J Clin Investig dermatology. 2015;3
64. Otomi Cho AT. Molecular characterization of the skin fungal microbiota in patients with seborrheic dermatitis. J Clin Exp Dermatol Res. 2015;05:5–8.
65. Nakabayashi A, Sei Y, Guillot J. Identification of *Malassezia* species isolated from patients with seborrhoeic dermatitis, atopic dermatitis, pityriasis versicolor and normal subjects. Med Mycol. 2000;38:337–41.
66. Tajima M, Sugita T, Nishikawa A, Tsuboi R. Molecular analysis of Malassezia microflora in seborrheic dermatitis patients: comparison with other diseases and healthy subjects. J Invest Dermatol. 2008;128:345–51.
67. Jing W. A retrospective survey of mucocutaneous manifestations of HIV infection in Malaysia: analysis of 182 cases. J Dermatol. 2000;27:225–32.
68. Kim TG, Lee KH, Oh SH. Skin disorders in Korean patients infected with human immunodeficiency virus and their association with a CD4 lymphocyte count: a preliminary study. J Eur Acad Dermatology Venereol. 2010;24:1476–80.
69. Wiwanitkit V. Prevalence of dermatological disorders in Thai HIV-infected patients correlated with different CD4 lymphocyte count statuses: a note on 120 cases. Int J Dermatol. 2004;43:265–8.
70. Rudramurthy SM, Honnavar P, Dogra S, Yegneswaran PP, Handa S, Chakrabarti A. Association of *Malassezia* species with dandruff. Indian J Med Res. 2014;139:431–7.
71. Honnavar P, Prasad GS, Ghosh A, Dogra S, Handa S, Rudramurthy SM. Malassezia arunalokei sp. nov., a novel yeast species isolated from seborrheic dermatitis patients and healthy individuals from India. J Clin Microbiol. 2016;54:1826–34.
72. Sunenshine PJ, Schwartz RA, Janniger CK. Tinea versicolor. Int J Dermatol. 1998;37:648–55.
73. Schwartz RA. Superficial fungal infections. Lancet. 2004;364:1173–82.
74. Gupta AK, Bluhm R, Summerbell R. Pityriasis versicolor. J Eur Acad Dermatol Venereol. 2002;16:19–33.
75. Karray M, Mckinney WP. Tinea, versicolor pathophysiology treatment/management. StatPearls Publ. 2019:1–5.
76. Zeinali E, Sadeghi G, Yazdinia F, Shams-Ghahfarokhi M, Razzaghi-Abyaneh M. Clinical and epidemiological features of the genus malassezia in iran. Iran J Microbiol. 2014;6:354–60.
77. Moallaei H, Namazi MJ, Bouchara JP, Pourhammed S. *Malassezia* species in students from universities of Sabzevar, Northeastern Iran. J Mycol Med. 2018;28:70–5.
78. He S, Du W, Yang S, Zhou S, Li W, Wang J, Xiao F, Xu S, Zhang X. The genetic epidemiology of tinea versicolor in China. Mycoses. 2008;51:55–62.
79. Krisanty RIA, Bramono K, Made Wisnu I. Identification of *Malassezia* species from pityriasis versicolor in Indonesia and its relationship with clinical characteristics. Mycoses. 2009;52:257–62.

80. Vijayanand S. Characterization of *Malassezia* species isolated from Pityriasis versicolor patients and healthy subjects of North-east India by PCR-RFLP. Int J Recent Sci Res. 2017;8:16624–31.
81. Biswas Pramanik S, Chakraborty A, Nandi A, Banerjee M, Ghosh R, Bandopadhyay M, Banerjee D. A Study of Prevalence of Different Species of Malassezia Causing Pityriasis Versicolor and Sites of Distribution of Lesion in a Tertiary Care Hospital in Kolkata, India. IntJCurrMicrobiolAppSci. 2015;4:471–8.
82. Sharma A, Rabha D, Choraria S, Hazarika D, Ahmed G, Hazarika NK. Clinicomycological profile of pityriasis versicolor in Assam. Indian J Pathol Microbiol. 2016;59:159–65.
83. Chaudhary R, Singh S, Banerjee T, Tilak R. Prevalence of different *Malassezia* species in pityriasis versicolor in central India. Indian J Dermatol Venereol Leprol. 2010;76:159–64.
84. Kindo AJ, Sophia SKC, Kalyani J, Anandan S. Identification of *Malassezia* species. Indian J Med Microbiol. 2004;22:179–81.
85. Prieto-Granada CN, Lobo AZC, Mihm MC. Skin infections. In: Diagnostic pathology of infectious disease. 1st ed. New York: Elsevier; 2010. p. 519–616.
86. Akaza N, Akamatsu H, Sasaki Y, Kishi M, Mizutani H, Sano A, Hirokawa K, Nakata S, Nishijima S, Matsunaga K. Malassezia folliculitis is caused by cutaneous resident Malassezia species. Med Mycol. 2009;47:618–24.
87. Durdu M, Güran M, Ilkit M. Epidemiological characteristics of Malassezia folliculitis and use of the May-Grünwald-Giemsa stain to diagnose the infection. Diagn Microbiol Infect Dis. 2013;76:450–7.
88. Sutton DA, Rinaldi MG, Sanche SE. Dematiaceous fungi. Elsevier, 329–54; 2009.
89. Sarangi G, Dash D, Chayani N, Patjoshi S, Jena S. Bilateral tinea nigra of palm: a rare case report from Eastern India. Indian J Med Microbiol. 2014;32:86–8.
90. Tilak R, Singh S, Prakash P, Singh D, Gulati A. A case report of tinea nigra from North India. Indian J Dermatol Venereol Leprol. 2009;75:538.
91. Noguchi H, Hiruma M, Inoue Y, Miyata K, Tanaka M, Ihn H. Tinea nigra showing a parallel ridge pattern on dermoscopy. J Dermatol. 2015;42:518–20.
92. Chen GY, Cheng YW, Wang CY, Hsu TJ, Hsu ML, Yang PT, Chen WC. Prevalence of skin diseases among schoolchildren in Magong, Penghu, Taiwan: A community-based clinical survey. J Formos Med Assoc. 2008;107:21–9.
93. Shivaprakash MR, Singh G, Gupta P, Dhaliwal M, Kanwar AJ, Chakrabarti A. Extensive white piedra of the scalp caused by Trichosporon inkin: a case report and review of literature. Mycopathologia. 2011;172:481–6.
94. Khandpur S, Reddy BS. Itraconazole therapy for white piedra affecting scalp hair. J Am Acad Dermatol. 2002;47:415–8.
95. Al-Sogair SM, Moawad MK, Al-Humaidan YM. Fungal infection as a cause of skin disease in the Eastern Province of Saudi Arabia: prevailing fungi and pattern of infection. Mycoses. 2010;34:333–7.
96. Kubec K, Dvorak R, Alsaleh QA. Trichosporosis (white piedra) in Kuwait. Int J Dermatol. 1998;37:186–7.
97. Adam BA, Soo-Hoo TS, Chong KC. Black piedra in west Malaysia. Australas J Dermatol. 1977;18:45–7.
98. Desai DH, Nadkarni NJ. Piedra: an ethnicity-related trichosis? Int J Dermatol. 2014;53:1008–11.
99. Venugopal PV, Venugopal TV. Superficial Mycoses in Saudi Arabia. Australas J Dermatol. 1992;33:45–8.
100. Thomas PA, Kaliamurthy J. Mycotic keratitis: epidemiology, diagnosis and management. Clin Microbiol Infect. 2013;19:210–20.
101. Radhakrishnan A (2011) Fungal Keratitis. 20–24.
102. Deorukhkar S, Katiyar R, Saini S. Epidemiological features and laboratory results of bacterial and fungal keratitis: A five-year study at a rural tertiary-care hospital in western Maharashtra, India. Singap Med J. 2012;53:264–7.
103. Bharathi MJ, Ramakrishnan R, Vasu S, Meenakshi R, Palaniappan R. Epidemiological characteristics and laboratory diagnosis of fungal keratitis. A three-year study. Indian J Ophthalmol. 2003;51:315–21.

104. Wang L, Sun S, Jing Y, Han L, Zhang H, Yue J. Spectrum of fungal keratitis in central China. Clin Exp Ophthalmol. 2009;37:763–71.
105. Thomas PA. Fungal infections of the cornea. Eye. 2003;17:852–62.
106. Ghosh AK, Gupta A, Rudramurthy SM, Paul S, Hallur VK, Chakrabarti A. Fungal keratitis in North India: spectrum of agents, risk factors and treatment. Mycopathologia. 2016;181:843–50.
107. Manikandan P, Abdel-hadi A, Randhir Babu Singh Y, Revathi R, Anita R, Banawas S, Bin Dukhyil AA, Alshehri B, Shobana CS, Panneer Selvam K, Narendran V. Fungal keratitis: epidemiology, rapid detection, and antifungal susceptibilities of fusarium and aspergillus isolates from corneal scrapings. Biomed Res Int. 2019;2019:1–9.
108. Khanal B, Kaini KR, Deb M, Badhu B, Thakur SK. Microbial keratitis in eastern Nepal. Trop Dr. 2001;31:168–9.
109. Dunlop AA, Wright ED, Howlader SA, Nazrul I, Husain R, McClellan K, Billson FA. Suppurative corneal ulceration in Bangladesh. A study of 142 cases examining the microbiological diagnosis, clinical and epidemiological features of bacterial and fungal keratitis. Aust N Z J Ophthalmol. 1994;22:105–10.
110. Xie L, Zhong W, Shi W, Sun S. Spectrum of Fungal Keratitis in North China. Ophthalmology. 2006;113:1943–8.
111. Hasika R, Lalitha P, Radhakrishnan N, Rameshkumar G, Prajna NV, Srinivasan M. Pythium keratitis in South India: Incidence, clinical profile, management, and treatment recommendation. Indian J Ophthalmol. 2019;67:42–7.
112. Thanathanee O, Enkvetchakul O, Rangsin R, Waraasawapati S, Samerpitak K, Suwan-apichon O. Outbreak of Pythium keratitis during rainy season: a case series. Cornea. 2013;32:199–204.
113. Lekhanont K, Chuckpaiwong V, Chongtrakool P, Aroonroch R, Vongthongsri A. Pythium insidiosum keratitis in contact lens wear: a case report. Cornea. 2009;28:1173–7.
114. Joseph J, Sridhar MS, Murthy S, Sharma S. Clinical and Microbiological Profile of Microsporidial Keratoconjunctivitis in Southern India. Ophthalmology. 2006;113:531–7.
115. Joseph J, Vemuganti GK, Sharma S. Microsporidia: emerging ocular pathogens. Indian J Med Microbiol. 2005;23:80–91.
116. Reddy AK, Balne PK, Garg P, Krishnaiah S. Is microsporidial keratitis a seasonal infection in India? Clin Microbiol Infect. 2011;17:1114–6.
117. Shivaprakash MR, Appannanavar SB, Dhaliwal M, Gupta A, Gupta S, Gupta A, Chakrabarti A. Colletotrichum truncatum: an unusual pathogen causing mycotic keratitis and endophthalmitis. J Clin Microbiol. 2011;49:2894–8.
118. Joseph J, Fernandes M, Sharma S. Colletotrichum dematium keratitis. J Postgrad Med. 2004;50:309–10.
119. Mendiratta D, Thamke D, Shukla A, Narang P. Keratitis due to Colletotrichum dematium - a case report. Indian J Med Microbiol. 2005;23:56.
120. Ali SY, Gajjala SR, Raj A. Study of prevalence of dermatophytes among human immunodeficiency virus/AIDS patients in Shadan Institute of Medical Sciences and Teaching Hospital and Research Centre, Hyderabad, Telangana, India. Indian J Sex Transm Dis AIDS. 2018;39:98–101.
121. Sen A, Bhunia D, Datta PK, Ray A, Banerjee P. A study of onychomycosis at a tertiary care hospital in Eastern Bihar. Indian J Dermatol. 2018;63:141–6.
122. Asifa N, Farhath K. Current mycological profile of onychomycosis in Kashmir valley: A hospital-based study. J Lab Physicians. 2017;9:190.
123. Dabas Y, Xess I, Singh G, Pandey M, Meena S. Molecular identification and antifungal susceptibility patterns of clinical dermatophytes following CLSI and EUCAST guidelines. J Fungi (Basel, Switzerland). 2017:3, 17–27.
124. Sharma R, Adhikari L, Sharma RL. Recurrent dermatophytosis: A rising problem in Sikkim, a Himalayan state of India. Indian J Pathol Microbiol. 2017;60:541–5.
125. Manjunath M. Clinicomycological study of Dermatomycosis in a tertiary care hospital. Indian J Microbiol Res. 2016;3:190–3.

126. Kaur R, Panda PS, Sardana K, Khan S. Mycological pattern of dermatomycoses in a tertiary care hospital. J Trop Med. 2015;2015:1–5.
127. Poluri LV, Indugula JP, Kondapaneni SL. Clinicomycological study of dermatophytosis in South India. J Lab Physicians. 2015;7:84–9.
128. Agarwal US, Saran J, Agarwal P. Clinico-mycological study of dermatophytes in a tertiary care centre in Northwest India. Indian J Dermatol Venereol Leprol. 2014;80:194–5.
129. Bhagra S, Ganju SA, Kanga A, Sharma NL, Guleria RC. Mycological pattern of dermatophytosis in and around shimla hills. Indian J Dermatol. 2014;59:268–70.
130. Surendran K, Bhat RM, Boloor R, Nandakishore B, Sukumar D. A clinical and mycological study of dermatophytic infections. Indian J Dermatol. 2014;59:262–7.
131. Yadav P, Singal A, Pandhi D, Das S. Clinicomycological study of dermatophyte toenail onychomycosis in New Delhi, India. Indian J Dermatol. 2015;60:153–8.
132. Kumari B, Randi K, Sharma R. The major etiological cause in human dermatophytoses in Chennai. Int J Mycol Plant Pathog. 2014;1:42–4.
133. Lone R, Bashir D, Ahmad S, Syed A, Khurshid S. A study on clinico-mycological profile, aetiological agents and diagnosis of onychomycosis at a government medical college hospital in kashmir. J Clin Diagn Res. 2013;7:1983–5.
134. Pandey A, Pandey M. Isolation and characterization of dermatophytes with tinea infections at Gwalior (MP), India. Int J Pharm Sci Inven. 2013;2:5–8.
135. Niranjan HP, Padmaja PB. Study of onychomycosis at a tertiary care hospital in South India. J Evol Med Dent Sci. 2012;1:823–9.
136. Sahai S, Mishra D. Change in spectrum of dermatophytes isolated from superficial mycoses cases: first report from Central India. Indian J Dermatol Venereol Leprol. 2011;77:335–6.
137. Patel P, Mulla S, Disha Patel GS. A Study of superficial mycosis in South Gujarat region. Natl J Community Med. 2010;1:85–8.
138. Adhikari L, Das Gupta A, Pal R, Singh TSK, Das GA, Pal R, TSK S. Clinico-etiologic correlates of onychomycosis in Sikkim. Indian J Pathol Microbiol. 2009;52:194–7.
139. Wu SX, Guo NR, Li XF, Liao WQ, Chen M, Zhang QQ, Li CY, Li RY, Bulmer GS, Li DM, Xi LY, Lu S, Liu B, Zheng YC, Ran YP, Kuan YZ. Human pathogenic fungi in China-emerging trends from ongoing National Survey for 1986, 1996, and 2006. Mycopathologia. 2011;171:387–93.
140. Zhu M, Li L, Wang J, Zhang C, Kang K, Zhang Q. Tinea capitis in Southeastern China: A 16-year survey. Mycopathologia. 2010;169:235–9.
141. Abastabar M, Haghani I, Shokohi T, Hedayati MT, Aghili SR, Jedi A, Dadashi S, Shabanzadeh S, Hosseini T, Aslani N, Meis JF, Badali H. Low in vitro antifungal activity of tavaborole against yeasts and molds from onychomycosis. Antimicrob Agents Chemother. 2018;62:e01632–18.
142. Farokhipor S, Ghiasian SA, Nazeri H, Kord M, Didehdar M. Characterizing the clinical isolates of dermatophytes in Hamadan city, Central west of Iran, using PCR-RLFP method. J Mycol Med. 2018;28:101–5.
143. Haghani I, Shams-Ghahfarokhi M, Dalimi Asl A, Shokohi T, Hedayati MT. Molecular identification and antifungal susceptibility of clinical fungal isolates from onychomycosis (uncommon and emerging species). Mycoses. 2019;62:128–43.
144. Babayani M, Salari S, Hashemi SJ, Ghasemi Nejad Almani P, Fattahi A. Onychomycosis due to dermatophytes species in Iran: Prevalence rates, causative agents, predisposing factors and diagnosis based on microscopic morphometric findings. J Mycol Med. 2018;28:45–50.
145. Khosravi AR, Shokri H, Vahedi G. Factors in etiology and predisposition of adult tinea capitis and review of published literature. Mycopathologia. 2016;181:371–8.
146. Chadeganipour M, Mohammadi R, Shadzi S. A 10-year study of dermatophytoses in Isfahan, Iran. J Clin Lab Anal. 2016;30:103–7.
147. Rashidian S, Falahati M, Kordbacheh P, Mahmoudi M, Safara M, Sadeghi Tafti H, Mahmoudi S, Zaini F. A study on etiologic agents and clinical manifestations of dermatophytosis in Yazd, Iran. Curr Med Mycol. 2015;1:20–5.
148. Naseri A, Fata A, Najafzadeh MJ, Shokri H. Surveillance of dermatophytosis in Northeast of Iran (Mashhad) and review of published studies. Mycopathologia. 2013;176:247–53.

149. Bassiri-Jahromi S. Epidemiological trends in zoophilic and geophilic fungi in Iran. Clin Exp Dermatol. 2013;38:13–9.
150. Ansar A, Farshchian M, Nazeri H, Ghiasian SA. Clinico-epidemiological and mycological aspects of tinea incognito in Iran: A 16-year study. Japanese J Med Mycol. 2011;52:25–32.
151. Pang SM, Pang JYY, Fook-Chong S, Tan AL. Tinea unguium onychomycosis caused by dermatophytes: a ten-year (2005-2014) retrospective study in a tertiary hospital in Singapore. Singap Med J. 2018;59:524–7.
152. Do NA, Nguyen TD, Nguyen KL, Le TA. Distribution of species of dermatophyte among patients at a dermatology Centre of Nghean Province, Vietnam, 2015–2016. Mycopathologia. 2017;182:1061–7.
153. Ramalingam R, Kunalan S, Tang MM. Mycology of onychomycosis: A 5-year retrospective review (2011 – 2015) in hospital Kuala Lumpur. Med J Malaysia. 2017;72:190–2.
154. Nussipov Y, Markabayeva A, Gianfaldoni S, Tchernev G, Wollina U, Lotti J, Roccia MG, Fioranelli M, Lotti T. Clinical and epidemiological features of dermatophyte infections in Almaty, Kazakhstan. Open Access Maced J Med Sci. 2017;5:409.
155. Khaled JM, Golah HA, Khalel AS, Alharbi NS, Mothana RA. Dermatophyte and non dermatophyte fungi in Riyadh City, Saudi Arabia. Saudi J Biol Sci. 2015;22:604–9.
156. Elmegeed A, Al Shimaa M, Ouf S, Moussa A, Tarek AA, Eltahlawi SMR. Dermatophytes and other associated fungi in patients attending to some hospitals in Egypt. Braz J Microbiol. 1973;46:799–805.
157. Abu Shaqra QM, Al Momani W. Cases of tinea capitis as encountered in a private practice laboratory from Jordan. J Mycol Med. 2011;21:24–7.
158. Akcaglar S, Ener B, Toker SC, Ediz B, Tunali S, Tore O. A comparative study of dermatophyte infections in Bursa, Turkey. Med Mycol. 2011;49:602–7.
159. Koksal F, Er E, Samasti M. Causative agents of superficial mycoses in Istanbul, Turkey: retrospective study. Mycopathologia. 2009;168:117–23.
160. Narang T, Manhas A, Aggarwal P, Bala M, Kaur M, Gupte S. Study of the distribution of Malassezia species in patients with pityriasis versicolor and healthy individuals in Tertiary Care Hospital, Punjab. Indian J Med Microbiol. 2013;31:270.
161. Jena DK, Sengupta S, Dwari BC, Ram MK. Pityriasis versicolor in the pediatric age group. Indian J Dermatol Venereol Leprol. 2005;71:259–61.
162. Dutta S, Bajaj AK, Basu S, Dikshit A. Pityriasis versicolor: socioeconomic and clinicomycologic study in India. Int J Dermatol. 2002;41:823–4.
163. Zhang H, Ran Y, Xie Z, Zhang R. Identification of malassezia species in patients with seborrheic dermatitis in China. Mycopathologia. 2013;175:83–9.
164. Mansouri P, Farshi S, Hashemi J, Khosravi AR, Saghazadeh M. Identification of Malassezia species isolated from patients with seborrheic dermatitis, atopic dermatitis, and normal subjects. J Mycol Med. 2010;20:279–82.
165. Rasi A, Naderi R, Behzadi AH, Falahati M, Farehyar S, Honarbakhsh Y, Akasheh AP. Malassezia yeast species isolated from Iranian patients with pityriasis versicolor in a prospective study. Mycoses. 2010;53:350–5.
166. Tarazooie B, Kordbacheh P, Zaini F, Zomorodian K, Saadat F, Zeraati H, Hallaji Z, Rezaie S. Study of the distribution of Malassezia species in patients with pityriasis versicolor and healthy individuals in Tehran, Iran. BMC Dermatol. 2004;4:5.
167. Lyakhovitsky A, Shemer A, Amichai B. Molecular analysis of Malassezia species isolated from Israeli patients with pityriasis versicolor. Int J Dermatol. 2013;52:231–3.
168. Rodoplu G, Saracli MA, Gümral R, Taner Yildiran S. Distribution of Malassezia species in patients with pityriasis versicolor in Turkey. J Mycol Med. 2014;24:117–23.
169. Karakaş M, Turaç-Biçer A, Ilkit M, Durdu M, Seydaŏlu G. Epidemiology of pityriasis versicolor in adana, Turkey. J Dermatol. 2009;36:377–82.
170. Kamalam A, Thambiah AS. A study of 3891 cases of mycoses in the tropics. Sabouraudia. 1976;14:129–48.
171. Kiken DA, Sekaran A, Antaya RJ, Davis A, Imaeda S, Silverberg NB. White piedra in children. J Am Acad Dermatol. 2006;55:956–61.

Epidemiology of Endemic Mycoses in Asia

3

Arunaloke Chakrabarti

Key Points

- Histoplasmosis, talaromycosis, and sporotrichosis are prevalent in Asian countries.
- With travel history to endemic zone, coccidioidomycosis and paracoccidioidomycosis may be suspected.
- Histoplasmosis and talaromycosis are more prevalent in AIDS patients and difficult to distinguish clinically in the overlapping endemic zone. Both diseases may be misidentified as tuberculosis.
- Always suspect endemic mycoses as differential diagnosis of pulmonary tuberculosis.
- Skin lesion is more common in talaromycosis.
- Histoplasma antigen in urine helps in diagnosis of histoplasmosis, though sensitivity of the test may be less in chronic pulmonary disease.
- *Histoplasma* cross-reacts with *Aspergillus* Galactomannan. In absence of *Histoplasma* antigen test, Galactomannan test can be performed.
- Mucosal ulcer and adrenal tumour are common in histoplasmosis of immunocompetent hosts.
- Sporotrichosis is common in China, India, and Japan and *S. globosa* is the causative agent.
- Outbreaks of sporotrichosis have been reported from contaminated hay and cornstalk.

A. Chakrabarti (✉)
Department of Medical Microbiology, Postgraduate Institute of Medical Education and Research (PGIMER), Chandigarh, India

A. Chakrabarti (ed.), *Clinical Practice of Medical Mycology in Asia*,
https://doi.org/10.1007/978-981-13-9459-1_3

3.1 Introduction

Endemic mycoses are a group of fungal diseases caused by diverse fungi having common characteristics like restricted ecological niche, dimorphic characters (yeast or spherule in the host at 37 °C and mycelial form in nature or culture at 25 °C), and capability producing infection in healthy hosts. The fungi classified under dimorphic pathogenic group are illustrated in Table 3.1. Among endemic mycoses, three diseases (histoplasmosis, penicilliosis, and sporotrichosis) are commonly seen in Asian countries [1]. The incidence of histoplasmosis and talaromycosis increased markedly with the rise of patients with AIDS in this region. After introduction of

Table 3.1 Dimorphic fungi causing human infections

Fungus	Disease	Natural habitat	Geographical distribution
Blastomyces dermatitidis	Blastomycosis	Poorly known, isolation from river and forest soil	(Mississippi and Ohio river valley)
Coccidioides immitis *C. posadasii*	Coccidioidomycosis	Soil of arid regions, animal burrows	Arid regions of southwest United States, parts of Central and South America
Histoplasma capsulatum var. capsulatum	Histoplasmosis	Soil enriched with avian or bat dung	Mississippi and Ohio river valley in United States, major parts of Latin America, focal distribution in Africa, Asia, few cases in Europe
H. capsulatum var. duboisii	Histoplasmosis duboisii	Rarely isolated from soil	Africa and Madagascar island
H. capsulatum var. farciminosum	Histoplasmosis farciminosi	Unknown	North Africa, East and West equatorial Africa, South Africa, Sudan, Middle East, India, Myanmar, Indonesia
Paracoccidioides brasiliensis	Paracoccidioidomycosis	Rarely isolated from soil	Central and South America
Sporothrix schenckii sensu lato	Sporotrichosis	Dead or senescent vegetation	Cosmopolitan with higher prevalence in tropical and subtropical regions
Emmonsia crescens	Adiaspiromycosis	118 animal species as host, rarely from soil	Worldwide except Africa and Australia
Emmonsia parva	Adiaspiromycosis	21 animal species as host, rarely from soil	Worldwide
Emergomyces pasteuriana	Emergomycosis	Unknown	India, Italy, and possibly China
Emergomyces africanus	Emergomycosis	Not known	South Africa, and possibly Canada
Sporotrichum pruinosum	Name not given	Soil	Solitary report from India, doubtful pathogenic potential

anti-retroviral therapy, it is expected that incidence of endemic mycoses would come down. However, the present status of such patients is not known due to paucity of data. Few indigenous blastomycosis cases have been reported from India and *Blastomyces dermatitidis* had been isolated from bats in India, but the disease is still rare in Asia [1–3]. The reported cases of coccidioidomycosis (few cases from India) and paracoccidioidomycosis (single case from Japan) are all imported cases.

The agents causing histoplasmosis, talaromycosis, and blastomycosis are acquired through the respiratory tract. They produce primary pulmonary infection and then disseminate in a suitable host. Due to common mode of acquisition, the epidemiology of these three diseases is discussed together. Sporotrichosis caused by *Sporothrix schenckii (*sensu *lato)* is predominantly acquired by inoculation of the organism across cutaneous barrier. Few pulmonary or systemic cases of sporotrichosis have been reported where the organism possibly entered the body through respiratory tract. A summary of these four endemic mycoses prevalent in Asia is described in Table 3.2.

A new dimorphic fungus (taxonomy not well characterized) has been found to produce infections (emergomycosis) in many HIV positive patients of South Africa. Initially the fungus was put under Genus *Emmonsia*, and later identified as *Emergomyces africanus* [4]. In India, few similar cases are identified and named the fungus as *Emergomyces pasteuriana* after molecular taxonomy [5]. However, the taxonomy of the fungus is still evolving and morphologically similar to *Blastomyces dermatitidis*.

3.2 Epidemiology of Histoplasmosis, Talaromycosis, and Blastomycosis in Asia

The detailed systematic epidemiological study of these three mycoses in Asia is not available due to possible misdiagnosis as tuberculosis, lack of awareness of fungal diseases in general and inadequate mycology laboratory facilities in this region. From the few centre-based data, it appears that the diseases have pocket distribution [1, 6–9].

Endemicity of histoplasmosis has been evaluated by few population-based histoplasmin skin test studies. Overall 5–14% of world population is histoplasmin skin test positive with higher rate (14%) in medical students and hospitalized patients [10]. In comparison, different studies from Asia reported 0–12.3% skin test positivity in India, 3% in Malaysia, 26% of long-term residents of Phillippines, and 19% in China. The skin test positivity is much higher in South-East region of China compared to North-East region [7, 8, 11–15]. These studies indicate that certain regions of Asia are possibly endemic for histoplasmosis. There is a single report of *H. capsulatum* isolation from environment in Asia. The fungus was isolated from an old building near Calcutta [16]. In a recent review of 204 cases from India, it is claimed that the histoplasmosis is prevalent in riverine belt (Ganges, Yamuna, and Brahmaputra) among males working in the agriculture field [17]. Contrary to this picture, another Indian study from Western India highlighted the presence of histoplasmosis cases in arid region of Rajasthan [18]. Possibly there is no non-endemic

Table 3.2 Endemic mycoses prevalent in Asia

	Histoplasmosis	Talaromycosis	Sporotrichosis	Blastomycosis
Endemic areas	Not clear but pocket distribution (microfoci) known Skin test positivity rate varies at 0–35% depending on endemicity. Cases have been reported from almost all countries in Asia. The case number has increased with the AIDS epidemic	South-east and Eastern Asia including Thailand, North-east India, China, Hong Kong, Laos, Cambodia, Malaysia, Myanmar, Vietnam, Taiwan. Case number increased after AIDS epidemic. Third most common opportunistic infection in AIDS in endemic areas	Most of the cases reported from China, India and Japan. The areas have a wide range of climatic and geographical variation	Only reported from India (few cases)
Favourable condition for exposure	Not clearly known, cosmopolitan distribution, single environmental isolation in India, so ecological niche is not clearly delineated	Environmental source not known, exposure to soil especially in rainy season may provide favourable condition for acquisition	Hay, corn stalk, and soil are possible sources. Persons engaged in farming, forestry, and horticultural work are susceptible	Isolated from lung and liver of bats in Delhi, but it is not known whether bats can be reservoir of human infection
Clinical presentation	Large numbers of cases remain asymptomatic and self-limiting. Three major clinical presentations—pulmonary, progressive disseminated, and primary cutaneous; 10% develop progressive disseminated infection, which manifest as chronic or acute progressive disease. Mucocutaneous lesions and adrenal tumours are common presentations in immunocompetent hosts	Fever, cough, anaemia, lymphadenopathy, hepatosplenomegaly, weight loss; skin lesions are common (60–85%) over face, upper trunk, extremities; lesions are necrotic or generalized papules or nodules, some are molluscum contagiosum like (central umbilication), Difficult to distinguish when both histoplasmosis and talaromycosis are endemic in same areas, though skin lesions are more common in talaromycosis	Subacute or chronic subcutaneous granulomatous disease. Two-third cases present as lympho-cutaneous variety, one-third fixed cutaneous, common on extremities, but may be seen at unusual sites like face. Primary pulmonary or multilocus varieties are very rare	Half of patients remain asymptomatic. Wide range of clinical manifestation including pulmonary disease and extra-pulmonary disseminated disease involving skin, soft tissue, bones, central nervous system

Diagnosis – Direct microscopy and Histopathology	H & E, GMS stain useful in progressive disseminate type (50% sensitivity for bone marrow). In AIDS-BAL—70%, in pulmonary— <25% Yeast cell (2–4 μ, budding) should be distinguished from other small yeasts (*Candida glabrata, Talaromyces marneffei*), Leishmania and Toxoplasma	Biopsy or scraping of skin lesion—typical elongated yeast cell (3–5 μ) with transverse septation. Microorganisms may be seen in other clinical specimen, depending on site of infection	Biopsy specimen may show cigar shaped yeast cells. But may be negative in large number of cases	Broad based budding, thick walled yeast in respiratory secretion or tissue
– Culture	Takes time—2–4 weeks Both macro- and microconidia (confirmed by molecular probe, conversion to yeast form, sequencing of ITS region of ribosomal DNA)	Blood culture and culture of biopsy or scraping specimen—colonies within 3–7 days, flat grey colony with red pigmentation on the background. Commonly associated with hyperbilirubinemia. **Simple skin scraping from lesion or blood culture to diagnose majority of the cases**	Best method of diagnosis, as direct microscopy may be negative, takes time to grow (1–2 weeks), typical thin hyphae with flower shaped arrangement of conidia. Confirmed by conversion to yeast form or molecular method especially to identify the new species	Sensitivity of BAL is higher. Identification difficult, should be differentiated from *Crysosporium* species (molecular probe, conversion to yeast form, molecular method by sequencing)
– Serology	Antigen detection very sensitive—90–95% in urine and serum. Antigen detection in acute pulmonary—80%, chronic pulmonary—20%, cross reaction with talaromycosis, blastomycosis, paracoccidioidomycosis. Antibody detection useful in chronic and subacute pulmonary histoplasmosis in immunocompetent host CF is better than ID	Many serological tests are of promise, but none is validated	No test commercialized	Antigen detection of urine and serum—90–98%, cross reaction on the histoplasmosis Ag detection, possible in BAL Most experts do not recommend antibody detection tests

(continued)

Table 3.2 (continued)

	Histoplasmosis	Talaormycosis	Sporotrichosis	Blastomycosis
Test for monitoring therapy	Antigen test can be used to monitor therapy	Smear and culture is the only method for monitoring therapy	Smear and culture are the only methods to monitor therapy	Antigen test can be used to monitor therapy
Treatment	Mild pulmonary—no therapy Acute and chronic pulmonary—amphotericin B lipid formulations (3–5 mg/kg/day) or amphotericin B deoxycholate (0.7–1 mg/kg/day for 1–2 weeks followed by itraconazole. (200 mg thrice daily × 3 day and then 200 mg twice daily for 12 weeks) – Methyl prednisolone for 1–2 weeks in respiratory complication. Progressive disseminated histoplasmosis—same as above (Therapeutic drug monitoring during itraconazole use) Mediastinal fibrosis—no antifungal, but if difficult to differentiate from granulomas—Itraconazole and may require surgery	Highly susceptible to itraconazole, fluconazole – amphotericin B deoxycholate (0.7–1 mg /kg/day) for 2 weeks, then itraconazole 400 mg/day for next 10 weeks. Mild disease—itraconazole. 400 mg/day for 8 weeks followed by 200 mg/day to prevent recurrence. Itraconazole tablet taken after food, whereas oral suspension on empty stomach	Cutaneous and lympho-cutaneous—itraconazole. 200 mg/day for 2–4 weeks to 3–6 months. Not responding to itraconazole – Higher dose of itraconazole. – Terbinafine (500 mg twice daily) – Saturated solution of potassium iodide—5 drops thrice daily, increased to 40–50 drops thrice daily. – Fluconazole occasionally. Osteo-articular and disseminated – Itraconazole for 12 months. – Amphotericin B may be used as initial therapy	Pulmonary blastomycosis—same as histoplasmosis, but itraconazole should be given for 6–12 months Extra-pulmonary—same as above

zone of histoplasmosis in Asia. In immunocompetent patients in this region histoplasmosis may present as mucosal ulcers and adrenal tumours [17].

Talaromycosis is the only endemic mycosis in South-East and Eastern Asia [1, 19–24]. The disease is considered as AIDS defining illness in this region as it is the third most common opportunistic infection after tuberculosis and cryptococcosis in AIDS [19]. The environmental source of the agent *T. marneffei* is not known. It has been isolated from four species of bamboo rats from many countries [24–29]. In a study from Guangxi province of China, isolates from bamboo rats and humans were compared by multilocus genotypes. The types of the isolates from humans were similar to those from infected rats and in some cases identical [30]. But it is highly unlikely that humans acquire the infection from bamboo rats, as these animals live in remote mountain region or in jungles. Rather, the disease is linked to soil exposure especially during rainy season [31]. The association of humidity with talaromycosis cases was further established in a recent multivariate analysis of patients admitted in a hospital in Vietnam and comparing it with cryptococcosis cases. It appeared that the patients acquired the infection within three weeks of exposure [32]. As an alternative source, the fungus was detected by two PCR methods in 13% of nasal swabs collected from dogs roaming on the streets and temples of Chiang Mai, Thailand, indicating that the dogs may be a potential source of *T. marneffei* [33]. In certain regions of Asia like Southeast of China, histoplasmosis and talaromycosis are prevalent in the same geographical location. As both the diseases have similar clinical presentation like fever, weight loss, anaemia, lymphadenopathy, and hepatosplenomegaly, it is difficult to distinguish the diseases clinically. Skin lesions are more common in talaromycosis [24, 34]. Patients with HIV infection associated with talaromycosis have a higher incidence of fungemia compared to HIV-negative patients [35].

All three diseases exhibit a spectrum of pulmonary manifestations ranging from mild self-limiting disease to acute invasive diseases. Histoplasmosis has most varied presentations. The mild pulmonary histoplasmosis may occasionally get complicated by pericarditis or rheumatologic manifestations. After heavy exposure to *H. capsulatum* spores in soil contaminated with bird or bat droppings, patients may present with severe acute pulmonary histoplasmosis needing hospitalization. Patients with underlying obstructive pulmonary disease may exhibit progressive chronic pulmonary histoplasmosis. Immunosuppressed patients usually present with progressive disseminated histoplasmosis, which manifests either as chronic or acute disease. In India, histoplasmosis patients present commonly with oropharyngeal lesions or adrenal tumour [1, 36]. Certain rare presentations like histoplasmosis at eyelid and epididymis have been reported from India [37, 38]. Blastomycosis patients may develop diffuse pneumonia accompanied by acute respiratory distress syndrome (ARDS). The fungus has been isolated from pulmonary, cutaneous, and cerebral lesion in India [39–42]. Patients with talaromycosis usually have symptoms and signs relating to the involvement of reticuloendothelial systems, pulmonary tract, skin, and gastrointestinal system. But occasionally the infection may spread to central nervous system and the patients present with subacute febrile syndrome and changes of mental status. The early diagnosis of such patients is important as CNS infections are medical emergencies and the presentation CNS talaromycosis is similar to viral encephalitis, tuberculosis, and cryptococcal meningitis, which are common infections in patients with AIDS [43].

3.3 Epidemiology of Sporotrichosis

Sporotrichosis is commonly seen as a chronic granulomatous disease of cutaneous and subcutaneous tissue caused by dimorphic fungus *Sporothrix schenckii sensu lato*. Rarely, systemic sporotrichosis has been reported (nearly 90 cases reported worldwide till date), and manifested as primary pulmonary sporotrichosis or multifocal sporotrichosis involving skin and joints [44]. An extremely rare case of pulmonary sporotrichosis due to *S. luriei (= S. schenckii* var. *luriei)* had been reported from India [45].

Sporothrix schenckii sensu lato requires a mean temperature of 26/27 °C and humidity 92–100% to grow. The fungus is isolated from decaying plant materials such as sphagnum moss, vegetation, hay and from soil. Many small outbreaks have been reported among people using sphagnum moss [46, 47]. Association of human cases with feline animals has been strongly claimed in South America [48]. However, the epidemiology of sporotrichosis in Asia appears different, as majority cases of India, China, and Japan have been reported under a wide range of climate and geographic conditions [49–55]. In contrast to Latin America, the disease is more prevalent in females possibly reflecting gender-related outdoor activities by woman in Asia [49–56]. Outbreaks in this region have been linked to contaminated hay and cornstalks instead of sphagnum moss. An outbreak of infant sporotrichosis in China was possibly due to contaminated cornstalk stored for cooking and heating purposes during winter [57]. The association with animals in patients with sporotrichosis has not been detected in Asian sporotrichosis except one rare case in India [58].

S. schenckii has been characterized recently by molecular method and is found to be a complex of many separate phylogenetic species: S. *brasiliensis, S. schenckii, S. globosa, S. mexicana, S. albicans,* and *S. inflata* [59]. The majority of Asian isolates from China, India and Japan belong to *S. globosa* and rarely *S. schenckii* [59, 60].

References

1. Chakrabarti A, Slavin MA. Endemic fungal infections in the Asia-Pacific region. Med Mycol. 2011;49:337–44.
2. Khan ZU, Randhawa HS, Lulla M. Isolation of *Blastomyces dermatitidis* from the lungs of a bat, *Rhinopoma hardwickei hardwickei* Gray, in Delhi. Sabouraudia. 1982;20: 137–44.
3. Randhawa HS, Chaturvedi VP, Kini S, Khan ZU. *Blastomyces dermatitidis* in bats: first report of its isolation from the liver of *Rhinopoma hardwickei hardwickei* Gray. Sabouraudia. 1985;23:69–76.
4. Schwartz IS, McLoud JD, Berman D, Botha A, Lerm B, Colebunders R, Levetin E, Kenyon C. Molecular detection of airborne Emergomyces africanus, a thermally dimorphic fungal pathogen, in Cape Town, South Africa. PLoS Negl Trop Dis. 2018;12:e0006174.

5. Malik R, Capoor MR, Vanidassane I, Gogna A, Singh A, Sen B, Rudramurthy SM, Honnavar P, Gupta S, Chakrabarti A. Disseminated Emmonsia pasteuriana infection in India: a case report and a review. Mycoses. 2016;59:127–32.
6. Padhye AA, Pathak AA, Katkar VJ, Hazare VK, Kaufman L. Oral histoplasmosis in India: a case report and an overview of cases reported during 1968-92. J Med Vet Mycol. 1994;32:93–103.
7. Wang TL, Cheah JS, Holmberg K. Case report and review of disseminated histoplasmosis in South-East Asia: clinical and epidemiological implications. Tropical Med Int Health. 1996;1:35–42.
8. Zhao B, Xia X, Yin J, et al. Epidemiological investigation of *Histoplasma capsulatum* infection in China. Chin Med J. 2001;114:743–6.
9. Nissapatorn V, Lee CK, Rohela M, Anuar AK. Spectrum of opportunistic infections among HIV-infected patients in Malaysia. Southeast Asian J Trop Med Public Health. 2004;35(Suppl 2):26–32.
10. Edwards PQ, Billings EL. Worldwide pattern of skin sensitivity to histoplasmin. Am J Trop Med Hyg. 1971;20:288–319.
11. Randhawa HS, Khan ZU. Histoplasmosis in India: current status. Indian J Chest Dis Allied Sci. 1994;36:193–213.
12. Ponnampalam JT. A review of histoplasmosis in Malaya. Med J Malaya. 1968;23:295–8.
13. Bulmer AC, Bulmer GS. Incidence of histoplasmin hypersensitivity in the Philippines. Mycopathologia. 2001;149:69–71.
14. Wen FQ, Sun YD, Watanabe K, Yoshida M, Wu JN, Baum GL. Prevalence of histoplasmin sensitivity in healthy adults and tuberculosis patients in southwest China. J Med Vet Mycol. 1996;34:171–4.
15. Zhao B, Yin J. Xia X. [Investigation on the epidemiology of *Histoplasma capsulatum* infection in Nanjing district]. Zhonghua Liu Xing Bing Xue Za Zhi. 1998;19:215–7. [Chinese]
16. Sanyal M, Thammayya A. *Histoplasma capsulatum* in the soil of Gangetic Plain in India. Indian J Med Res. 1975;63:1020–8.
17. Gupta A, Ghosh A, Singh G, Xess I. A Twenty-First-Century Perspective of Disseminated Histoplasmosis in India: Literature Review and Retrospective Analysis of Published and Unpublished Cases at a Tertiary Care Hospital in North India. Mycopathologia. 2017;182:1077–93.
18. Patel AK, Patel KK, Toshniwal H, Gohel S, Chakrabarti A. Histoplasmosis in non-endemic North-Western part of India. Indian J Med Microbiol. 2018;36:61–4.
19. Supparatpinyo K, Khamwan C, Baosoung V, Nelson KE, Sirisanthana T. Disseminated *Penicillium marneffei* infection in southeast Asia. Lancet. 1994;344:110–3.
20. Duong TA. Infection due to *Penicillium marneffei*, an emerging pathogen: review of 155 reported cases. Clin Infect Dis. 1996;23:125–30.
21. Nittayananta W. Penicilliosis marneffei: another AIDS defining illness in Southeast Asia. Oral Dis. 1999;5:286–93.
22. Ranjana KH, Priyokumar K, Singh TJ, et al. Disseminated *Penicillium marneffei* infection among HIV-infected patients in Manipur state, India. J Infect. 2002;45:268–71.
23. Wu TC, Chan JW, Ng CK, Tsang DN, Lee MP, Li PC. Clinical presentations and outcomes of *Penicillium marneffei* infections: a series from 1994 to 2004. Hong Kong Med J. 2008;14:103–9.
24. Vanittanakom N, Cooper CR Jr, Fisher MC, Sirisanthana T. *Penicillium marneffei* infection and recent advances in the epidemiology and molecular biology aspects. Clin Microbiol Rev. 2006;19:95–110.
25. Deng ZL, Yun M, Ajello L. Human penicilliosis marneffei and its relation to the bamboo rat *(Rhizomys pruinosus)*. J Med Vet Mycol. 1986;24:383–9.
26. Wei XG, Ling YM, Li C, Zhang FS. Study of 179 bamboo rats carrying *Pennicillium marneffei*. China Journal of Zoonoses. 1987;3:34–5. [Chinese]
27. Ajello L, Padhye AA, Sukroongreung S, Nilakul CH, Tantimavanic S. Occurrence of *Penicillium marneffei* infections among wild bamboo rats in Thailand. Mycopathologia. 1995;131:1–8.

28. Chariyalertsak S, Vanittanakom P, Nelson KE, Sirisanthana T, Vanittanakom N. *Rhizomys sumatrenensis* and *Cannomys badius*, new natural animal hosts of *Penicillium marneffei*. J Med Vet Mycol. 1996;34:105–10.
29. Gugnani H, Fisher MC, Paliwal-Johsi A, Vanittanakom N, Singh I, Yadav PS. Role of *Cannomys badius* as a natural animal host of *Penicillium marneffei* in India. J Clin Microbiol. 2004;42:5070–5.
30. Cao C, Liang L, Wang W, Luo H, Huang S, Liu D, Xu J, Henk DA, Fisher MC. Common reservoirs for *Penicillium marneffei* infection in humans and rodents, China. Emerg Infect Dis. 2011;17:209–14.
31. Chariyalertsak S, Sirisanthana T, Supparatpinyo K, Praparattanapan J, Nelson KE. Case-control study of risk factors for *Penicillium marneffei* infection in human immunodeficiency virus-infected patients in northern Thailand. Clin Infect Dis. 1997;24:1080–6.
32. Bulterys PL, Le T, Quang VM, Nelson KE, Lloyd-Smith JO. Environmental predictors and incubation period of AIDS-associated *Penicillium marneffei* infection in Ho Chi Minh City, Vietnam. Clin Infect Dis. 2013;56:1273–9.
33. Chaiwun B, Vanittanakom N, Jiviriyawat Y, Rojanasthien S, Thorner P. Investigation of dogs as a reservoir of *Penicillium marneffei* in northern Thailand. Int J Infect Dis. 2011;15:e236–9.
34. Mootsikapun P, Srikulbutr S. Histoplasmosis and penicilliosis: comparison of clinical features, laboratory findings and outcome. Int J Infect Dis. 2006;10:66–71.
35. Wong SS, Wong KH, Hui WT, et al. Differences in clinical and laboratory diagnostic characteristics of penicilliosis marneffei in human immunodeficiency virus (HIV)- and non-HIV-infected patients. J Clin Microbiol. 2001;39:4535–40.
36. Goswami RP, Pramanik N, Banerjee D, Raza MM, Guha SK, Maiti PK. Histoplasmosis in eastern India: the tip of the iceberg? Trans R Soc Trop Med Hyg. 1999;93:540–2.
37. Sen S, Bajaj MS, Vijayaraghavan M. Histoplasmosis of the eyelids--a case report. Indian J Pathol Microbiol. 1999;42:495–7.
38. Randhawa HS, Chaturvedi S, Khan ZU, et al. Epididymal histoplasmosis diagnosed by isolation of *Histoplasma capsulatum* from semen. Mycopathologia. 1995;131:173–7.
39. Randhawa HS, Khan ZU, Gaur SN. *Blastomyces dermatitidis* in India: first report of its isolation from clinical material. Sabouraudia. 1983;21:215–21.
40. Shukla S, Singh S, Jain M, Kumar SS, Chander R, Kawatra N. Paediatric cutaneous blastomycosis: a rare case diagnosed on FNAC. Diagn Cytopathol. 2009;37:119–21.
41. Goel A, Bhayani R, Desai AP, Goel N. Extensive extraaxial blastomycosis granuloma at the skull base—case report. Neurol Med Chir (Tokyo). 1996;36:393–5.
42. Desai AP, Pandit AA, Gupte PD. Cutaneous blastomycosis. Report of a case with diagnosis by fine needle aspiration cytology. Acta Cytol. 1997;41:1317–9.
43. Le T, Huu Chi N, Kim Cuc NT, et al. AIDS-associated *Penicillium marneffei* infection of the central nervous system. Clin Infect Dis. 2010;51:1458–62.
44. Aung AK, Teh BM, McGrath C, Thompson PJ. Pulmonary sporotrichosis: case series and systematic analysis of literature on clinico-radiological patterns and management outcomes. Med Mycol. 2013;51:534–44.
45. Padhye AA, Kaufman L, Durry E, et al. Fatal pulmonary sporotrichosis caused by *Sporothrix schenckii var.* luriei in India J Clin Microbiol. 1992;30:2492–4.
46. Bustamante B, Campos PE. Endemic sporotrichosis. Curr Opin Infect Dis. 2001;14:145–9.
47. Quintal D. Sporotrichosis infection on mines of the Witwatersrand. J Cutan Med Surg. 2000;4:51–4.
48. Borges TS, Rossi CN, Fedullo JD, Taborda JP, Larsson CE. Isolation of *Sporothrix schenckii* from the claws of domestic cats (Indoor and Outdoor) and in captivity in São Paulo (Brazil). Mycopathologia. 2013;176(1–2):129–37.
49. Verma S, Verma GK, Singh G, et al. Sporotrichosis in sub-himalayan India. PLoS Neg Trop Dis. 2012;6:e1673.
50. Song Y, Li SS, Zhong SX, Liu YY, Yao L, Huo SS. Report of 457 sporotrichosis cases from Jilin province, northeast China, a serious endemic region. J Eur Acad Dermatol Venereol. 2011;27:313. https://doi.org/10.1111/j.1468-3083.2011.04389.x. [Epub ahead of print].

51. Haldar N, Sharma MK, Gugnani HC. Sporotrichosis in north-east India. Mycoses. 2007;50:201–4.
52. Ghosh A, Chakrabarti A, Sharma VK, Singh K, Singh A. Sporotrichosis in Himachal Pradesh (north India). Trans R Soc Trop Med Hyg. 1999;93:41–5.
53. Chakrabarti A, Roy SK, Dhar S, Kumar B. Sporotrichosis in north-west India. Indian J Med Res. 1994;100:62–5.
54. Itoh M, Okamoto S, Kariya H. Survey of 200 cases of sporotrichosis. Dermatologica. 1986;172:209–13.
55. Devi KR, Devi MU, Singh TN, et al. Emergence of sporotrichosis in Manipur. Indian J Med Microbiol. 2006;24:216–9.
56. Umemoto N, Demitsu T, Osawa M, Toda S, Kawasaki M, Mochizuki T. Sporotrichosis in a husband and wife. J Dermatol. 2005;32:569–73.
57. Song Y, Yao L, Zhong SX, Tian YP, Liu YY, Li SS. Infant sporotrichosis in northeast China: a report of 15 cases. Int J Dermatol. 2011;50:522–9.
58. Yegneswaran PP, Sripathi H, Bairy I, Lonikar V, Rao R, Prabhu S. Zoonotic sporotrichosis of lymphocutaneous type in a man acquired from a domesticated feline source: report of a first case in southern Karnataka, India. Int J Dermatol. 2009;48:1198–200.
59. Marimon R, Cano J, Gene J, Sutton DA, Kawasaki M, Guarro J. *Sporothrix brasiliensis*, *S. globosa*, and *S. mexicana*, three new *Sporothrix* species of clinical interest. J Clin Microbiol. 2007;45:3198–206.
60. Arunaloke C, Alexandro B, Clara G-GM, Takashi M, Li S. Global epidemiology of sporotrichosis. Med Mycol. 2015;53:3–14.

Epidemiology of Opportunist Fungal Infections in Asia

4

Arunaloke Chakrabarti

Key Points

- Multidrug resistant *Candida auris* infection is an emerging threat in tertiary care hospitals in Asia.
- The infection has been reported from Japan, South Korea, Singapore, China, India, Pakistan, Kuwait, and Qatar.
- The burden of opportunist fungal infections is much higher in Asian countries compared to developed countries due climatic condition, over-capacity patient population in hospital, compromise in healthcare, misuse/abuse of antibiotic and steroids.
- Limited studies show distinct epidemiology of opportunist mycoses in this continent, which warrant to have more studies in each country to know local epidemiology.
- New species and new susceptible hosts for opportunist fungal infections demand awareness campaign among clinicians and development of competent diagnostic mycology laboratories in Asian countries.
- The incidence of chronic pulmonary aspergillosis and mucormycosis is very high in those countries.
- Availability and affordability of antifungal drugs are major challenges in management of opportunist fungal infections.

4.1 Introduction

Systemic fungal infections are caused by pathogenic fungi, which can adapt human body. Pathogenic fungi are few. Majority of the fungi remain as saprobes and do not cause human infections as they fail to grow at 37 °C and resist low redox potential

A. Chakrabarti (✉)
Department of Medical Microbiology, Postgraduate Institute of Medical Education and Research (PGIMER), Chandigarh, India

A. Chakrabarti (ed.), *Clinical Practice of Medical Mycology in Asia*,
https://doi.org/10.1007/978-981-13-9459-1_4

in tissue. However, some of those saprobes can cause infections when the host is compromised either in immunity or due to co-morbidities. Those organisms are called opportunist that utilizes the opportunity offered by weakened defense of host to inflict damage. However, this distinction of pathogens and opportunists is getting blurred with the adaptation of more fungi on host and acquisition of virulence. Further, the global warming allows number of saprobe fungi to overcome the temperature restriction zone between host and environment. Simultaneously the understanding of host immunity clarifies that fungi may not necessarily require overt immunosuppression of host to cause invasive disease; specific defect in signal transduction pathway (like CARD 9, STAT 1) may make the host susceptible for fungal infections [1]. Underlying illness or risk factors for opportunistic fungal infections include human immunodeficiency virus (HIV) infection, hematological malignancies undergoing chemotherapy, hematopoietic stem cells and solid organ transplant recipients, burns, prematurity, and patients having indwelling devices. However, the spectrum of susceptible hosts has increased in recent years. Opportunistic fungal infections have been recorded in patients with post-influenza episode, chronic liver failure, diabetes, and obstructive pulmonary disease and staying in intensive care units (ICUs) [2].

Among opportunistic fungal infections invasive candidiasis is commonest disease, followed by aspergillosis and mucormycosis. Cryptococcosis, histoplasmosis, and talaromycosis are important in patients with HIV/AIDS. With the change of epidemiology many new fungi are gaining importance to cause infections in compromised hosts and those include *Fusarium, Scedosporium,* dematiaceous fungi, and many rare fungi. We are facing the following challenges due to emergence of rare fungi causing human infections [3, 4]:

- Epidemiology of those infections is not well understood with regard to environmental reservoirs, modes of transmission, and ways to detect them.
- Because of their relative rarity, laboratory diagnosis of these potential pathogens is challenging.
- Specific identification requires expertise.
- In vitro Antifungal susceptibility testing is difficult to perform without standard methodology, and antifungal breakpoints are not available. It is therefore difficult to choose appropriate antifungal therapy.
- Quality-assured diagnosis requires reference laboratories.
- Reference laboratory facilities are not available in all regions and countries.

The epidemiology and disease burden of opportunistic fungal infections are well studied and estimated in Western world, but the picture in Asian countries is largely unknown due to lack of study, awareness, and adequate diagnostic laboratory facilities. The available limited data indicate high incidence and unique epidemiology of opportunistic mycoses in this region due to large population at risk, broad spectrum of fungal agents, and distinct clinical entities [5, 6]. Separate chapters in the book deal with systemic and opportunist fungal disease under different risk groups. This chapter summarizes the present status of opportunist fungal infections in Asia among patients in general (Table 4.1).

Table 4.1 Opportunistic fungal infections in Asian countries

Disease	Incidence/Prevalence	Autopsy data	Epidemiology in Asia	Spectrum of agents
Candidiasis	• 1–12/1000 admission	• 0.6% of all cases • 22% of invasive fungal infections (IFIs)	• High incidence in patients admitted in ICUs. • Outbreaks due to rare yeasts and Candida auris • High hand carriage among healthcare providers (45–80%) • Intra-abdominal candidiasis especially *Candida* pancreatitis is an emerging problem • Young patients with less morbidity acquire the infection early while admitted in ICU	• 70–90% non-*albicans Candida* spp. • *C. tropicalis* commonest (35–40%) followed by C. parapsilosis and C. albicans. • Outbreak due to *Kodamaea ohmeri, Pichia anomala, C. auris*.
Aspergillosis	• No systematic data available	• 1% of all cases • 42% of IFIs	• 6–14% cases in immunocompetent hosts • Endophthalmitis, invasive fungal rhinosinusitis, and central nervous system aspergillosis are common in immunocompetent hosts • Outbreaks of endophthalmitis reported due to presumably contaminated infusion • Chronic aspergillosis in post-tuberculosis patients.	• *A. fumigatus* is common species in lung infection • *A. flavus* common in tropical climate in rhinosinusitis and endophthalmitis • *A. terreus* (amphotericin B resistant) is emerging in ICU.

(continued)

Table 4.1 (continued)

Disease	Incidence/Prevalence	Autopsy data	Epidemiology in Asia	Spectrum of agents
Mucormycosis	• 1.6/1000 diabetics • 0.14/1000 population (very high incidence)	• 0.6% of all cases • 23% of IFIs.	• High incidence is associated with uncontrolled diabetes (diabetes with high number in adults of India, China, Japan) • Renal failure, a new risk factor • Isolated renal mucormycosis in apparently healthy individual, a new clinical entity in India and China. • Cutaneous mucormycosis due *to Mucor irregularis* among farmers in South-East China and India—a new clinical entity.	• *Rhizopus oryzae* commonest. *Apophysomyces variabilis* next common species in India. • Comparatively antifungal resistant *R. microsporus* emerging • *Rhizopus homothallicus,* a new pathogenic agent. • Susceptibility variation among isolates under same species.
Cryptococcosis	• 1–9% of AIDS patients (very high incidence in Chiang Mai, Thailand and Ho Chi Minh city in Vietnam)	• 0.1% of all cases • 5% of IFIs	• Second most common AIDS defining illness in Chiang Mai, Thailand and fifth most common in Ho Chi Minh City of Vietnam. • The incidence has reduced after introduction of HAART therapy, but reduction is not substantial. • Incidence in immunocompetent host rising	• *C. neoformans* var. grubii commonest • *C. gattii* predominantly in immunocompetent host, reported from India, Malaysia, Hong Kong, China. • *C gattii* infection—more serious with high intracranial pressure. • *C. gattii*—hetero-resistance to fluconazole
Scedosporiosis and fusariosis	• Rarely reported	• No data available	• Post-tsunami *S. apiospermum* infection reported. • Post-transplantation fusariosis recorded in China and India. • Low incidence of both diseases may be due to lack of awareness and difficulty in diagnosis.	• *S. prolificans* (resistant to almost all antifungal agents—Voriconazole and terbinafine combination may be used) • The reports of these infections are increasing.

Disease	Incidence/Prevalence	Autopsy data	Epidemiology in Asia	Spectrum of agents
Pneumocystosis	• 5–69% of patients with AIDS. • 6.5% in NHL undergoing chemotherapy. • <1% of renal transplant recipients after chemoprophylaxis (6–12 months post transplant)	• 0.03% of all cases • 1% of IFIs.	• The incidence is low compared to western world—reason may be difficulty in diagnosis. • New risk groups emerged—pediatric population at risk.	• *Pneumocystis jiroveci*
Pythiosis	• No data	• No data	• Large number of cases reported from Thailand • Keratitis cases are reported from India in recent years • Localized keratitis, cutaneous, disseminated, and vascular form reported. • Vascular form commonly occurs in extremities of patients with underlying hemoglobinopathies	• *Pythium insidiosum*

4.1.1 Incidence/Prevalence

The global estimates indicate >700,000 cases of invasive candidiasis, >200,000 cases of invasive aspergillosis, >220,000 cases of cryptococcosis in HIV/AIDS, ~500,000 cases of *Pneumocystis jiroveci* pneumonia, ~100,000 cases of disseminated histoplasmosis occurring annually [6]. Though such estimates are not available in Asian countries, invasive candidiasis and mucormycosis rate appear very high in this region [7–9] and it relates to large patient load, compromise in healthcare, unabated construction activities in the hospital without covering the site from patient area, and largely tropical environment that helps fungi to thrive [7, 10–12].

A comparison of incidence of candidemia shows 1 to 12 cases/1000 admission in India [7] compared to 0.05 to 0.36/1000 admission, 0.8/1000 discharges, and 0.2–0.5/1000 discharges in Australia [13], United States [14], and European countries [15, 16], respectively; this means that the rate of candidemia in India is 20–30 times higher as compared to the developed world. In a cross-sectional study at 25 tertiary care centers of six Asian countries, the overall incidence of candidemia was 1.22 episodes per 1000 discharges and varied among the hospitals (range 0.16–4.53 per 1000 discharges) and countries (range 0.25–2.93 per 1000 discharges) [17]. Neonatal candidemia rate was ~46 cases/1000 admission in a tertiary care center in North India, which is nearly three times higher than the incidence reported by National Nosocomial Infection Surveillance in the USA. Multi-center prospective study on ICU acquired candidemia covering 27 ICUs across India, reported 6.5 candidemia cases/1000 ICU admission [8].

Similarly, a very high incidence of mucormycosis has been reported in diabetics (1.6 cases/1000 diabetics) from India [18]. Rhinocerebral mucormycosis is most common presentation. In one center, gastrointestinal mucormycosis has been reported at a rate of 20% of all operated cases of enterocolitis in neonates [19]. All cases autopsy data reported mucormycosis at the rate of 0.6% (23% of all invasive fungal infections) in India (personal communication with Dr. Ashim Das, Professor of Pathology at our Center) which is six times higher than national registry from Japan [20]. Analyzing the reported literature and development of a computational model, the prevalence rate of mucormycosis was estimated at 0.14 cases per 1000 population in India, which is 70 times higher than the incidence of western world [21].

However, such projected data is not possible for invasive aspergillosis as reported case series are limited. A recent multi-center ICU data from India reported 9.5 cases of invasive mold infection per 1000 ICU admission and majority are due to invasive aspergillosis [22]. All cases autopsy data from our center reflects invasive aspergillosis at a rate of 1% (42% of all invasive mycosis). Though majority cases of invasive aspergillosis are known to occur in immunosuppressed patients, 6–14% of Indian patients are apparently immunocompetent especially with clinical presentation of central nervous system aspergillosis, endophthalmitis, and invasive fungal rhinosinusitis [23]. Post-tuberculosis chronic pulmonary aspergillosis (CPA) is a common disease in Asian countries and significantly higher than other continents. Among Asian countries, the highest burden of CPA is from India (209,147) followed by Pakistan (72,438), Philippines (77,172), and Vietnam (55,509) [6].

Before AIDS era, the prevalence of cryptococcosis was nearly equal in immunocompetent and immunosuppressed patients. The balance shifted to immunosuppressed patients with the advent of AIDS. Cryptococcosis is the second most common AIDS defining illness in Chiang Mai Province of Thailand and has been reported at a rate of 1–2% of HIV infected population. Despite the availability of generic fluconazole and highly active antiretroviral therapy, the incidence of cryptococcosis has not decreased substantially in Asian AIDS population. The reason may be poor affordability and compliance to therapy [5].

Pneumocystis pneumonia is a well-known disease in patients with AIDS. Though HIV infection is a major public health problem in Asian Countries, the reported incidence of pneumocystis pneumonia is not as high as developed countries. This low to moderate incidence may be due to difficulty to diagnose this infection rather than actual low prevalence of the organism in this geographical region [24]. A rise in talaromycosis and histoplasmosis cases was recorded during HIV epidemic in restricted geographic regions of Asia. However, the incidence is going down with the introduction of antiretroviral therapy [25].

Many emerging fungi caused outbreaks in Asian countries. Several unusual yeast species (*Pichia anomala*, *P. fabianii*, and *Kodamaea ohmeri*) were isolated in outbreaks in India affecting large number of patients [26, 27]. *C. africana*, a cryptic species of *C. albicans*, has recently been reported to cause infection in China [28]. Trichosporonosis due to multidrug resistant *Trichosporon asahii* is frequently encountered in China, India, Japan, Taiwan, and Thailand [29, 30]. Other uncommon yeasts reported from Asia include *Geotrichum*, *Malassezia*, *Rhodotorula*, and *Saccharomyces* species [30, 31]. The emergence of multidrug resistant *C. auris* is the latest threat in Asia. It started from Japan in 2009, spread to South Korea, then India and Pakistan. The infection is also reported from China and Singapore [32, 33]. The magnitude of the infection can only be accessed from the study conducted in India covering 27 ICUs. *C. auris* accounted for 5.3% of 1400 *Candida* blood isolates [8]. *Saccharomyces* fungemia related to use of probiotics has raised concern in critically ill patients of India [34]. Among the black fungi, *Cladophialophora bantiana* is an emerging fungus in Asia and causes brain abscess even in immunocompetent patients. More than 50% cases reported from the world are from Asia, especially India [35].

4.1.2 Risk Factors/Underlying Illness

Considerable variations of underlying disease/risk factors have been observed in opportunistic mycoses from Asian countries. In the hospitals, outbreaks have been reported due to sub-optimal hospital care practices and contaminated environment [26, 36], whereas outbreaks in the community is related to spurious practices by untrained healthcare providers [37]. Easy availability of antibiotics and steroids over the counters, intravenous drug abuse, and contaminated infusion bottles contribute further in the rise of these infections [7]. Other than classical risk factors like hematological malignancies, transplant recipients, and immunosuppressive therapy, opportunistic fungal infections are also recorded in critically ill patients with tuberculosis, chronic liver failure, diabetes, chronic obstructive pulmonary diseases, and renal failure. Invasive aspergillosis is also recorded in patients with H1N1 influenza infections [38]. Nearly 10–14% of the patients with opportunistic fungal infections have no predisposing factor. The risk factors for opportunistic fungal infections are tabulated in Tables 4.2 and 4.3. During the suppression of cell-mediated immunity (HIV infection) cryptococcosis, histoplasmosis, pneumocystis pneumonia, and mucosal candidiasis are prevalent, while in neutropenic patients (hematological

Table 4.2 Fungi causing opportunistic fungal infections in different risk groups

Risk groups	Fungi and diseases	Comments
HIV infected patients	• Oropharyngeal candidiasis (up to 75%) • Esophageal candidiasis (10–15%) • Cryptococcosis • PCP pneumonia • Talaromycosis • Histoplasmosis	• Cryptococcosis—second most common AIDS defining illness in Chiang Mai Province, Thailand. • Talaromycosis—third most common AIDS defining illness in the same area. • Histoplasmosis incidence increased in India with the advent of AIDS. • PCP pneumonia incidence seems to be lower in Asian countries (may be due to lack of diagnosis)
Transplant patients • *HSCT (3–20% IFIs)*	• Invasive candidiasis (30–70%) • Aspergillosis (20–45%) • Mucormycosis (8%)	• Fusariosis and scedosporiosis are emerging in developed countries, no large series reported from Asian countries • The incidence of invasive aspergillosis is rising
• *Kidney (0–20%)*	• Invasive candidiasis (50%), cryptococcosis (10–20%) • Aspergillosis (10–15%) • Mucormycosis (2%) • Hyalohyphomycosis, phaeohyphomycosis (rare to 3%)	• The incidence of cryptococcosis was higher before tacrolimus use (cyclosporine was used) • PCP pneumonia after 1 year post-transplant when prophylaxis stopped • Rare dematiaceous fungal infections reported
• *Liver (5–40%)*	• Candidiasis (70%) • Aspergillosis (10%) • Mucormycosis (2%) • Other fungal infections rarely	• Invasive fungal infections common when MELD score > 30 • Complexity of surgery and duration • Intra-operative transfusion • Renal and hepatic failure
• *Lung (8–35%)*	• Aspergillosis (40–60%) • Candidiasis (20–25%) • Mucormycosis (3%) • Other fungal infections rarely.	• Rate of lung transplantion is rising in Asian countries, but data on invasive fungal infections is still limited.

Table 4.2 (continued)

Risk groups	Fungi and diseases	Comments
• *Heart (5–20%)*	• Candidiasis (50–60%) • Aspergillosis (25%) • Mucormycosis (3%) • Other fungal infections rarely.	• Rate of Heart transplantation is rising in Asian countries, but data on ivasive fungal infectios is still limited.
• *Small bowel (12–60%)*	• Candidiasis (80%) • Aspergillosis (2%) • Other fungal infections rarely.	• Small bowel transplantation is rare in Asia.
• *Pancreas (3–35%)*	• Candidiasis (75%) • Aspergillosis (10–15%) • Other fungal infections rarely.	• Pancreas transplantation is rare in Asia
Hematological malignancy undergoing chemotherapy (5–30%)	• Aspergillosis (45–55%) • Candidiasis (25–50%) • Mucormycosis (9–10%) • Cryptococcosis (5%) • Trichosporonosis (5%) • Other fungal infections are rare.	• AML patients have highest rate of IFIs followed by ALL and CML.
Chronic granulomatous disease (20–40%)	• Aspergillosis (40%) • Candidiasis (10–15%) • Other fungal infection rarely	
Exogenous steroid therapy	• Aspergillosis • Candidiasis • Mucormycosis • Other fungal infections are rare	
Diabetes	• Candidiasis (most common) • Mucormycosis (1.6/1000 diabetics)	• Very high incidence in India and China
Anti-TNF therapy	• Histoplasmosis (30%) • Aspergillosis (24%) • Candidiasis (23%) • Cryptococcosis (10%) • Mucormycosis (1.5%)	• Figures are from western world • No data from Asian countries.

malignancies under chemotherapy, transplant recipients) invasive candidiasis, aspergillosis, and mucormycosis are common diseases. Invasive candidiasis and aspergillosis may be seen occasionally in patients with AIDS when CD4 count goes <50 cells/cm and neutropenia develops [2, 5].

4.1.2.1 Spectrum of Agents

The spectrum of fungal agents causing opportunistic fungal infections has widened in Asia over the years. Many new agents have been reported only from this continent. The spectrum varies from other continents and even between the countries in

Table 4.3 Opportunistic fungal infections associated with different risk factors

Disease	Underlying disease	Healthcare-related facts
Candidiasis	Prematurity, neutropenia due to any disease, burn (>50%), APACHE SEORE II >20, diabetes, renal failure, extremes of age, pancreatitis	Colonization at multiple sites, antibiotics, major abdominal injury, total parenteral nutrition, hemodialysis, central venous catheters, multiple transfusion, immunosuppressive therapy, ICU stay.
Aspergillosis	Acquired/primary neutrophil defect, neoplastic diseases with persistent neutropenia, transplant recipients, chronic granulomatous diseases, Job's syndrome, aplastic anemia/ myelodysplastic syndrome/ myelofibrosis, rheumatoid arthritis **Non-neutropenic causes** Chronic obstructive pulmonary disease, chronic and acute liver disease, post-influenza, alcoholism, sepsis, diabetes, burns.	High dose of steroid, immunosuppressive therapy, surgery, ICU stay, building construction.
Mucormycosis	Uncontrolled diabetes with or without ketoacidosis, hematological malignancies under chemotherapy, transplant recipients, prematurity, protein-calorie malnutrition, renal failure, trauma	Deferoxamine therapy, intravenous drug abusers, intramuscular injection, adhesive tapes, tongue depressor, building construction, natural disasters steroid, voriconazole/echinocandins therapy.
Cryptococcosis	HIV infection, transplant recipients, hematological malignancies Immunocompetent host may also acquire the disease	Anti-TNF factor use.
Pneumocystosis	HIV infection, renal transplant recipients, non-Hodgkin lymphoma, premature neonates	
Scedosporiosis and fusariosis	Transplant recipients, hematological malignancy, trauma, burn.	Surgery

Asia. Among *Candida* species causing invasive candidiasis, the prevalence of infections caused by *C. albicans* drastically has come down in certain countries like India, though it is still >40% in 13 of 25 tertiary care centers studied in six countries in Asia [17]. *C. tropicalis* is commonest species in India, Malaysia, Singapore, Thailand, and the countries situated in tropical region. In ICU study in India, 31 yeast species were found to cause fungemia [8]. Besides, multidrug resistant *C. auris* is an emerging species in many Asian countries. The major challenge is that those rare Candida species can not be identified by phenotypic methods commonly practiced in laboratories in Asian countries [32]. Contrary to *A. fumigatus, A. flavus* is the commoner agent causing infection in some of the Asian countries [23]. Though *Aspergillus* spp. are the common mycelial fungi causing infection in critically ill patients, in a recent multi-center study mucormycosis has been recorded in

24% of invasive mold infections [22]. Among *Mucorales, R. arrhizus* is the commonest species isolated. *Apophysomyces variabilis, R. microsporus, R. homothallicus, and Rhizomucor variabilis* are the emerging agents in Asian countries [22, 38–40]. The details of the fungal species prevalent in Asian countries are provided in Table 4.1. Like other countries, antifungal resistance to *Candida* spp. is evolving. Even azole resistance has been noted in so-called susceptible *C. albicans* and *C. tropicalis* [8]. However, azole resistance in *A. fumigatus* is still not a major problem in Asian countries [41].

4.2 Conclusions

Opportunistic fungal infections are serious problem in the management of immunocompromised and seriously ill patients in Asian countries. While managing a patient with systemic infection, a low threshold to include opportunistic fungal infections in differential diagnosis is desirable due to its high incidence in those countries. Study on local epidemiology is essential, as the risk factors and spectrum of agents vary in those countries. The available literature shows several unique features in epidemiology of opportunistic mycoses in Asian countries: a) high incidence, b) high yeast carriage rate in the hands of healthcare providers, c) high fungal spore burden in the air in the vicinity of susceptible patients, d) emergence of new risk factors, e) systemic fungal infections even in apparently healthy hosts, f) unique spectrum of etiological agents and resistance pattern. The epidemiology also indicates the need of adequate understanding of disease, source limitation, and early diagnosis to control opportunistic fungal infections in Asian countries.

References

1. Vaezi A, Fakhim H, Abtahian Z, Khodavaisy S, Geramishoar M, Alizadeh A, Meis JF, Badali H. Frequency and geographic distribution of CARD9 mutations in patients with severe fungal infections. Front Microbiol. 2018;9:2434.
2. Richardson MD. Changing patterns and trends in systemic fungal infections. J Antimicrob Chemother. 2005;56(Suppl 1):i5–i11.
3. Perfect JR. Fungal diagnosis: how do we do it and can we do better? Curr Med Res Opin. 2013;29(Suppl 4):3–11.
4. Perusquía-Ortiz AM, Vázquez-González D, Bonifaz A. Opportunistic filamentous mycoses: aspergillosis, mucormycosis, phaeohyphomycosis and hyalohyphomycosis. J Dtsch Dermatol Ges. 2012;10:611–21.
5. Slavin MA, Chakrabarti A. Opportunistic fungal infections in the Asia-Pacific region. Med Mycol. 2012;50:18–25.
6. Bongomin F, Gago S, Oladele RO, Denning DW. Global and multi National Prevalence of fungal diseases—estimate precision. J Fungi. 2017;3:57.
7. Chakrabarti A, Chatterjee SS, Shivaprakash MR. Overview of opportunistic fungal infections in India. Nippon Ishinkin Gakkai Zasshi. 2008;49:165–72.
8. Chakrabarti A, Sood P, Rudramurthy SM, Chen S, Kaur H, Capoor M, Chhina D, Rao R, Eshwara VK, Xess I, Kindo AJ, Umabala P, Savio J, Patel A, Ray U, Mohan S, Iyer R, Chander J, Arora A, Sardana R, Roy I, Appalaraju B, Sharma A, Shetty A, Khanna N, Marak R, Biswas

S, Das S, Harish BN, Joshi S, Mendiratta D. Incidence, characteristics and outcome of ICU-acquired candidemia in India. Intensive Care Med. 2015;41:285–95.
9. Kaur H, Chakrabarti A. Strategies to reduce mortality in adult and neonatal candidemia in developing countries. J Fungi. 2017;3:E41. https://doi.org/10.3390/jof3030041.
10. Kumar S. Batra R. a study of yeast carriage on hands of hospital personnel. Indian J Pathol Microbiol. 2000;43:65–7.
11. Huang YC, Lin TY, Leu HS, Wu JL, Wu JH. Yeast carriage on hands of hospital personnel working in intensive care units. J Hosp Infect. 1998 May;39(1):47–51.
12. Chakrabarti A, Chatterjee SS, Rao KLN, Zameer MM, Shivaprakash MR, Singhi S, Singh R, Varma SC. Recent experience with fungaemia: change in species distribution and azole resistance. Scand J Infect Dis. 2009;41:275–84.
13. Chen S, Slavin M, Nguyen Q, et al. Active surveillance for candidemia, Australia. Emerg Infect Dis. 2006;12:1508–16.
14. Hajjeh RA, Sofair AN, Harrison LH, et al. Incidence of bloodstream infections due to Candida species and in vitro susceptibilities of isolates collected from 1998 to 2000 in a population-based active surveillance program. J Clin Microbiol. 2004;42:1519–27.
15. Almirante B, Rodríguez D, Park BJ, et al. Epidemiology and predictors of mortality in cases of Candida bloodstream infection: results from population-based surveillance, Barcelona, Spain, from 2002 to 2003. J Clin Microbiol. 2005;43:1829–35.
16. Arendrup MC, Fuursted K, Gahrn-Hansen B, et al. Seminational surveillance of fungemia in Denmark: notably high rates of fungemia and numbers of isolates with reduced azole susceptibility. J Clin Microbiol. 2005;43:4434–40.
17. Tan BH, Chakrabarti A, Li RY, Patel AK, Watcharananan SP, Liu Z, Chindamporn A, Tan AL, Sun PL, Wu UI, Chen YC. Asia fungal working group (AFWG); Asia fungal working group AFWG. Incidence and species distribution of candidaemia in Asia: a laboratory-based surveillance study. Clin Microbiol Infect. 2015;21:946–53.
18. Bhansali A, Bhadada S, Sharma A, et al. Presentation and outcome of rhino-orbital-cerebral mucormycosis in patients with diabetes. Postgrad Med J. 2004;80:670–4.
19. Patra S, Vij M, Chirla DK, et al. Unsuspected invasive neonatal gastrointestinal mucormycosis: a clinicopathological study of six cases from a tertiary care hospital. J Indian Assoc Pediatr Surg. 2012;17:153–6.
20. Yamazaki T, Kume H, Murase S, et al. Epidemiology of visceral mycoses: analysis of data in annual of the pathological autopsy cases in Japan. J Clin Microbiol. 1999;37:1732–8.
21. Chakrabarti A, Sood P, Denning D. Estimating fungal infection burden in India using computational models: Mucormycosis burden as a case study [poster number 1044]. Presented at the 23rd ECCMID conference. Berlin. Germany; April. 2013:27–30.
22. Chakrabarti A, Kaur H, Savio J, et al. Epidemiology and clinical outcomes of invasive mould infections in Indian Intensive Care Units (FISF study). J Crit Care. 2019;51:64–70.
23. de Armas Rodríguez Y, Wissmann G, Müller AL, et al. Pneumocystis jirovecii pneumonia in developing countries. Parasite. 2011;18:219–28.
24. Chakrabarti A, Slavin MA. Endemic fungal infections in Asia-Pacific region. Med Mycol. 2011;49:337–44.
25. Chakrabarti A, Singh K, Narang A, et al. Outbreak of Pichia anomala in the pediatric service of a tertiary care center in northern India. J Clin Microbiol. 2001;39:1702–6.
26. Chakrabarti A, Rudramurthy SM, Kale P, Hariprasath P, Dhaliwal M, Singhi S, Rao KL. Epidemiological study of a large cluster of fungaemia cases due to Kodamaea ohmeri in an Indian tertiary care Centre. Clin Microbiol Infect. 2014;20:O83–9.
27. Hu Y, Yu A, Chen X, Wang G, Feng X. Molecular characterization of Candida africana in genital specimens in Shanghai, China. Biomed Res Int. 2015;2015:185387. https://doi.org/10.1155/2015/185387.
28. Miceli MH, Díaz JA, Lee SA. Emerging opportunistic yeast infections. Lancet Infect Dis. 2011;11:142–51.
29. Liao Y, Lu X, Yang S, et al. Epidemiology and outcome of Trichosporon Fungemia: a review of 185 reported cases from 1975 to 2014. Open Forum Infect Dis. 2015;2:ofv141.

30. Wirth F, Goldani LZ. Epidemiology of Rhodotorula: an emerging pathogen. Interdiscip Perspect Infect Dis. 2012;2012:465717.
31. Cortegiani A, Misseri G, Fasciana T, Giammanco A, Giarratano A, Chowdhary A. Epidemiology, clinical characteristics, resistance, and treatment of infections by Candida auris. J Intensive Care. 2018;6:69. https://doi.org/10.1186/s40560-018-0342-4.
32. Tan YE, Tan AL. Arrival of Candida auris fungus in Singapore: report of the first 3 cases. Ann Acad Med Singap. 2018;47:260–2.
33. Roy U, Jessani LG, Rudramurthy SM, Gopalakrishnan R, Dutta S, Chakravarty C, Jillwin J, Chakrabarti A. Seven cases of Saccharomyces fungaemia related to use of probiotics. Mycoses. 2017;60:375–80.
34. Chakrabarti A, Kaur H, Rudramurthy SM, Appannanavar SB, Patel A, Mukherjee KK, Ghosh A, Ray U. Brain abscess due to Cladophialophora bantiana: a review of 124 cases. Med Mycol. 2016;54:111–9.
35. Chowdhary A, Becker K, Fegeler W, et al. An outbreak of candidemia due to Candida tropicalis in a neonatal intensive care unit. Mycoses. 2003;46:287–92.
36. Gupta A, Gupta V, Dogra MR, et al. Fungal endophthalmitis after single intravenous administration of presumably contaminated dextrose infusion fluid. Retina. 2000;20:262–8.
37. Chakrabarti A, Das A, Mandal J, et al. The rising trend of invasive zygomycosis in patients with uncontrolled diabetes mellitus. Med Mycol. 2006;44:335–42.
38. Diwakar A, Dewan RK, Chowdhary A, et al. Zygomycosis—a case report and overview of the disease in India. Mycoses. 2007;50:247–54.
39. Chakrabarti A, Singh R. Mucormycosis in India: unique features. Mycoses. 2014;57(Suppl 3):85–90.
40. Prakash H, Ghosh AK, Rudramurthy SM, Singh P, Xess I, Savio J, Pamidimukkala U, Jillwin J, Varma S, Das A, Panda NK, Singh S, Bal A, Chakrabarti A. A prospective multicenter study on mucormycosis in India: Epidemiology, diagnosis, and treatment. Med Mycol. 2018;57:395. https://doi.org/10.1093/mmy/myy060.
41. Arikan-Akdagli S. Azole resistance in Aspergillus: global status in Europe and Asia. Ann N Y Acad Sci. 2012;1272:9–14.

Part II

Special Population

5 Mycoses in Intensive Care Units

Subhash Todi

Key Points

- The incidence of candidemia is 6.5 cases/1000 ICU admission in India.
- Candidemia should always be regarded as pathological warranting treatment.
- The mean age of patients with opportunistic mycoses is relatively younger in the Indian study.
- Candidemia occurs relatively early during the ICU stay.
- Candidemia occurred in less sicker group of patients than the western counterpart.
- *Candida tropicalis* and *Candida albicans* are the most common *Candida* species isolated.
- Fluconazole sensitivity is still high among *C. tropicalis* and *C. albicans*, though resistance is increasing in those species.
- *Candida glabrata* is rare.
- Multidrug resistant *Candida auris* is being increasingly recognized.
- Risk prediction scoring system has a very low positive predictive value.
- Experience with beta-D-glucan is limited but may be used to limit empirical antifungal therapy.
- Source control and removal of invasive lines is of paramount importance in management of candidemia.
- Crude mortality of candidemia can be as high as 40%.

5.1 Introduction

Invasive fungal infections (IFIs) in Intensive Care Units (ICUs) are increasingly being recognized globally in critically ill patients [1, 2]. With increasing growth of ICUs in the developing world, the prevalence of IFI is exponentially increasing in

S. Todi (✉)
Director Critical Care, AMRI Hospitals, Kolkata, India

A. Chakrabarti (ed.), *Clinical Practice of Medical Mycology in Asia*,
https://doi.org/10.1007/978-981-13-9459-1_5

this part of the world. The most common IFI encountered in ICU is invasive candidiasis but other severe invasive fungal infections like invasive aspergillosis, mucormycosis, cryptococcal meningitis, and pneumocystis pneumonia are also encountered in specific subset of ICU population [3]. The increased prevalence of IFIs is partly real due to more life sustaining treatments offered to this vulnerable group, but it may be partly artiefactual due to increasing awareness, recognition, and availability of modern diagnostic tools in the developing world. The epidemiology of IFIs in ICU specifically the species of different fungi may be different in Asia Pacific region as compared to Western hemisphere. The reason for this is not entirely clear and may be environmental due to the tropical climate and/or genetic. *Candida auris* for example is being increasingly reported from the South Asia region [3]. New risk factors for developing IFIs are being recognized, with uncontrolled diabetes being one of them. Due to increasing prevalence of diabetes in India, mucormycosis is being increasingly reported. In general, infection control practices are below par in the ICUs of developing world, which facilitates the spread of IFIs within the unit. Antibiotic stewardship practice is not very common in the developing world, which also leads to overuse of broad-spectrum antibiotics in ICUs leading to secondary fungal sepsis. This chapter will highlight recent advances in the epidemiology of IFIs in Asia with emphasis on original research on this aspect from this part of the world.

5.2 Invasive Candidiasis (IC)

Candida growth in the blood culture should always be regarded as pathological warranting treatment and should not be disregarded as a colonizer or contaminant. Two-thirds of patients with IC in ICU will have candidemia and most of the other non-candidemic patients will have deep seated candidiasis like intra-abdominal candidiasis [4, 5]. Although candiduria is detected in 20% of ICU patients, it seldom leads to secondary candidemia [6]. A seminal study was conducted by Chakrabarti et al. in 27 ICUs across India, to observe the epidemiological pattern of candidemia [3]. During the eighteen month study period, 1400 candidemia cases were reported from the ICUs which gave an incidence of 6.51 cases/1000 ICU admission. There was regional variation among the incidence of candidemia and a higher incidence was noted in the public hospital as opposed to private hospital, which is a phenomenon peculiar to the developing world due to the overcrowding of public hospitals and less stringent infection control policies. In a survey of other published research on global epidemiological studies of candidemia maintained by Leading International Fungal Education (LIFE) portal, it was noticed that fifty percent of the global cases of candidemia were reported in Asia followed by Americas and Europe [7]. The highest prevalence of candidemia was reported in Pakistan (21 cases per 100,000) followed by Brazil (14.9 cases per 100,000) and Russia (8.29 cases per 100,000).

In the Indian study, the mean age of patients with ICU acquired candidemia was much lower (49.7 years) than in other countries (mean 59–66.2 years). This may be reflective of the general population census in the developing world. ICU acquired candidemia was noted to occur significantly earlier (8 days) than in other studies (11–15 days), which may be a reflection of delayed hospital admission of critically ill patients in resource limited setting. Severity of illness scores like APACHE was relatively less in this study. One of the reasons could be the younger age of study population lowering the APACHE score, or it could be due to the excessive noted exposure of broad-spectrum antibiotics and corticosteroids to a relatively less sick ICU population and inadequate infection control practices make them prone to acquire nosocomial candidemia.

Very high prevalence (41.6%) of *Candida tropicalis* was noted in this study which was also observed in studies from other Asian countries. *Candida albicans* and *Candida parapsilosis* affected 20% and 10% of the study population, respectively. This is in contrast to studies in western population where *Candida tropicalis* is less common (5–10%) and *Candida albicans* and *Candida glabrata* are more common [8]. The reason for this change in epidemiology is unclear. In a survey of health care personnel in the study centers, 82% were carrier of yeast on their hands of which 80% were *Candida tropicalis* [9]. Prior azole exposure is not probably an explanation of increased incidence of *Candida tropicalis* as the species was mostly susceptible to fluconazole. On the other hand, low incidence of *Candida glabrata* was noted in spite of prior fluconazole exposure in many patients, a finding contrary to the observation from the West.

Candida auris, a rapidly emerging multidrug resistant Candida comprised 5.2% of all *Candida* isolates [10]. This organism which is difficult to detect and treat is increasingly being reported from intensive care units worldwide and more so from the developing world. In a recent study from a neurosurgical unit, axillary temperature probe contaminated with *Candida auris* was reported as a cause of outbreak of these fungi in the unit, which emphasizes the need for strict infection control as a measure to control the spread of these dreaded fungi. Many of the current fungal identification systems misidentify *Candida auris* and a close collaboration with the reference microbiology laboratory is required to properly identify this fungi.

Various scoring systems which include risk prediction models have been derived for predicting IC in ICU population. These models have a very low positive predictive value and cannot be relied upon solely to start empiric antifungal therapy. In an observational study to externally validate the various candida scoring system in a medical/surgical ICU in India, it was observed that more than 90% of patients get colonized during their stay in the ICU and many of the risk factors for candidemia are present in these patients, but the overall incidence of candidemia is low and relying on the predictive model was subjecting a majority of patients to an unnecessary antifungal exposure [11].

Biomarkers like beta-D-glucan (BDG) has been increasingly used for empiric/preemptive therapy for IC in ICU. In general, the availability of this biomarker is low in the developing world. In a cost effective analysis from India, BDG levels were significantly higher in septic patients with IC than in non-septic patients, but the values overlapped with bacterial septic patients. Discontinuation of empiric antifungal therapy based on a value <80 resulted in cost savings of 14,000 INR per day per patient [12].

Appropriate antifungal choice is imperative for a successful outcome of this lethal disease. Although species can predict drug susceptibility, local epidemiological patterns vary and affect the value of species prediction. Overall, more than 95% of *C. albicans* and *C. parapsilosis* isolates remain azole-susceptible. In the Indian study, fluconazole resistant was noted in 2–9% of *C. albicans, C. tropicalis,* and *C. parapsilosis*. In a similar study from China, 10% of *C. albicans* isolates and 19% of *C. parapsilosis* isolates were azole-resistant [13]. *C. glabrata, C. krusei*, and *C .auris* are less susceptible than other species to fluconazole. Resistance to echinocandins among *Candida* species like *C. auris* and *C. parapsilosis* is increasingly being reported.

Candiduria should only be treated if symptomatic in ICU patients and the drug of choice is fluconazole as it attains high levels in the urinary tract. For azole-resistant urinary tract infection, high dose fluconazole, amphotericin deoxycholate (not liposomal amphotericin B as they have poor penetration in the urinary tract), micafungin, flucytosine, and local amphotericin bladder wash have been tried [14]. An attempt should be made to remove indwelling urinary catheters, nephrostomy tubes, and stents. Echinocandins are the preferred first line of agent in ICU patients with IC, though this can be de-escalated rapidly for azole sensitive strains. The reason for superiority of echinocandins over azoles is their rapid fungicidal action, safety profile, less drug interaction, and ability to penetrate biofilms, as indwelling catheters are one of main sources of IC in ICU patients. Lipid amphotericin B formulations should be considered in patients with CNS involvement and endocarditis, whereas azoles are the preferred choice for endophthalmitis as echinocandins do not penetrate vitreous well. Repeated blood cultures should be performed and antifungal therapy should be continued for two weeks after the last negative culture. In culture negative patient, shortening the antifungal use by following biomarkers and stopping rules have been successfully tried in recent studies. This approach substantially reduces antifungal burden in ICU [15].

The volume of distribution is high in many ICU patients due to aggressive volume resuscitation in sepsis; moreover, some of these patients have augmented renal clearance which leads to reduced therapeutic drug levels for fluconazole and echinocandins. This in combination with higher minimum inhibitory concentration of many *Candida* species for these antifungals has led to an optimization of pharmacokinetic and pharmacodynamics parameters by advocating higher doses of these dugs which have a high safety margin. (e.g., 12 mg/kg of fluconazole loading followed by 4 mg/kg of maintenance, double the loading dose of caspofungin) resulting in a better therapeutic level leads to a satisfactory therapeutic drug level [16].

Empirical antifungal therapy in symptomatic patients at risk of developing IC is a common practice in ICUs, though effectiveness of this strategy has not been proven in recent studies. This may be due to overall low incidence of IC in general medical/surgical ICUs and number needed to treat will be very high to show a decrease in mortality [17].

Source control is a key factor in managing candidemia in ICU and removal of central venous lines has been recommended in such cases. In the study from India, it was clearly demonstrated that removal of central line was clearly associated with decreased mortality, but this was performed in only one-third of cases. This highlights the need for protocolized care and proper implementation of guidelines and infectious disease physician involvement which is unfortunately lacking in many developing countries.

Candidemia is a lethal disease with crude mortality of up to 50% in some studies. As most of the ICU patients with candidemia have underlying significant comorbidity, attributable mortality is difficult to compute and varies between 5 and 49% in various studies. In the study from India, crude and attributable mortality from candidemia was noted to be 44% and 20%, respectively. In other studies, intra-abdominal candidiasis was associated with high attributable mortality of 26–60% in cases of secondary or tertiary peritonitis [18].

5.2.1 Invasive Mold Infection (IMI)

Invasive infections by filamentous fungi are increasingly being reported from ICUs worldwide. Due to the increasing use of Candida prophylaxis, infections with molds are being increasingly reported from transplant patients [19]. The epidemiology of IMIs is not well studied in developing countries in spite of the fact that risk factors for developing these infections like diabetes are prevalent in this part of the world. Moreover it has been shown that the spore count of aspergillus was found to be high (average of 82 CFU/m^3) [20] in an ICU from India. Newer risk factors for developing IMIs like chronic obstructive pulmonary disease, chronic liver and kidney failure and use of corticosteroids is common in ICUs; moreover, the diagnostic criteria for IMIs is not well defined as opposed to that of hemato/oncology and classical immunosuppressed patients. In ICU patients, classical radiological signs like halo or crescent sign are not seen most of the time and nonspecific infiltrates and nodules are more common. Presence of aspergillus in the respiratory tract cannot be taken as a feature of invasive aspergillosis as this may be mere colonization [21, 22]. Commonly used biomarkers like galactomannan may be falsely high and nonspecific in this patient population. Obtaining a tissue sample which is the gold standard for IMI diagnosis is difficult in ICU patients due to many contraindications like coagulopathy and thrombocytopenia. Moreover, lack of availability and experienced personnel, inertia on the part of physicians, cost involved, and difficulty in obtaining informed consent for biopsy compound to the problem.

In a global epidemiological survey, it was found that 50% of invasive aspergillosis cases are reported from Asia (excluding India and China) [7]. Approximately 95% of invasive aspergillosis is due to the *Aspergillus fumigatus* complex. In a recently published multicentric prospective, observational study conducted by Fungal Infection Study Forum (FISF) from India, risk factors, epidemiology, and outcome of IMIs in Indian ICUs were studied [23]. Over a eighteen months period, eleven tertiary care centers participated in the study. EORTC/MSG criteria was applied for diagnosis of IMI in classical immunocompromised patient, Bulpa et al. criteria applied for COPD patients and Blot et al. criteria for general medical/surgical ICU patients. Patients with "Proven" or "Probable/Putative" IMIs were only included for the study purpose.

During the study period, 398 cases (proven 96, probable 302) of IMI were diagnosed with a prevalence of 9.5 cases per 1000 ICU admissions. Similar to candidemia study conducted in India cases, the severity of illness was low (APACHE mean of 14), younger age at presentation (average age 45 years) and early presentation (average 4 days since ICU admission) as compared to the western counterpart. Nonclassical groups consisting of diabetes, COPD, and H1N1 influenza constituted majority of IMIs (63.6%). Though *Aspergillus* species were the commonest (82.1%) mold isolated, Mucorales were isolated from a considerable number (14.4%) of subjects. The most common radiological finding on CT chest was consolidation followed by nodule and pleural effusion. Majority (80%) of patients had pulmonary disease. The IMI patients were treated with various antifungals both empiric and targeted. Majority (n = 321, 80.7%) of the subjects had pulmonary disease. The crude mortality was 64%, despite the fact that majority of patients received targeted therapy. This may reflect severity of underlying disease, suboptimal or delayed medical therapy, and underutilization of surgical debridement.

5.2.2 *Pneumocystis jirovecii Pneumonia (PCP)* [7]

PCP occurs mainly in patients with HIV/AIDS infection. Global prevalence is thought to be higher than 400,000 annually cases reported worldwide. Though the incidence has come down with highly active antiretroviral therapy (HAART), it still remains high in patients with inadequately treated HIV or noncompliance with HAART therapy. Mortality of PCP ranges from 10 to 30% and can be even higher if the diagnosis is delayed. Increasing incidence of PCP is noticed in non-HIV patients with classical immunocompromised states. Achieving early diagnosis remains the main challenge in treating PCP. A low index of suspicion, CT scan of chest, early bronchoalveolar lavage with proper staining, polymerase chain reaction (PCR) and judicious interpretation of serum galactomannan are the mainstay of early diagnosis of this infection. As per LIFE program, 77% of the cases were reported in Africa, followed by America (10%), Europe (7%), and Asia (6%). Differences in the estimations across countries can be associated to differences in the HIV prevalence in the different countries and the accessibility to highly active antiretroviral therapy. Moreover diagnosis may depend on experience and competence of the laboratory.

5.3 Conclusion

High index of suspicion for opportunistic invasive fungal infection should be maintained in ICU patients. Persistent sepsis in spite of broad-spectrum antibiotics should prompt rapid diagnostic tests to rule out IFI should be done. Empiric treatment against invasive candidiasis though not proven to decrease mortality in ICU patient is still practiced widely. Judicious use of biomarker, and targeted therapy where appropriate should be practiced. Rapid de-escalation and shortening the duration of antifungal based on biomarkers will reduce the antifungal burden in the ICU.

References

1. Vincent JL, Sakr Y, Sprung CL, Ranieri VM, et al. Sepsis in European intensive care units: results of the SOAP study. Crit Care Med. 2006;34:344–53.
2. Vincent JL, Rello J, Marshall J, et al. International study of the prevalence and outcomes of infection in intensive care units. JAMA. 2009;302:2323–9.
3. Chakrabarti A, Sood P, Rudramurthy SM, et al. Incidence, characteristics and outcome of ICU-acquired candidemia in India. Intensive Care Med. 2015;41:285–95.
4. Kullberg BJ, Arendrup MC. Invasive candidiasis. N Engl J Med. 2015;373:1445–56.
5. Bassetti M, Righi E, Ansaldi F, et al. A multicenter multinational study of abdominal candidiasis: epidemiology, outcomes and predictors of mortality. Intensive Care Med. 2015;41: 1601–10.
6. Hollenbach E. To treat or not to treat—critically ill patients with candiduria. Mycoses. 2008;51(suppl 2):12–24.
7. Bongomin F, Gago S, Oladele RO, Denning DW. Global and multi-National Prevalence of fungal diseases-estimate precision. J Fungi (Basel). 2017;3(4):57.
8. Playford EG, Marriott D, Nguyen Q, et al. Candidemia in nonneutropenic critically ill patients: risk factors for non-albicans *Candida* spp. Crit Care Med. 2008;36:2034–9.
9. Chakrabarti A, Chatterjee SS, Rao KL, et al. Recent experience with fungaemia: change in species distribution and azole resistance. Scand J Infect Dis. 2009;41(4):275–84.
10. Chowdhary A, Sharma C, Meis JF. Candida auris: a rapidly emerging cause of hospital-acquired multidrug-resistant fungal infections globally. PLoS Pathog. 2017;13(5): e1006290.
11. Ahmed A, Baronia AK, Azim A, Marak RS, Yadav R, Sharma P, et al. External validation of risk prediction scores for invasive candidiasis in a medical/surgical intensive care unit: an observational study. Indian J Crit Care Med. 2017;21:514–20.
12. Bansal N, Gopalakrishnan R, Sethuraman N, Ramakrishnan N, Nambi PS, Kumar DS, et al. Experience with β-D-glucan assay in the management of critically ill patients with high risk of invasive candidiasis: an observational study. Indian J Crit Care Med. 2018;22:364–8.
13. Liu W, Tan J, Sun J, et al. Invasive candidiasis in intensive care units in China: in vitro antifungal susceptibility in the China-SCAN study. J Antimicrob Chemother. 2014;69:162–7.
14. Sullivan KA, Caylor MM, Lin F-C, Campbell-Bright S. Comparison of amphotericin B bladder irrigations versus fluconazole for the treatment of candiduria in intensive care unit patients. J Pharm Pract. 2017;30:347–52.
15. Pappas PG, Kauffman CA, Andes DR, et al. Clinical practice guideline for the management of candidiasis: 2016 update by the Infectious Diseases Society of America. Clin Infect Dis. 2016;62:e1–50.
16. Cornely OA, Bassetti M, Calandra T, et al. ESCMID guideline for the diagnosis and management of candida diseases 2012: non-neutropenic adult patients. Clin Microbiol Infect. 2012;18(suppl 7):19–37.
17. Timsit JF, Azoulay E, Schwebel C, Charles PE, et al. Empirical micafungin treatment and survival without invasive fungal infection in adults with ICU-acquired Sepsis, Candida colonization, and multiple organ failure: the EMPIRICUS randomized clinical trial. JAMA. 2016;316(15):1555–64.
18. Lortholary O, Renaudat C, Sitbon K, et al. Worrisome trends in incidence and mortality of candidemia in intensive care units (Paris area, 2002–2010). Intensive Care Med. 2014;40: 1303–12.
19. Baddley JW, Stephens JM, Ji X, Gao X, Schlamm HT, Tarallo M. Aspergillosis in intensive care unit (ICU) patients: epidemiology and economic outcomes. BMC Infect Dis. 2013; 13:29.
20. Rudramurthy SM, Singh G, Hallur V, et al. High fungal spore burden with predomi- nance of Aspergillus in hospital air of a tertiary care hospital in Chandigarh. Indian J Med Microbiol. 2016;34:529–32.

21. He H, Ding L, Li F, Zhan Q. Clinical features of invasive bronchial-pulmonary aspergillosis in critically ill patients with chronic obstructive respiratory diseases: a prospective study. Crit Care. 2011;15:R5.
22. Crum-Cianflone NF. Invasive aspergillosis associated with severe influenza infections. Open Forum Infect Dis. 2016;3:71.
23. Chakrabarti A, Kaur H, Savio J, Rudramurthy SM. Atul Patel epidemiology and clinical outcomes of invasive mould infections in Indian intensive care units (FISF study). J Crit Care. 2019;51:64–70.

6 Mycoses in AIDS

Atul K. Patel

Key Points

- Due to defective cell mediated immune system in HIV infected patients- histoplasmosis, talaromycosis, cryptococcosis, pneumocystis jirovecii pneumonia and mucosal candidiasis are prevalent especially when CD4 cell count <200/micro/L.
- With the advent of ART therapy, fungal infection rate has come down in patients with AIDS; however, fungal infections remain significant cause of morbidity and mortality in developing countries especially sub-Saharan Africa.
- Limited data from Asian countries report high rate of fungal infections in patients with AIDS.
- Other than usual opportunist fungal infections in patients with AIDS, talaromycosis is prevalent in Southeast Asian countries, and emmonsiosis is possible new entrant in Asia after South Africa.
- TMP-SMX prophylaxis is highly effective in preventing *Pneumocystis jirovecii* pneumonia.
- Combination antifungal therapy consisting of amphotericin B (conventional or liposomal) with flucytosine is associated with rapid sterilization of CSF and improved survival compared to amphotericin B monotherapy in patients with cryptococcal meningitis.
- Uncontrolled raised intracranial pressure is an important cause of in-hospital mortality in patients with cryptococcal meningitis.
- *Histoplasma* antigen testing from urine, blood, and broncho-alveolar lavage is a sensitive and rapid diagnostic test for patients with disseminated histoplasmosis.
- Distinction of fungal infections from immune reconstitution inflammatory syndrome (IRIS) is important for optimal management.

A. K. Patel (✉)
Infectious Diseases Clinic, "VEDANTA" Institute of Medical Sciences, Ahmedabad, India

A. Chakrabarti (ed.), *Clinical Practice of Medical Mycology in Asia*,
https://doi.org/10.1007/978-981-13-9459-1_6

6.1 Introduction

Invasive and superficial fungal infections remained major causes of morbidity and mortality in the early years of human immunodeficiency virus (HIV) epidemic. Though with the change in treatment guideline and large cover of antiretroviral treatment, the incidence of fungal infection has come down, the disease still contributes to high mortality in late diagnosed and untreated HIV-infected patients. [1] Progressive loss of CD4 cells in untreated HIV-infected patients renders the patient susceptible to opportunistic mycoses. Invasive mycoses in AIDS can be divided into two broad groups: endemic and opportunistic mycoses. Endemic mycoses caused by dimorphic fungi including histoplasmosis and coccidioidomycosis are prevalent in AIDS patients in respective endemic area. In Asian region, histoplasmosis and talaromycosis (formerly penicilliosis) are prevalent. A new endemic mycosis, emmonsiosis is prevalent in AIDS patients of South Africa. The disease has also been reported from India [8, 9]. Among opportunistic mycoses, cryptococcosis and *Pneumocystis jirovecii* pneumonia are prevalent worldwide. Other less common opportunistic mycoses including aspergillosis, pseudallescheriasis, and mucormycosis occur in patients with very low CD4 count. Though superficial *Candida* infection is common in AIDS patients, invasive candidiasis is rare.

During initial years of HIV epidemic, mucosal candidiasis, *Pneumocystis jirovecii* pneumonia (PJP), and cryptococcosis were the most common mycotic diseases. In the later period, endemic mycoses like histoplasmosis, coccidioidomycosis, blastomycosis, and talaromycosis have gained importance in HIV positive patients in respective endemic area. The mycotic disease burden in HIV is not clearly ascertained in Asian countries. However, it is estimated nearly one million invasive fungal infections (IFIs) occur every year in AIDS patients worldwide, and the diseases include cryptococcosis, pneumocystosis, histoplasmosis, and talaromycosis, with overall mortality of 500,000 per year [2]. Autopsy study carried out between 1984 and 2002 in Italy identified invasive fungal infections (IFIs) in 297 (18.2%) of 1630 autopsies in patients who died with AIDS. IFIs prevalence significantly decreased over time (from 25.0% in 1984–1988 to 15% in 1998–2002; $P = 0.004$). PJP was the most frequent IFI (131 cases [44.1%]), followed by aspergillosis (83 [27.9%]), cryptococcosis (62 [20.9%]), candidiasis (15 [5.1%]), histoplasmosis (4 [1.3%]), and zygomycosis (mucormycosis) (2 [0.7%]). The lung was the most frequently affected organ (83.5% of cases), followed by the central nervous system (CNS) (22.6%) and kidneys (13.1%); disseminated disease was observed in 83 cases (27.9%) [3]. Despite the advancement in medical science, patients from developing countries in Asia and Africa continue to get invasive mycoses especially PJP, cryptococcal meningitis, and mucosal candidiasis including *Candida* esophagitis due to late diagnosis and poor treatment compliance. Studies from different geographic locations reported mortality of 30–70% in cryptococcal meningitis (African countries) [4], 50% at one year with histoplasmosis (French Guiana) [5], 20% with pneumocystosis (Uganda) [6], and 28% with talaromycosis

(Vietnam) [7]. With the advancements in antiretroviral treatment (ART) and opportunistic infection prophylaxis, patients with HIV infection have significant improvement in quality of life, survival benefit and dramatic reduction in all opportunistic infections including fungal diseases. The geographic location, diagnosis, and management of common fungal diseases in AIDS are summarized in Table 6.1.

Table 6.1 Common fungal infections and it's management in AIDS

Disease	CD4 count	Geographic distribution	Diagnosis	Management	Comment
Pneumocystis jirovecii pneumonia	<200	Worldwide	BAL examination, CT scan thorax, serum BDG	TMP-SMX	Preventable by TMP-SMX prophylaxis
Cryptococcosis	<100	Worldwide	CSF examination, CrAg, culture	Amphotericin B + 5 flucytosine	Risk of IRIS, ART should be delayed by 2–10 weeks after induction therapy or achieving sterile culture
Talaromycosis	<100	South East Asia including northeast India, Myanmar, northern Thailand, Cambodia, Vietnam, Taiwan and southern China, and Indonesia	Culture from biological sample, histopathology especially of skin biopsies	Amphotericin B, Itraconazole, Posaconazole, Voriconazole	High mortality
Histoplasmosis	<200	North and Latin America, South east Asia, Africa, and Australia	Culture from biological sample, histopathology, Histoplasma antigen test	Amphotericin B, Itraconazole, Posaconazole, Voriconazole	Mimick tuberculosis, IRIS is uncommon, significant drug interactions with ART
Mucosal candidiasis	<200	Worldwide	Clinical examination, culture	Fluconazole, topical nystatin	Early HIV diagnosis and ART has significantly reduced mucosal candidiasis

6.1.1 *Pneumocystis jirovecii* Pneumonia

PJP was increasingly recognized after HIV epidemic. The incidence of pneumocystis pneumonia in HIV-infected patients in developed countries has greatly decreased after introduction of primary prophylaxis with trimethoprim-sulfamethoxazole (TMP-SMX) and widespread use of ART. However, PJP is one of the common presenting illnesses for HIV patients in developing countries including India. Study published from TAHOD database from Asian countries reported higher mortality in HIV positive patients without prophylaxis, even in the era of combination ART [8]. In sub-Saharan Africa, access to these interventions remains limited for the 23 million people living with HIV infection; recent estimate indicates that the prevalence of PJP among HIV-infected patients with pneumonia may be as high as 27% in some African countries [9]. PJP generally occurs in HIV-infected patients once CD4 count drops to below 200/cmm; incidence of 0.5% reported in patients with CD4 counts of 200–350/cm^3. In HIV-infected patients, PJP has gradual onset mainly involving pulmonary system with classical triad of symptoms—fever, dry cough (95%), and progressive worsening dyspnea. Approximately 7% of the patients are asymptomatic. Atypical manifestations and extrapulmonary PJP are seen in patients receiving inhalation pentamidine prophylaxis. Uncommon extrapulmonary manifestations include lesions within the liver, spleen, kidney, and brain [10]. Physical examination may be entirely normal in patients with PJP except fever and tachypnea. Chest examination may be normal or few crackles may be heard. TMP-SMX is drug of choice for treatment. For mild to moderate disease, oral treatment is generally adequate. Patient should receive oral treatment for severe disease in case of non-availability of intravenous formulation. Corticosteroids are recommended in patients with severe disease. Patients with PJP typically deteriorate after two to three days of therapy, due to increased alveolitis in response to dying organisms. Mutations associated with resistance to sulfa drugs have been documented in *Pneumocystis jirovecii*, but their effect on clinical outcome is uncertain [11, 12]. Patients who have PJP despite TMP-SMX prophylaxis can be treated effectively with standard doses of TMP-SMX. Other agents useful in the treatment of PJP are TMP-dapsone, clindamycin-primaquine, pentamidine, and atovaquone. In study by Rabodonirina et al., *P. jirovecii* type 7 and mechanical ventilation at PJP diagnosis were associated with increased risk of death due to PJP [13]. ART should be initiated, when possible, within two weeks of diagnosis of PJP. Management of PJP associated immune reconstitution inflammatory syndrome (IRIS) is not well defined; some experts would consider corticosteroids in patients with respiratory deterioration if other causes were ruled out.

6.1.2 Cryptococcosis

Cryptococcal meningoencephalitis is a life-threatening opportunistic fungal infection with a prevalence rate of 6–30% in HIV-infected patients. Among all fungi causing infection in AIDS patients, the ubiquitous fungus *Cryptococcus neoformans* is the leading cause of high morbidity and mortality. The disease is highly prevalent in sub-Saharan Africa. Current estimates indicate that every year, nearly one million cases of cryptococcal meningitis are diagnosed worldwide and the disease accounts for more than 600,000 deaths [14]. A low CD4 cell count (<100/cm^3) is the main predictor of risk of cryptococcal meningoencephalitis in HIV-infected patients. Cryptococcosis commonly presents as subacute meningitis or meningoencephalitis with fever, malaise, and headache in HIV-infected patients. Seizures, altered mental status, and focal neurological deficits are less commonly found especially in patients with late diagnosis or patients with high fungal load and associated with poor outcome. Classical features of meningitis like photophobia and neck stiffness are generally absent in HIV-infected patients and seen in one-third to one-quarter only. Diagnosis is commonly arrived by CSF examination with India ink preparation, cryptococcal antigen and culture. Prior to a lumbar puncture, all AIDS patients with suspected cryptococcal meningoencephalitis must have neuroimaging especially patients who presented with focal neurological deficit and/or altered sensorium. For the risk of herniation, lumber puncture should be avoided in patients with evidence of increased ICP, like effacement cerebral sulci. In other patients even with high opening pressure, 25–30 cm^3 of CSF can be safely removed to control raised intracranial pressure without the risk of herniation.

Poor prognostic factors for cryptococcal meningitis includes
1. Abnormal mental status
2. Cerebrospinal fluid (CSF) antigen titer >1:1024
3. CSF white blood cell count <20/μL
4. High opening pressure

Treatment: Amphotericin B (conventional or liposomal) combining with flucytosine is clearly a regimen of choice in treatment of HIV-infected patients with cryptococcal meningitis. The addition of flucytosine to amphotericin B is associated with rapid sterilization of CSF [15] and improved survival compared to the same dose of amphotericin B alone without flucytosine [16]. Fluconazole at the dose of 800 mg/day is inferior but acceptable alternative to flucytosine in combination with amphotericin B when accessibility is an issue [16, 17]. Patients, who are intolerant to amphotericin B and cannot afford liposomal amphotericin B, oral regimen containing fluconazole (400–800 mg daily) in combination with flucytosine (100mg/kg/day) is a potential alternative for treatment of CM [18]. Fluconazole alone is inferior to amphotericin B for induction therapy and is recommended only for patients who cannot tolerate or do not respond to standard treatment [19]. If it is used for primary induction therapy, the starting daily dose should be 1200 mg [20]. Optimal timing for initiation of ART in patients with acute cryptococcal meningitis is not well defined. Cryptococcal Optimal ART Timing (COAT) trial reported that survival was better in delayed ART arm as compared to simultaneous treatment arm while receiving anti-*Cryptococcus* drugs [21]. Additionally, early ART is not associated with improved CSF cryptococcal clearance but leads to higher risk of development of IRIS [22]. It may be prudent to delay initiation of ART until induction (the first 2 weeks) or till completion of the total induction/consolidation phase (i.e., 10 weeks).

Patients should be carefully followed up for development of IRIS after initiation of ART. Clinicians need to differentiate IRIS from relapse of cryptococcal meningitis by CSF examination and culture. Paradoxical HIV associated cryptococcal meningitis (CM)-IRIS occurs in 6–45% of patients, who received ART [23]. Clinically it is difficult to differentiate relapse vs paradoxical CM-IRIS and there is no laboratory test available for diagnosis of paradoxical CM-IRIS and it remains a diagnosis of exclusion. Risk factors for paradoxical CM-IRIS are a high organism/antigen load at baseline, acellular CSF, and early initiation of ART with rapid immune restoration [24].

CSF examination in patients with IRIS may show evidence of inflammations with raised white cells, proteins, and opening pressure with reduced glucose and sterile CSF. India ink and a cryptococcal antigen (CrAg) test of CSF have limited diagnostic utility for distinguishing IRIS from relapse. CrAg titers generally remain positive and slow decline over months to years at variable rates after successful CM treatment [24]. Patients who has four-fold rise in CSF CrAg titer can be early indication of relapse.

Secondary prophylaxis generally can be discontinued in patients who achieved >100/cmm CD4 counts with undetectable HIV viral load for more than three months on ART and who received one year of fluconazole suppressive treatment. Antifungal prophylaxis should be restarted in such patients who experience decline in CD4 counts to <100/cm^3.

6.1.3 Talaromycosis (Formerly Penicilliosis)

Talaromycosis caused by *Talaromyces marneffei* is an endemic disease restricted to South East Asia including Northeast India, Myanmar, Northern Thailand, Cambodia, Vietnam, Taiwan and Southern China, and Indonesia [25]. Cases are increasingly reported after HIV pandemic, and talaromycosis is the third most common AIDS-defining illness (after tuberculosis and cryptococcosis) in South East Asia. Most cases of talaromycosis are observed in patients who have CD4 T lymphocyte (CD4) cell counts <100 cells/mm^3 [26]. Disseminated disease is thought to be universally fatal if untreated. The common clinical manifestations include fever, anemia, weight loss, and papular lesions with central umbilication resembling molluscum contagiosum. Skin lesions are commonly seen on the face, ears, extremities, and occasionally the genitalia. As clinical presentations of histoplasmosis and talaromycosis are similar (skin lesion is more common in talaromycosis), the two diseases should be distinguished by proper diagnostic tests in regions where both the diseases are prevalent like south China. The definitive diagnosis of talaromycosis is based on isolation of organisms from cultures of blood or other clinical specimens and/or by histopathologic demonstration of organisms in biopsy material. The fungus is multiplied by central division, contrary to budding in other yeasts. The fungus is susceptible to amphotericin B, itraconazole, voriconazole, ketoconazole, miconazole, terbinafine, and 5-fluorocytosine; and resistant to fluconazole. Primary prophylaxis is indicated for HIV-infected patients with CD4 counts <100 cells/cmm who reside or stay for a long period in endemic area. Itraconazole 200 mg once a day is preferred over fluconazole 400 mg once a week. Initial treatment regimen for talaromycosis includes two weeks of liposomal amphotericin B followed by eight weeks of oral itraconazole. This should be followed by secondary prophylaxis consisting of 200 mg/day of itraconazole to prevent recurrence. Secondary prophylaxis can be discontinued after successful immune reversal following ART maintaining CD4 counts >100 cm^3 for at least six months. The antifungal treatment failure rates (defined as persistent fungemia, lack of clinical improvement, or clinical deterioration) were 22.8% for amphotericin B, 25% for itraconazole, and 63.6% for fluconazole in a case series study from Thailand [27].

6.1.4 Histoplasmosis

Histoplasmosis is caused by inhalation of the microconidia of *Histoplasma capsulatum*, a thermally dimorphic fungus. The mold form of the fungus may be found in moist and enriched soils containing bird/bat droppings [28]. Histoplasmosis is endemic in north and south America, Southeast Asia, Africa, and Australia. Histoplasmosis represents the first AIDS-defining illness in 50–75% of HIV patients in endemic area with mortality ranges from 10 to 60%. Disseminated form is the most common clinical presentation of histoplasmosis in AIDS. Fever, weakness, weight loss, cough, breathlessness, abdominal pain, diarrhea, mucocutaneous lesions, lymphadenopathy, and hepatosplenomegaly are common clinical presentations. In tuberculosis endemic region, it is difficult to differentiate histoplasmosis and tuberculosis based on clinical and radiological findings [29]. Diagnosis can be arrived by direct examination with special staining (Giemsa, periodic acid–Schiff, and methenamine-silver) and culture of all tissues or body fluids including bone marrow and blood culture. *Histoplasma* antigen testing from urine, blood, and broncho-alveolar lavage is a sensitive and rapid diagnostic test for patients with disseminated histoplasmosis [30]. The availability of molecular diagnostic tests for diagnosis of histoplasmosis in clinical care is still evolving [31].

Treatment: Amphotericin B ([liposomal amphotericin B (L-AmB) 3–4 mg/kg/day or amphotericin B deoxycholate (ABDC) 0.7 mg/kg/day] for first two weeks or until improvement in clinical features is the treatment of choice for induction therapy for patients with progressive disseminated form, and moderate to severe disease followed by itraconazole for 1 year in standard dosage, i.e., 200 mg three times a day for first three days followed by twice a day. L-AmB 3 mg/kg is found to be more effective compared to ABDC due to rapid and complete response, less toxicity with low mortality. Patient with single organ involvement and mild disease can be treated by itraconazole alone [32, 33]. Other triazole antifungals, posaconazole and voriconazole are also effective for treatment of HIV patients with histoplasmosis. Antiretroviral treatment should be considered within a month of starting antifungal treatment or once patient achieves clinical response. IRIS is rarely reported with histoplasmosis in HIV patients following ART [33]. Clinicians should be careful of significant drug–drug interactions between antiretroviral agents and itraconazole. Therapeutic drug monitoring is encouraged in all patients receiving itraconazole. Long-term secondary prophylaxis or chronic suppressive therapy with itraconazole 200 mg/day is recommended in HIV patients. Diagnosis and management of histoplasmosis in HIV patients remained a big challenge in TB endemic and low-middle income countries [29].

6.1.5 Mucosal Candidiasis

Oropharyngeal and esophageal candidiasis are the commonest opportunistic fungal disease in HIV-infected patients worldwide. The occurrence of oropharyngeal or esophageal candidiasis is recognized as an indicator of immune suppression and is often observed in patients with CD4 T lymphocyte (CD4) cell counts <200 cells/mm^3. ART has led to a dramatic decline in the prevalence of mucosal candidiasis.

6.1.6 Aspergillosis

Invasive aspergillosis is rare and less frequently diagnosed infection in HIV-infected individuals. However, the autopsy series from Italy reported invasive aspergillosis as the second most frequently identified invasive mycosis in fatal cases and 88% of the cases were diagnosed only in postmortem examination. Aspergillosis has been reported in patients with advanced HIV infection (CD4 < 100/cm^3) and not receiving ART [3, 34]. Lung is commonest organ involved in invasive aspergillosis. The extrapulmonary manifestation includes sinusitis, cutaneous disease, osteomyelitis, and brain abscess [35].

References

1. Brown GD, Denning DW, Gow NA, Levitz SM, Netea MG, White TC. Hidden killers: human fungal infections. Sci Transl Med. 2012;4:165rv13.
2. Armstrong-James D, Meintjes G, Brown GD. A neglected epidemic: fungal infections in HIV/AIDS. Trends Microbiol. 2014;22:120–7.
3. Antinori S, Nebuloni M, Magni C, et al. Trends in the postmortem diagnosis of opportunistic invasive fungal infections in patients with AIDS: a retrospective study of 1,630 autopsies performed between 1984 and 2002. Am J Clin Pathol. 2009;132:221–7.
4. Park BJ, Shetty S, Ahlquist A, et al. Long-term follow-up and survival of antiretroviral-naive patients with cryptococcal meningitis in the pre-antiretroviral therapy era, Gauteng Province, South Africa. Int J STD AIDS. 2011;22:199–203.
5. Nacher M, Adenis A, Sambourg E, et al. Histoplasmosis or tuberculosis in HIV-infected patients in the amazon: what should be treated first? PLoS Negl Trop Dis. 2014;8:e3290.
6. Koss CA, Jarlsberg LG, den Boon S, et al. A clinical predictor score for 30-Day mortality among HIV-infected adults hospitalized with pneumonia in Uganda. PLoS One. 2015;10:e0126591.

7. Le T, Wolbers M, Chi NH, et al. Epidemiology, seasonality, and predictors of outcome of AIDS-associated Penicillium marneffei infection in Ho Chi Minh City. Viet Nam Clinical infectious diseases : an official publication of the Infectious Diseases Society of America. 2011;52:945–52.
8. Lim PL, Zhou J, Ditangco RA, et al. Failure to prescribe pneumocystis prophylaxis is associated with increased mortality, even in the cART era: results from the treat Asia HIV observational database. J Int AIDS Soc. 2012;15(1):1.
9. Hartung TK, Chimbayo D, van Oosterhout JJ, et al. Etiology of suspected pneumonia in adults admitted to a high-dependency unit in Blantyre. Malawi Am J Trop Med Hygiene. 2011;85:105–12.
10. Ng VL, Yajko DM, Hadley WK. Extrapulmonary pneumocystosis. Clin Microbiol Rev. 1997;10:401–18.
11. Alvarez-Martinez MJ, Miro JM, Valls ME, et al. Prevalence of dihydropteroate synthase genotypes before and after the introduction of combined antiretroviral therapy and their influence on the outcome of Pneumocystis pneumonia in HIV-1-infected patients. Diagn Microbiol Infect Dis. 2010;68:60–5.
12. Crothers K, Beard CB, Turner J, et al. Severity and outcome of HIV-associated Pneumocystis pneumonia containing Pneumocystis jirovecii dihydropteroate synthase gene mutations. AIDS. 2005;19:801–5.
13. Rabodonirina M, Vaillant L, Taffe P, et al. Pneumocystis jirovecii genotype associated with increased death rate of HIV-infected patients with pneumonia. Emerg Infect Dis. 2013;19:21–8. quiz 186
14. Park BJ, Wannemuehler KA, Marston BJ, Govender N, Pappas PG, Chiller TM. Estimation of the current global burden of cryptococcal meningitis among persons living with HIV/AIDS. AIDS. 2009;23:525–30.
15. van der Horst CM, Saag MS, Cloud GA, et al. Treatment of cryptococcal meningitis associated with the acquired immunodeficiency syndrome. National Institute of Allergy and Infectious Diseases mycoses study group and AIDS Clinical Trials Group. N Engl J Med. 1997;337:15–21.
16. Day JN, Chau TT, Wolbers M, et al. Combination antifungal therapy for cryptococcal meningitis. N Engl J Med. 2013;368:1291–302.
17. Pappas PG, Chetchotisakd P, Larsen RA, et al. A phase II randomized trial of amphotericin B alone or combined with fluconazole in the treatment of HIV-associated cryptococcal meningitis. Clin Infect Dis. 2009;48:1775–83.
18. Larsen RA, Bozzette SA, Jones BE, et al. Fluconazole combined with flucytosine for treatment of cryptococcal meningitis in patients with AIDS. Clin Infect Dis. 1994;19:741–5.
19. Bicanic T, Meintjes G, Wood R, et al. Fungal burden, early fungicidal activity, and outcome in cryptococcal meningitis in antiretroviral-naive or antiretroviral-experienced patients treated with amphotericin B or fluconazole. Clin Infect Dis. 2007;45:76–80.
20. Nussbaum JC, Jackson A, Namarika D, et al. Combination flucytosine and high-dose fluconazole compared with fluconazole monotherapy for the treatment of cryptococcal meningitis: a randomized trial in Malawi. Clin Infect Dis. 2010;50:338–44.
21. Boulware D, Muzoora C, et al. ART initiation within the first 2 weeks of cryptococcal meningitis is associated with higher mortality: a multisite randomized trial. Program and abstracts of the 20th Conference on Retroviruses and Opportunistic Infections Atlanta, Georgia 2013.
22. Bisson GP, Molefi M, Bellamy S, et al. Early versus delayed antiretroviral therapy and cerebrospinal fluid fungal clearance in adults with HIV and cryptococcal meningitis. Clin Infect Dis. 2013;56:1165–73.
23. da Cunha Colombo ER, Mora DJ, Silva-Vergara ML. Immune reconstitution inflammatory syndrome (IRIS) associated with Cryptococcus neoformans infection in AIDS patients. Mycoses. 2011;54:e178–82.
24. Longley N, Harrison TS, Jarvis JN. Cryptococcal immune reconstitution inflammatory syndrome. Curr Opin Infect Dis. 2013;26:26–34.

25. Supparatpinyo K, Khamwan C, Baosoung V, Nelson KE, Sirisanthana T. Disseminated Penicillium marneffei infection in Southeast Asia. Lancet. 1994;344:110–3.
26. Chariyalertsak S, Supparatpinyo K, Sirisanthana T. Nelson KE. A controlled trial of itraconazole as primary prophylaxis for systemic fungal infections in patients with advanced human immunodeficiency virus infection in Thailand. Clin Infect Dis. 2002;34:277–84.
27. Supparatpinyo K, Nelson KE, Merz WG, et al. Response to antifungal therapy by human immunodeficiency virus-infected patients with disseminated Penicillium marneffei infections and in vitro susceptibilities of isolates from clinical specimens. Antimicrob Agents Chemother. 1993;37:2407–11.
28. Woods JP. Revisiting old friends: developments in understanding Histoplasma capsulatum pathogenesis. J Microbiol. 2016;54:265–76.
29. Nacher M, Adenis A, Aznar C, et al. How many have died from undiagnosed human immunodeficiency virus-associated histoplasmosis, a treatable disease? Time to act. Am J Trop Med Hyg. 2014;90:193–4.
30. Theel ES, Harring JA, Dababneh AS, Rollins LO, Bestrom JE, Jespersen DJ. Reevaluation of commercial reagents for detection of Histoplasma capsulatum antigen in urine. J Clin Microbiol. 2015;53:1198–203.
31. Adenis AA, Aznar C, Couppie P. Histoplasmosis in HIV-infected patients: a review of new developments and remaining gaps. Curr Trop Med Rep. 2014;1:119–28.
32. Benson CA, Kaplan JE, Masur H, et al. Treating opportunistic infections among HIV-infected adults and adolescents: recommendations from CDC, the National Institutes of Health, and the HIV medicine association/Infectious Diseases Society of America. MMWR Recomm Rep. 2004;53:1–112.
33. Panel on Opportunistic Infections in HIV-Infected Adults and Adolescents. Guidelines for the prevention and treatment of opportunistic infections in HIV-infected adults and adolescents: recommendations from the Centers for Disease Control and Prevention, the National Institutes of Health, and the HIV Medicine Association of the Infectious Diseases Society of America. Accessed 28 June 2018.
34. Mylonakis E, Barlam TF, Flanigan T, Rich JD. Pulmonary aspergillosis and invasive disease in AIDS: review of 342 cases. Chest. 1998;114:251–62.
35. Mylonakis E, Paliou M, Sax PE, Skolnik PR, Baron MJ, Rich JD. Central nervous system aspergillosis in patients with human immunodeficiency virus infection. Report of 6 cases and review. Medicine. 2000;79:269–80.

Mycoses in Neonates and Children

7

Tanu Singhal

Key Points

- The main risk groups for paediatric IFI include neonates, critically sick children in the intensive care unit and those on cancer chemotherapy.
- Neonates with invasive candidiasis commonly have CNS involvement. The drug of choice is amphotericin B deoxycholate. Prophylaxis should be considered in babies with birth weight <1000 gms in NICUs where incidence of candidemia is higher than 10%.
- Invasive candidiasis should be considered as a cause of sepsis in critically sick children in PICUs. Empiric therapy should be started early based on risk factor assessment and choices include fluconazole, amphotericin B and echinocandins.
- Children on cancer chemotherapy are at high risk for invasive fungal infection especially molds. The principles for diagnosis and management are same as adults. Antifungal prophylaxis is indicated in recipients of HSCT, AML and relapsed ALL.

7.1 Introduction

Children at risk for invasive fungal infections (IFI) include neonates, critically sick children, children on cancer chemotherapy/stem cell transplant and those with primary or acquired immunodeficiency (Table 7.1). Like adults, the incidence of IFI in children is also increasing due to increase in the 'at-risk group'. But limited trial data and non-availability of many paediatric antifungal formulations complicate treatment of IFI in children even more than adults. The burden and outcome of paediatric IFI in Asian countries are likely to be worse than resource-rich settings due

T. Singhal (✉)
Kokilaben Dhirubhai Ambani Hospital and Medical Research Institute, Mumbai, India

Department of Paediatrics, Kokilaben Hospital, Mumbai, India
e-mail: tanu.singhal@relianceada.com

A. Chakrabarti (ed.), *Clinical Practice of Medical Mycology in Asia*,
https://doi.org/10.1007/978-981-13-9459-1_7

Table 7.1 Children at risk for invasive fungal infections

Neonates
Children in the critical care unit
Children on cancer chemotherapy or who have undergone haematopoietic stem cell transplant (HSCT)
Children with primary immunodeficiency (PID) [chronic granulomatous disease (CGD), severe combined immunodeficiency disorder (SCID), etc.]
Children with acquired immunodeficiency [HIV, receipt of steroids and other immunosuppressive drugs, solid organ transplant (SOT)]

to poor infection control practices in neonatal and paediatric intensive care units, overuse of antibiotics, increased mold spore counts in the hospital environment and residential dwellings, tropical climate, malnutrition, advanced disease at diagnosis, reduced awareness, lack of appropriate diagnostic facilities and cost/availability of antifungal drugs. This write-up gives a bird's eye view of IFI in children from an Asian perspective. While knowledge and attention to guidelines is essential, what is more important is to formulate diagnostic and treatment algorithms based on local epidemiology, resources and availability.

7.2 Neonates

7.2.1 Epidemiology

Invasive candidiasis (IC) is a common and serious infection in premature and low birth weight newborns and is associated with death or poor neurodevelopmental outcomes in more than half the infected infants. Colonization of the infant skin and gastrointestinal tract is common and the immaturity of the epithelial and mucosal barriers in preterm babies predisposes to candidiasis. The major risk factors are low Apgar score, prolonged antibiotics (cephalosporin), male, parenteral nutrition, CVC, H2 blockers, mechanical ventilation, long hospital stay, DIC, shock, etc. [1]. The incidence varies between centres and has been reported to be between 2 and 28% [2]. Incidence has declined in the last decade due to the use of antifungal prophylaxis. In a study from Central India, the reported incidence between 2010 and 2015 was 3.6% of total admissions; 4.9% in very low birth weight (<1500 gms) and 11.2% in extremely low birth weight (<1000 gms) neonates [3]. In a recent study from a hospital in New Delhi which included 2588 neonates (between 2011 and 2015) both outborn and inborn as well as some who were delivered at home, high rates of sepsis were noted. *Candida* was isolated in 22.7% of septic neonates but >¾ were babies born at 32 weeks above the weight of 1500 gms [4]. A study from a tertiary care hospital in Pakistan including 45 cases of neonatal candidiasis between 1996 and 2006 reported the incidence of candidemia to be 0.9% with most cases occurring in newborns less than 1500 gms, *C. albicans* as the predominant isolate and mechanical ventilation, positive bacterial blood culture and prolonged length of NICU stay as the major risk factors [5].

Contrary to *C. parapsilosis* in western world, *C. tropicalis* is the most common species isolated from Asian countries, followed closely by *C. albicans*, *C. parapsilosis*, *C. glabrata* and *C. krusei* in that order. *C. auris* will soon be knocking at the doors of NICUs (2 isolates in the author's institution in neonates who underwent cardiac surgery in the year 2018; unpublished data).

Apart from *Candida*, infection with rare yeast including *Kodamaea*, *Trichosporon*, *Malassezia*, *Rhodotorula*, and *Pichia* species has been described in NICUs. Large outbreaks with *Pichia anomala* and *Pichia kudriavzevii* have been reported from India [5]. Apart from yeast, gastrointestinal mucormycosis has also been described in newborns presenting with necrotizing enterocolitis [6, 7]. Kaur et al. in their review paper have proposed that a high degree of suspicion for gastrointestinal mucormycosis should be kept in preterm neonates exposed to broad spectrum antibiotics and formula/spoon feeding presenting with a syndrome complex of abdominal distension, bilious vomiting and abdominal mass [8].

7.2.2 Clinical Presentation and Diagnosis

Infection with *Candida* and other yeast generally causes late onset sepsis (3–42 days). Rarely, candidiasis of the maternal genital tract can cause early onset sepsis with rash in vaginally delivered infants. The clinical manifestations are usually subtle and include feed intolerance, respiratory deterioration, abdominal distension, temperature instability and hypotension [9]. Thrombocytopenia is more common in candida-related sepsis in newborns than bacterial sepsis [10]. *Candida* in neonates is known to invade every organ including brain, retina, kidneys, liver, spleen, bones and the heart. Sometimes the course may be so indolent that the organ localizations may appear long after the infectious episode.

Newborns with suspected candidiasis should have a set of blood fungal cultures sent (0.5–1 mL of blood is sufficient). The culture positivity is 50% and same as adults. Urine should be examined and presence of budding yeast on Grams stain or growth in culture is more often a sign of invasive candidiasis rather than colonization. USG examination may show fungal balls in the kidneys. All newborns with positive blood or urine cultures for *Candida* should undergo CSF examination to detect haematogenous candida meningoencephalitis (HCME). There is limited data supporting the use of serum beta D glucan in diagnosis of neonatal candidiasis.

7.2.3 Treatment [11]

Empirical therapy for invasive candidiasis should be considered in very low birth weight (VLBW)/extremely low birth weight (ELBW) babies with late onset neonatal sepsis with risk factors, when there is no clinical response to antibacterials especially if these babies have not been on prophylaxis. Amphotericin B deoxycholate is the drug of choice. Details of drug therapy are listed in Table 7.2. Central lines should be removed as soon as possible.

Table 7.2 Therapy of neonatal candidiasis [11, 12]

Drug (IDSA grading)	Dose	Comments
Amphotericin B deoxycholate (AII)	1 mg/kg/day	Preferred drug for neonatal IC Minimal adverse effects Penetrates meninges (40–90%) and kidneys well
Liposomal amphotericin B (CIII)	3–5 mg/kg/day	Recent study showed increased mortality as compared to AMB-D Does not eradicate renal infection Superiority for CNS infection may be offset by poor renal penetration
Fluconazole (AII)	Loading of 25 mg/kg/day and then 12 mg/kg/day as single dose	As efficacious as AMB if susceptible Can be used for switch over therapy Penetrates the CNS and kidneys well Possible resistance and cannot be used empirically if baby on fluconazole prophylaxis
Flucytosine (CIII)	25 mg/kg 6 hourly	Only as add on/salvage therapy for CNS candidiasis or endocarditis in patients not responding to standard therapy Serious risk of adverse effects
Echinocandins (CIII) Caspofungin Micafungin Anidulafungin	25–50 mg/m^2/day 4–10 mg/kg/day 3 mg/kg/day loading and then 1.5 mg/kg/day	Not the preferred agents Lack of dosing and pharmacokinetic data Poor meningeal and urinary levels Should be used only if resistance to/failure of other agents High doses of micafungin 10 mg/kg/day in babies with HCME

CSF analysis and brain imaging, urine analysis and culture should be done for all babies with candidemia. Blood cultures should be repeated every 48–72 h to demonstrate clearance from the blood. Babies with persistent positive blood cultures should undergo echocardiography and imaging of liver, spleen and kidneys. Fundoscopy should be done in all infected babies.

The duration of therapy is 2 weeks after last negative blood culture provided there is complete resolution of signs and symptoms and there are no metastatic complications. Therapy can be stepped down to fluconazole if the isolate is susceptible. In babies with HCME, therapy should be continued till resolution of clinical, CSF and radiologic abnormalities and can even be months (oral fluconazole if isolate is susceptible). All shunts and reservoirs must be removed. Routine addition of flucytosine in babies with HCME is not recommended. In babies with osteomyelitis, treatment up to 6 months may be needed.

7.2.4 Prevention

Randomized controlled trials have shown 80–90% reduction in the risk of invasive candidiasis with the use of fluconazole in VLBW/ELBW babies. Some of these trials have been criticized widely for various reasons including that they did not demonstrate impact on mortality, neurodevelopmental outcome and antifungal resistance, and were single centre studies with very high rate of baseline invasive candidiasis, etc. [12]. A recent meta-analysis using individual patient data from six trials conducted in the USA concluded that use of fluconazole reduces the risk of invasive candidiasis or death (but not death alone) with no adverse effects and risk of emergence of resistant strains [13]. The IDSA guidelines therefore recommend that nurseries with >10% risk of invasive candidiasis should consider using intravenous fluconazole in ELBW babies (<1000 gms) in dose of 3–6 mg/kg twice weekly for 6 weeks (AI) [11].

Equally important apart from using fluconazole are other infection control measures such as hand hygiene, implementation of central line care bundles, restricting the use of antibiotics, steroids, antacids, H2 blockers and promotion of early feeding.

7.3 Children in the Critical Care Unit

7.3.1 Epidemiology

Like adults, children in the paediatric intensive care unit (PICU) are an emerging risk group for IC. The National Nosocomial Surveillance System of the USA, in its data from 1992 to 1997, reported Candida as the fifth commonest pathogen causing nosocomial blood stream infection [14]. In another study at the Children Hospital of Philadelphia between 1997 and 2004, there were 101 episodes of candidemia with a rate of 3.4/1000 PICU admissions and 30 day mortality of 44% [15]. Closer home, a study from India reported 70% of PICU patients as being colonized with *Candida* and Candida accounting for roughly 8% of all nosocomial blood stream infections [16]. A prospective study on ICU acquired candidemia in India between 2011 and 2012 reported 1400 episodes of candidemia in 215,122 patients, leading to a rate of 6.51/1000 admissions of which 35% were children below 18 years of age [17]. The commonest species in adult patients were *C. tropicalis* (41%), *C. albicans* (20%), *C. parapsilosis* (11%) and *C. auris* (5.2%).The emergence of *C. auris* in critically ill patients is of particular concern since this fungus is commonly misidentified, is highly drug resistant and can cause outbreaks. In the author's own institution, in a 10 bedded paediatric ICU of the 25 episodes of nosocomial BSI in past 8 years (2010–2017), 9 were due to *Candida* (36%), with one isolate being *C. auris*.

The incidence of other invasive fungal infections including *Aspergillus, Mucorales* and other rare filamentous fungi is significantly lower in non-immunocompromised critically ill children and will not be discussed further.

7.3.2 Risk Factors, Clinical Features and Diagnosis of IC

Risk factors for IC in critically ill children are more or less similar to adults and include prolonged ICU stay, use of broad spectrum antibiotics, presence of central venous catheter, use of steroids, total parenteral nutrition (TPN), dialysis, pancreatitis, gut surgery, multiple transfusion and multifocal colonization with *Candida* [15].

In a study specifically looking at risk factors for candidemia in PICU patients, presence of CVC, malignancy, administration of vancomycin/antibiotics with anaerobic coverage and use of TPN were independent risk factors for candidemia with presence of CVC associated with a 30-fold risk of candidemia [15].

Candida sepsis is clinically indistinguishable from bacterial sepsis. The gold standard for diagnosis is fungal cultures; if a central line is present, then paired cultures should be sent. The sensitivity of blood cultures is around 50%. In adults, 1,3 beta D glucan estimation has been found to be useful for diagnosing invasive candidiasis with high negative predictive value; in children, data is still emerging with preliminary studies showing significant false positivity [11, 18].

7.3.3 Therapy

Empiric therapy is indicated for children with suspected invasive candidiasis since cultures are positive in only 50% of the instances and delay in therapy is associated with increased mortality. In adults, several scoring systems including the candida colonization index, Candida score, Ostrovsky Zeichner score have been proposed to identify adult patients who are candidates for empiric antifungal therapy [19]. These scores have good negative predictive value but poor positive predictive values and may lead to overtreatment with antifungals. There are no studies systematically evaluating these scores in children. Hence empiric therapy in children should be based on careful assessment of risk factors.

Recent ESCMID and IDSA guidelines recommend echinocandins as the drugs of choice for empiric antifungal therapy in adults (AI) [11]. Data on echinocandins in children is emerging. Children also tolerate amphotericin B deoxycholate much better than adults. Hence the choice of antifungals in children depends on several factors including local epidemiology, azole exposure, degree of sickness, cost of treatment, and includes fluconazole, amphotericin B (deoxycholate/ liposomal) and echinocandins.

The IDSA guidelines recommend that if the cultures are negative for *Candida*, antifungal therapy should be continued for 2 weeks in patients showing a clinical response [11]. In those patients with no clinical response or negative biomarkers or emergence of an alternative diagnosis, therapy can be stopped earlier.

If the cultures are positive, then therapy should be optimized depending on susceptibility. Central venous catheters should be removed (AII). Cultures should be repeated every 3–4 days and therapy should be continued till 2 weeks of culture negativity. A fundoscopic examination should be done in all patients before stopping therapy.

7.3.4 Prevention

The issue of antifungal prophylaxis in the ICU is controversial with the benefits of prophylaxis pitted against adverse effects, cost and emergence of resistance. While meta-analysis in adult patients has shown prophylaxis to reduce candidemia/IC (but not mortality), they did not address issues of adverse effects and ecologic changes. The number needed to treat varied from 9 in high risk to 188 in low risk patients [11]. Though there are no studies in critically ill paediatric patients assessing the impact of antifungal prophylaxis, a single study by Zaoutis et al. has recommended prophylaxis in children with multiple risk factors and high probability of IC [15].

It is more important to implement the central venous catheter care bundles including daily chlorhexidine bathing of the patients with central lines and implement antimicrobial stewardship to reduce IC. The use of probiotics has been shown to reduce candida colonization and candiduria in critically ill children in one randomized controlled trial and needs further investigation [20]. The administration of probiotics in critically ill children especially neonates has been reportedly associated with probiotic fungemia; hence caution should be exercised [21].

7.4 Children on Cancer Chemotherapy/HSCT

7.4.1 Epidemiology

The risk of IFI in children on cancer chemotherapy or those with HSCT depends largely on the type of cancer or HSCT status (Table 7.3) and is further modified by the intensity of the chemotherapy regime, local factors including the health care set-up where the children are undergoing chemotherapy and the use of antifungal prophylaxis [22]. Basically prolonged and profound neutropenia (absolute neutrophil count of ≤500/μL), defects in cell-mediated immunity (lymphopenia due to T cell cytotoxic agents and steroids) and disruption of mucosal barriers (mucositis, presence of central venous catheters) are the main risk factors. The commonest fungi causing IFI in this risk group include *Candida, Aspergillus* and *Mucorales*; the incidence of other moulds including *Fusarium* and *Scedosporium* is also increasing. The key differences from adults include the accuracy of the available diagnostic tests as well as the choice and dosing of antifungal drugs for treatment/prophylaxis. The outcomes of IFI in children like adults are poor with mortality rates ranging from 10 to 80%.

Table 7.3 Approximate risk of IFI in children on cancer chemotherapy/HSCT [22]

Group	Risk of IFI
Allogenic HSCT with GVHD, allogenic HSCT (especially umbilical cord blood transplant, partially matched related donor), AML/MDS treated as AML, relapsed acute lymphatic leukaemia, severe aplastic anaemia, congenital immunodeficiency	≥ 10%
Non-Hodgkin's lymphoma, autologous HSCT, new acute lymphatic leukaemia	<5%
Hodgkin's lymphoma, solid tumours	Sporadic/ rare

In a study from Northern India, the prevalence of IFI in children (as defined by EORTC/MSG criteria) with acute leukaemia and febrile neutropenia who were not on antifungal prophylaxis was significantly high (23%) with a relatively low mortality rate of 9.5% [23]. In a study from Taiwan in children with acute myeloid leukaemia between 2005 and 2014, the incidence of invasive fungal infections was 20.5%. *Candida* was the commonest cause of IFI (60%). However unlike the Indian data, the overall mortality was very high (53%) with IPA having the highest mortality of 80% [24].

7.4.2 **Diagnosis** [22, 25]

The standard EORTC/MSG criteria may also apply to diagnosis and classification of IFI in children into proven, probable and possible categories [25]. The gold standards for microbiologic diagnosis are cultures from blood/tissue/bronchoalveolar lavage for fungi. Serum galactomannan using a cut-off defined as ≥0.5 has been found to have good sensitivity (76%) and specificity (86%) for diagnosis of invasive aspergillosis in children as in adults. In children with high risk of mold infection twice weekly galactomannan estimation is recommended (A II) but is usually not possible due to high cost and availability. The use of antifungal prophylaxis also reduces the performance of the serum galactomannan assay. A positive BAL galactomannan (≥1) is a good diagnostic test for invasive pulmonary aspergillosis. In suspected CNS aspergillosis, a CSF galactomannan may be estimated (cut-off of ≥0.5), though it is not yet approved by FDA. There is limited data about the sensitivity and specificity of the beta D glucan test in diagnosis of invasive candidiasis and aspergillosis in children with some current studies showing high rates of false positivity [18]. CT imaging of chest and if indicated sinuses is of value in diagnosis of invasive mold infection. However, the characteristic signs including the halo/crescent and reverse halo signs are seen infrequently in children especially those below 5 years. The usual findings in young children are non-specific nodules, masses, consolidations and infiltrates.

7.4.3 **Treatment** [22]

The management principles have been largely extrapolated from adult studies and are more or less same as adults. These include reducing/withdrawing immunosuppression as far as possible and attention to source control. The drugs recommended for managing IFI in children with cancer include mainly amphotericin B, voriconazole and the echinocandins (Table 7.4). While liposomal amphotericin B is preferred, the deoxycholate preparation can be used in resource limited setting; children have much lower rates of nephrotoxicity as compared to adults. Posaconazole is approved in children above 13 years and anidulafungin is not yet approved in children. If voriconazole or posaconazole is used, then advice about interactions with food and therapeutic drug monitoring is a must. The recommended therapeutic level

Table 7.4 Management of IFI in children on cancer chemotherapy and undergoing HSCT [22]

Condition	Drug choices (ECIL grading)	Comments
Febrile neutropenia Empiric therapy for those with fever lasting for 4 or more days despite broad spectrum antibiotics (B II)	Liposomal amphotericin B (AI) Caspofungin (AI) AMB-D if cost is an issue	Send cultures, biomarkers and CT imaging Stop when neutropenia resolves/alternate diagnosis made/diagnosis of IFD made Preemptive therapy not studied in children but may be considered if quick access to CT/biomarkers
Invasive candidiasis	Echinocandins (BII) LAMB (BII) Fluconazole/ Voriconazole (BII) AMB-D (resource limited)	Remove central lines if possible (BII) Data on echinocandins emerging in children Can step down to fluconazole/ voriconazole if susceptible Addition of flucytosine for CNS infections, endocarditis Treat for 2 weeks after last negative culture
Invasive aspergillosis	Voriconazole in age ≥2 (AI) LAMB (B III) AMB-D (resource limited)	For salvage therapy posaconazole/ caspofungin or combination of voriconazole/amphotericin B with echinocandins Duration till resolution of signs and symptoms and stabilization of CT findings and continue secondary prophylaxis if patient on intense immunosuppression
Mucormycosis	LAMB (BII) LAMB with caspofungin/ posaconazole (CIII)	Aggressive and urgent surgical debridement Correction of underlying predisposing factors Hyperbaric therapy if available on site
Fusariosis/Scedosporiosis	Voriconazole ≥2 years (BII) LAMB (no grading) Posaconazole ≥13 years (no grading)	Attempt antifungal susceptibility testing

for voriconazole is 1–5 mg/L and for posaconazole is 0.7–1.5 mg/L. Though there are no studies in paediatric patients in India, studies in adults show wide variability in the levels owing to polymorphisms in the CYP2C19 enzymes that metabolize voriconazole [2]. Drug interactions should also be kept in mind especially with voriconazole. Switch in class is recommended on those patients who develop break-through IFI on prophylaxis. Combination therapy is not recommended as routine but may be considered in special settings. The duration of therapy is variable but is usually till resolution of clinical and radiologic signs and symptoms. Secondary prophylaxis may need to be continued in many patients till immunosuppressive therapy is withdrawn or lowered.

7.4.4 Prevention/Prophylaxis [22, 26, 27]

The general measures to prevent IFI in this group of patients include implementation of the prevention bundle for central venous catheters, avoiding areas of construction, dampness and seepage, potted plants. Patients undergoing HSCT and even those patients on cancer chemotherapy with severe and prolonged neutropenia should be treated in rooms with positive pressure and HEPA filters.

Given the high incidence of IFI, problems associated with treating IFI and the poor outcomes, antifungal prophylaxis seems to be an attractive option. Systematic review suggests that antifungal prophylaxis in allogenic HSCT patients reduces incidence of IFI as well as fungus attributable and all cause mortality, whereas in acute leukaemia it reduces IFI and fungus attributable mortality. There is a general consensus that children undergoing allogenic HSCT, AML, relapsed ALL, and severe aplastic anaemia should be given antifungal prophylaxis. Patients undergoing autologous HSCT should also receive anti-yeast prophylaxis during the neutropenic phase. Newly diagnosed ALL and solid tumours do not merit routine prophylaxis.

Studies on fluconazole prophylaxis in allogenic HSCT recipients have demonstrated reduced risk of both early and late candidiasis, gut-related GVHD and mortality. However, the main limitation of fluconazole is no effect on molds. Subsequently, several agents including amphotericin B deoxycholate, aerosolized amphotericin B, LAMB, itraconazole, voriconazole, posaconazole, micafungin and caspofungin have been evaluated against fluconazole. All these agents have limitations of cost, adverse effects, need for TDM, drug interactions and non-availability of paediatric data. There is no one size fits all drug. Hence choice of antifungal prophylaxis varies between centres. Indian studies report a high incidence of mold infections in this predisposed population and hence need for a mold active agent is important. In a study from New Delhi, India in paediatric acute leukaemia (ALL and AML) oral voriconazole was as effective as intravenous low dose amphotericin B deoxycholate as prophylaxis [28]. Table 7.5 discusses the choices for antifungal prophylaxis in children. In HSCT, the duration of prophylaxis is variable with either stopping prophylaxis with engraftment or continuing till immunosuppression is stopped [in patients with GVHD or high risk for GVHD (mismatched, unrelated, haploidentical or umbilical cord transplants)].

Patients with acute lymphoblastic leukaemia, lymphoma and those undergoing HSCT are also at risk for infection with *Pneumocystis jirovecii* and hence need to be put on cotrimoxazole prophylaxis.

7.5 Children with Primary and Acquired Immunodeficiency

Children with primary immunodeficiency disorders involving cell-mediated immunity and phagocytic defects are at significant risk for fungal infections [29]. The risk is highest in patients with hyper IgE syndrome and chronic granulomatous disease (CGD) followed by severe combined immunodeficiency disorder

Table 7.5 Suggested antifungal prophylaxis for children on cancer chemotherapy/undergoing HSCT [22, 27]

Drug choices	Dose	Comments
Fluconazole	8–12 mg/kg/day (max 400 mg) once daily	Most commonly recommended drug for children No protection against molds Interactions with vincristine/other anticancer drugs
Itraconazole	5 mg/kg/day Q 12 hourly	Superior to fluconazole but more side effects Food interactions, need for TDM Drug interactions Non-availability of syrup/IV formulation in majority of Asian countries Not commonly used
Voriconazole	As in Table 7.6	No protection against Mucor Need for TDM Drug interactions with many drugs chiefly cyclosporine and tacrolimus The only oral mold active agent for children Adverse effects with prolonged therapy
Posaconazole (above 13 years)	Oral: 200 mg thrice daily IV: 300 mg twice daily on day 1 and then 300 mg once daily	Superior to fluconazole and itraconazole in adults with AML/MDS but more serious adverse effects Cannot be given in children below 13 Food interactions and unpredictable pharmacokinetics for syrup Tablet form not available in India IV posaconazole better Cost Adverse effects and drug interactions
Amphotericin B deoxycholate	0.2 mg/kg/day	Non-inferior to fluconazole But significantly more toxic May be an option in resource limited setting
Liposomal amphotericin B	1 mg/kg alternate day 2.5 mg/kg twice weekly	Non-inferior to fluconazole More toxic Cost Administration problems
Aerosolized amphotericin B	12.5 mg on two consecutive days of week	Only effective for pulmonary molds Need for special nebulizer Cough may interrupt therapy Needs to be combined with IV fluconazole for protection against *candida*
Micafungin	1 mg/kg/day (max dose 50 mg)	Non-inferior to fluconazole Minimal adverse effects, no drug interactions Cost, IV route
Caspofungin	70 mg/m^2 day 1 and then 50 mg/m^2/day	Non-inferior to itraconazole Minimal adverse effects, no drug interactions Cost, IV route

(SCID), Hyper IgM syndrome, Wiskott–Aldrich syndrome, Di George syndrome, common variable immunodeficiency, disorders of gamma interferon-IL12 axis and idiopathic CD4 lymphocytopenia. The usual pathogens are *Aspergillus, Candida, Cryptococcus and Pneumocystis jirovecii*. It is important for clinicians to maintain a high index of suspicion for these pathogens in patients with these disorders and conversely these disorders in patients presenting with these infections with no obvious immunodeficiency. The usual principles for diagnosis and management apply. There is also a role for prophylaxis with itraconazole in patients with CGD, cotrimoxazole in patients with SCID and idiopathic CD4 lymphocytopenia.

Patients with acquired immunodeficiency are also at high risk for fungal infections [30]. Children living with HIV and severe immunodeficiency are at risk for cryptococcosis and pneumocystis infections; those on long-term steroids and other immunosuppressive agents including those having undergone solid organ transplant are at risk for invasive mold infections (*Aspergillus, Mucorales*), *Cryptococcus, Histoplasma* and *Pneumocystis jirovecii*. The usual principles for diagnosis apply. The sensitivity for galactomannan in diagnosis of invasive aspergillosis in the non-neutropenic setting is low; BAL galactomannan may be more useful. Treatment recommendations are same as other settings. Primary prophylaxis for PCP is recommended in many settings. Secondary prophylaxis may need to be continued in many till immunocompetence is restored or immunosuppression is withdrawn.

7.6 Conclusions

It can thus be seen that IFI in children are more similar than different to their adult counterparts. The dosing of antifungal drugs in children is summarized in Table 7.6. There is a huge unmet need to increase awareness among clinicians about the diagnosis, treatment and prevention of these infections in children. At the same time, there is a research requirement for more studies and trials in children with IFI along with development of paediatric formulations of antifungal drugs.

Table 7.6 Therapeutic dosing of antifungal drugs in children

Drug	Dose	Comment
Fluconazole	12 mg/kg loading (max 800 mg) followed by 6 mg/kg/day (max 400 mg)	
Voriconazole		
2–12 years 12–14 years (weight <50 kg)	IV 9 mg/kg/dose twice daily day 1 and then 8 mg/kg/dose twice daily Oral 9 mg/kg twice daily	TDM needed Level: 1–6
12–14 years >50 kg ≥15 years	6 mg/kg twice daily on day 1 And then 4 mg/kg twice daily or 200 mg twice daily	

Table 7.6 (continued)

Drug	Dose	Comment
Posaconazole (children more than 13 years)		
Oral suspension	Prophylaxis 200 mg thrice daily Treatment 200 mg four times daily/400 mg twice daily	Give full stomach with fatty meal TDM necessary Prophylactic level ≥0.7 Therapeutic ≥1
Intravenous (approved only for prophylaxis)	300 mg twice daily on day 1 and then 300 mg once daily	
Amphotericin B deoxycholate	0.7–1 mg/kg/day	Monitor creatinine, K, Mg Slow infusion in 5% dextrose
Liposomal amphotericin B	Candidiasis/Aspergillosis (3 mg/kg/day) Mucormycosis (5–7.5 mg/kg/day)	
Flucytosine	100 mg/kg/day given 6 hourly (maximum dose 6 gm)	Renal dose adjustments needed
Caspofungin	70 mg/m^2 day 1 (max dose 70 mg) and then 50 mg/m^2 daily (max dose 50 mg)	
Micafungin	2–4 mg/kg/day (100–200 mg daily) (4–10 mg/kg/day in neonates)	
Anidulafungin	3 mg/kg/day loading and 1.5 mg/kg/day maintainence	Not yet approved for children

References

1. Saiman L, Ludington E, P faller M, et al. Risk factors for candidemia in neonatal intensive care unit patients. The National Epidemiology of Mycosis Survey study group. Pediatr Infect Dis J. 2000;19:319.
2. Benjamin DK Jr, Stoll BJ, Fanaroff AA, et al. Neonatal candidiasis among extremely low birth-weight infants: risk factors, mortality rates, and neurodevelopmental outcomes at 18 to 22 months. Pediatrics. 2006;117:84–92.
3. Basu S, Kumar R, Tilak R, Kumar A. Candida blood stream infection in neonates: experience from a Tertiary Care Teaching Hospital of Central India. Indian Pediatr. 2017;54(7):556–9.
4. Jajoo M, Manchanda V, Chaurasia S, Sankar MJ, Gautam H, Agarwal R, et al. Investigators of the Delhi Neonatal Infection Study (DeNIS) Collaboration, New Delhi, India. Alarming rates of antimicrobial resistance and fungal sepsis in outborn neonates in North India. PLoS One. 2018;13(6):e0180705.
5. Ariff S, Saleem AF, Soofi SB, Sajjad R. Clinical spectrum and outcomes of neonatal candidiasis in a tertiary care hospital in Karachi, Pakistan. J Infect Dev Ctries. 2011;5:216–23.
6. Chakrabarti A, Singh K, Narang A, Singhi S, Batra R, Rao KL, et al. Outbreak of Pichia anomala infection in the pediatric service of a tertiary-care center in Northern India. J Clin Microbiol. 2001;39:1702–6.
7. Patra S, Vij M, Chirla DK, Kumar N, Samal SC. Unsuspected invasive neonatal gastrointestinal mucormycosis: a clinicopathological study of six cases from a tertiary care hospital. J Indian Assoc Pediatr Surg. 2012;17:153–6.
8. Kaur H, Ghosh A, Rudramurthy SM, Chakrabarti A. Gastrointestinal mucormycosis in apparently immunocompetent hosts—a review. Mycoses. 2018;61(12):898–908.

9. Castagnola E, Buratti S. Clinical aspects of invasive candidiasis in paediatric patients. Drugs. 2009;69(Suppl 1):45–50.
10. Manzoni P, Mostert M, Galletto P, et al. Is thrombocytopenia suggestive of organism-specific response in neonatal sepsis? Pediatr Int. 2009;51:206–10.
11. Pappas PG, Kauffman CA, Andes DR, Clancy CJ, Marr KA, Ostrosky-Zeichner L, et al. Clinical practice guideline for the management of candidiasis: 2016 update by the Infectious Diseases Society of America. Clin Infect Dis. 2016;62(4):409–17.
12. Kaufman DA. Challenging issues in neonatal candidiasis. Curr Med Res Opin. 2010;26:1769–78.
13. Ericson JE, Kaufman DA, Kicklighter SD, Bhatia J, Testoni D, Gao J, et al. Fluconazole Prophylaxis Study Team on behalf of the Best Pharmaceuticals for Children Act–Pediatric Trials Network Steering Committee; Fluconazole Prophylaxis Study Team on behalf of the Best Pharmaceuticals for Children Act–Pediatric Trials Network Steering Committee. Fluconazole prophylaxis for the prevention of candidiasis in premature infants: a meta-analysis using patient-level data. Clin Infect Dis. 2016;63:604–10.
14. Richards MJ, Edwards JR, Culver DH, Gaynes RP. Nosocomial infections in pediatric intensive care units in the United States. National Nosocomial Infections Surveillance System. Pediatrics. 1999;103(4):e39.
15. Zaoutis TE, Prasad PA, Localio AR, Coffin SE, Bell LM, Walsh TJ, Gross R. Risk factors and predictors for candidemia in pediatric intensive care unit patients: implications for prevention. Clin Infect Dis. 2010;51:e38–45.
16. Singhi S, Rao DS, Chakrabarti A. Candida colonization and candidemia in a pediatric intensive care unit. Pediatr Crit Care Med. 2008;9:91–5.
17. Chakrabarti A, Sood P, Rudramurthy SM, Chen S, Kaur H, Capoor M, et al. Incidence, characteristics and outcome of ICU-acquired candidemia in India. Intensive Care Med. 2015;41:285–95.
18. Calitri C, Caviglia I, Cangemi G, Furfaro E, Bandettini R, Fioredda F, et al. Performance of 1,3-β-D-glucan for diagnosing invasive fungal diseases in children. Mycoses. 2017;60:789–95.
19. Eggimann P, Bille J, Marchetti O. Diagnosis of invasive candidiasis in the ICU. Ann Intensive Care. 2011;1(1):37.
20. Kumar S, Bansal A, Chakrabarti A, Singhi S. Evaluation of efficacy of probiotics in prevention of candida colonization in a PICU—a randomized controlled trial. Crit Care Med. 2013;41:565–72.
21. Romanio MR, Coraine LA, Maielo VP, Abramczyc ML, Souza RL, Oliveira NF. Saccharomyces cerevisiae fungemia in a pediatric patient after treatment with probiotics. Rev Paul Pediatr. 2017;35(3):361–4.
22. Groll AH, Castagnola E, Cesaro S, Dalle JH, Engelhard D, Hope W, et al. Fourth European Conference on Infections in Leukaemia (ECIL-4): guidelines for diagnosis, prevention, and treatment of invasive fungal diseases in paediatric patients with cancer or allogeneic haemopoietic stem-cell transplantation. Lancet Oncol. 2014;15:e327–40.
23. Kumar J, Singh A, Seth R, Xess I, Jana M, Kabra SK. Prevalence and predictors of invasive fungal infections in children with persistent febrile neutropenia treated for acute leukemia—a prospective study. Indian J Pediatr. 2018;85:1090–5. https://doi.org/10.1007/s12098-018-2722-0.
24. Lin GL, Chang HH, Lu CY, Chen CM, Lu MY, Lee PI, et al. Clinical characteristics and outcome of invasive fungal infections in pediatric acute myeloid leukemia patients in a medical center in Taiwan. J Microbiol Immunol Infect. 2018;51:251–9.
25. De Pauw B, Walsh TJ, Donnelly JP, Stevens DA, Edwards JE, Calandra T, et al. European Organization for Research and Treatment of Cancer/Invasive Fungal Infections Cooperative Group; National Institute of Allergy and Infectious Diseases Mycoses Study Group (EORTC/MSG) Consensus Group. Revised definitions of invasive fungal disease from the European Organization for Research and Treatment of Cancer/Invasive Fungal Infections Cooperative Group and the National Institute of Allergy and Infectious Diseases Mycoses Study Group (EORTC/MSG) Consensus Group. Clin Infect Dis. 2008;46:1813–21.

26. Dvorak CC, Fisher BT, Sung L, Steinbach WJ, Nieder M, Alexander S, Zaoutis TE. Antifungal prophylaxis in pediatric hematology/oncology: new choices & new data. Pediatr Blood Cancer. 2012;59:21–6.
27. Tomblyn M, Chiller T, Einsele H, Gress R, Sepkowitz K, Storek J, et al. Guidelines for preventing infectious complications among hematopoietic cell transplantation recipients: a global perspective. Biol Blood Marrow Transplant. 2009;15:1143–238.
28. Mandhaniya S, Swaroop C, Thulkar S, Vishnubhatla S, Kabra SK, Xess I, Bakhshi S. Oral voriconazole versus intravenous low dose amphotericin B for primary antifungal prophylaxis in pediatric acute leukemia induction: a prospective, randomized, clinical study. J Pediatr Hematol Oncol. 2011;33:e333–41.
29. Antachopoulos C. Invasive fungal infections in congenital immunodeficiencies. Clin Microbiol Infect. 2010;16:1335–42.
30. Siberry GK, Abzug MJ, Nachman S. Panel on Prevention and Treatment of Opportunistic Infections in HIV-Exposed and HIV-Infected Children. Executive summary: 2013 update of the guidelines for the prevention and treatment of opportunistic infections in HIV-exposed and HIV-infected children. Pediatr Infect Dis J. 2013;32:1303–7.

8 Mycoses in Transplant

Subramanian Swaminathan

8.1 Fungal Infections in Solid Organ Transplant

- Invasive candidiasis is most common IFI in SOT
- Aspergillosis risk is elevated in liver and lung recipients
- The commonest manifestation seen in intra-abdominal transplant is candidemia and intra-abdominal fungal infection
- *C. albicans* still commonest species
- Most common risk factors for invasive candidiasis are re-transplant, post-transplant dialysis, antibiotic prophylaxis, advanced underlying organ dysfunction, CMV viremia and bacteraemia in liver recipients
- Renal transplant carries the lowest risk for IFI
- Heart transplant risk of IFI is less understood, with *Candida* being more common

Invasive fungal infection (IFI) is an important cause of morbidity and mortality in patients undergoing solid organ transplant. Better understanding of the risk factors, clinical presentation and management have resulted in better outcomes. Based on the largest collaborative consortium, the risk of IFI was noted to range from 1.3% in renal recipients to 11.6% in small bowel recipients. Overall, invasive candidiasis was the most common (53%), followed by invasive aspergillosis (19%), cryptococcosis and non-*Aspergillus* mould infections (9% each), endemic mycoses (5%) and mucormycosis (2%) [1].

Invasive candidiasis is the commonest IFI in solid organ recipients (except heart and lung transplant recipients—it is invasive Aspergillosis). Candidemia and intra-abdominal fungal infections are the commonest manifestation [2]. It is most commonly seen in intra-abdominal transplants and occurs within 3 months post-transplant. The commonest species was *C.albicans* in that cohort of patients.

S. Swaminathan (✉)
Gleneagles Global Hospitals, Chennai, India

Gleneagles Global Hospitals, Bengaluru, India

A. Chakrabarti (ed.), *Clinical Practice of Medical Mycology in Asia*,
https://doi.org/10.1007/978-981-13-9459-1_8

The risk factors have been extensively studied in liver transplant recipients. Earlier data [3] suggested that operative time and use of blood products were important risk factors; subsequent studies have confirmed that those factors are no longer important [4]. The most important risk factors for invasive candidiasis are re-transplantation, post-transplant dialysis and use of antibiotic prophylaxis for prevention of bacterial peritonitis. This shift in the importance of risk factors is more likely due to better surgical procedures and intervention—shorter surgical time, shorter cold ischaemia time and more judicious use of blood products. Recent studies have identified few additional risk factors including patients with more advanced underlying organ dysfunction, cytomegalovirus (CMV) and bacterial infections [5].

Renal transplant recipients are considered to have the lowest risk for IFI—according to the TRANSNET data, only 1.3% patients develop IFI [2], in contrast to earlier studies which had shown up to 45% of renal recipients developing IFI [6]. The usual risk factors identified are aged population, underlying diabetes, pre-transplant dialysis, CMV disease, allograft dysfunction and treatment of rejection.

The risk factors for IFI in heart transplant recipients are less well understood. Studies have shown that nearly half the infections are due to *Candida* though mould and Cryptococcus infections are also important concerns [2]. More recent data suggests a cumulative incidence of IFI at 10.7% [7]. Infection with vancomycin resistant *Enterococcus*, rejection and use of thymoglobulin and renal replacement therapy are noted as risk factors. Post-transplant ECMO use is also noted to be an important risk factor [8].

Lung transplant recipients are at elevated risk for IFI. The risk is more for *Aspergillus* and mould infections as compared to invasive candidiasis [2]. The risk factors include mould colonization of the respiratory tract, graft dysfunction, rejection and CMV disease.

8.2 Epidemiology

- The risk of IFI seems to be significantly higher in the developing world as compared to the Western data. There is also concern for earlier onset disease. The incidence rates are almost similar to the Western data 15–20 years back, suggesting a learning curve. Many factors that were identified as risk are no longer a concern, as they have been eliminated by better practices like reduction in blood use and shortening of operative time.
- Outcomes also seem to be poorer in developing countries. This could be due to a combination of more dangerous infection, delayed identification, resource restriction, and patients with more morbidity.
- The fungal risk and the epidemiology appear to be related to the understanding and the use of appropriate risk reduction strategies. As a result, higher resource countries or centres with greater experience have a lower incidence overall, and the risk is more for *Candida* than for moulds.

- There is a changing epidemiology in terms of pathogens identified and possibly emergence of drug resistance, which could be a greater challenge in the future.
- With greater transplant tourism in developing countries, awareness of the epidemiology of the host country is imperative in optimizing empiric care of illness in a returning recipient.

The epidemiology of fungal infections in developing nations seems to be significantly different. For example, as compared to developed countries, some studies have shown more mould infection compared to invasive candidiasis, and a significantly lower risk for Cryptococcosis [9, 10].

Data from the developing world is relatively sparse with respect to thoracic transplantation related IFI. One publication from Brazil on heart recipients noted mucocutaneous candidiasis early after transplant; *Aspergillus* and *Pneumocystis* infections were recorded in the later period [11]. With respect to lung transplant, data is available only from Brazil, and they have noted invasive aspergillosis as a major concern [12].

The data in renal transplant recipients is quite robust and shows a significant heterogeneity based on region of origin. Australian data from Sydney shows IFI in 2.1% of their renal recipients, with 50% of them being due to *Cryptococcus*; no invasive candidiasis was reported, and the median time to infection was 33 months post-transplant [13]. An older study from India analysing 1476 renal transplant recipients noted 110 IFI in 98 patients—*Aspergillus, Cryptococcus* and *Candida* constituted 61% of the pathogens. CMV infection, diabetes, tuberculosis and liver disease were noted as risk factors, and the factors impacted survival significantly [14]. Another study from India on 1900 renal transplant recipients showed incidence of IFI in 30 (1.56%) patients, about 13 months after transplant; aspergillosis in 13, invasive candidiasis in 16 and mucormycosis in 1 patient. Diabetes, CMV infection, organ rejection, use of broad-spectrum antibiotics and triple immune suppression were noted as risk factors [10]. In a recent publication, subcutaneous phaeohypomycosis is reported in 7 of 84 renal transplant recipients within a year of transplant [15]. The transplant experience has also uncovered rare infection like blastomycosis in a renal transplant recipient from India and Tunisia [16, 17]. The importance of regional epidemiology was highlighted in a single centre study from Brazil, which showed IFI in 4.6% of their renal transplant recipients; the majority (36.3%) was cryptococcosis; histoplasmosis and invasive candidiasis were next important IFIs [18]. Data from Africa is relatively limited; one study from Tunisia has shown IFI risk at 3.4%, which included pneumocystosis, aspergillosis, candidiasis, cryptococcosis and mucormycosis. Majority of IFIs occurred more than 3 months after transplant [19]. With transplant tourism becoming more common in Asian countries, it is important that centres be aware of regional epidemiology and management of IFIs in transplant recipients. Experience from Oman revealed no IFI in the 36 patients who were transplanted within the country, but 13 of 142 patients developed IFIs limited to graft kidney who went to Pakistan for renal transplantation—9 patients developed aspergillosis, 3 mucormycosis and 1 *Paecilomyces* infection [20]; 3 patients died, and 7 returned to dialysis; the graft was salvageable with some loss of function in 3 others. A similar experience has been published by a Turkish group who reported a significant number of IFI in renal recipients who underwent the procedure at Russia or India, with Aspergillus fumigatus being the most common pathogen [21].

With regard to liver transplants, more data are evolving in recent years from many parts of the world. The importance of IFI in this population has been better characterized. In fact, in a study from Uruguay, IFI remained an important predictor of mortality in their population, although the rates of IFIs are comparable to global standards—invasive candidiasis at 3.6% and aspergillosis at <1% [22]. A 6-year data analysis from a single centre at Brazil showed 40 IFI cases in 596 liver transplants among 540 patients; 67% invasive candidiasis and majority due to non-albicans *Candida* species, and 17% aspergillosis [23]. A recent publication analysing 64 liver transplant recipients from India showed candidiasis as the only IFI in 7 patients, with *C.albicans* and *C.tropicalis* as common etiological agents [24]. In fact, this changing epidemiology has also been coupled with rising antifungal drug resistance in those isolates. In a recent multi-centre study assessing 42 patients with invasive candidiasis in post-liver transplant recipients, *C.albicans* was found to be the most common agent, and azole resistance rate rose to 16.7% and caspofungin resistance at 4.8% [25]. Data from a Chinese group indicates a high rate of IFI in liver transplant recipients—13.5% with 70.8% case fatality, mostly due to *C.albicans*. The risk factors noted were TPN use, high blood sugars, long-term mechanical ventilation and antibiotic use [26]. Another group from China has also reported IFI rate at 15.9% among 232 liver transplant recipients, all within 5 weeks of transplant—23 due to *Candida* species and 12 due to *Aspergillus* species [27]. One Japanese centre reported IFI at 12.2% of 156 patients; the majority was due to *Candida* species, with a few cases due to *Pneumocystis* and *Aspergillus* species [28].

8.3 Reported Studies on IFI In Renal Transplant Recipients

Study	TRANSNET [1]	Australia [13]	India [10]	Brazil [18]	Tunisia [19]	Iran [9]	Kuwait [29]
IFI rate	1.3%	2.1%	1.56%	4.6%	3.4%	0.87%	3.5%
Causative agent as per frequency	Candida	Cryptococcus	Candida	Crypto	Pneumocystis	Mucor	Candida
	Crypto	Aspergillus	Aspergillus	Histoplasma	Candida Aspergillus Crypto	Candida	Aspergillus
	Aspergillus	Pseudallescheria	Mucor	Candida		Aspergillus	Crypto
	Endemic fungi	Mucor				Histo	Zygo
	Other mould				Mucor		
	Pneumocystis						

8.4 Reported Studies on IFI in Liver Transplant Recipients

Study	TRANSNET (!)	Uruguay [22]	Brazil [23]	India [24]	China [27]	Japan [28]	Japan [30]
IFI rate	4.7%		7%	11%	15.9%	12.2%	5.4%
Causative agent as per frequency	Candida	Candida	Candida	Candida	Candida	Candida	Aspergillus
	Aspergillus	Aspergil-lus	Aspergillus		Aspergillus	Pneu-mocystis	Candida
	Crypto		Crypto Histo Fusarium			Asper-gillus	
	Endemic						
	Mould						
	Pneumocystis						

From these studies, it is possible to make the following conclusions.

8.5 Presentation of IFI in Solid Organ Transplant

- Biphasic onset
  - Early onset (graft site/surgical site infection, lung)
    Preexistent disease
    Donor derived
  - Late onset

As noted earlier, there is an early onset of disease, possibly reflecting unrecognized preexistent disease or early exposure to pathogens, or a donor derived transmission in developing countries. Unlike Western literature, the unique aspects of IFI in developing countries include the increased risk of infection at graft site or at the surgical site. This could indicate a donor-derived infection, contamination at the time of preservation and transport, and poor infection control measures. Both *Candida* and mould infections are noted in this setting. Other than above two sites, lung is commonly infected organ, and this tends to be more due to mould infection. Late presentation may be by endemic mycoses, which may present only with fever. The other situation with late presentation in the developing world appears to be the cutaneous presentation with dematiaceous fungi.

Given the biphasic onset of disease, the typical "vulnerable" patient is of two types. The patients who develop early disease are usually have advanced disease (usually liver, and acute liver failure being very high risk), requiring a long and complex surgery, with significant blood product need, renal dysfunction requiring dialysis and poor graft function. The patients who develop late disease usually are older hosts who have poor graft function, recent increase in immune suppression in response to rejection and CMV disease. It should be noted that not all recipients who develop late onset fungal infection have any of the risk factors noted above, suggesting the possibility of exposures and environmental influences.

8.6 Evaluation of Patient with Possible IFI

- Pulmonary (most common presentation)
  - Aspergillus most common
  - Pneumocystis incidence is decreased due to cotrimoxazole prophylaxis
  - Do radiological assessment, bronchoscopy, biopsy and galactomannan assay as needed
- CNS
  - Presents as meningitis and space occupying lesion
  - Candida presents as multiple small abscess
  - Consider radiological assessment, culture and histopathology, Cryptococcus antigen assay, urine histoplasma antigen
- Cutaneous
  - Consider Cryptococcus as a cause of necrotizing fasciitis
  - Mucor mycosis with IV catheter injury/infection
  - Do biopsy
- Sepsis
  - Candidemia most common
  - Consider blood culture, BD glucan and Cryptococcus antigen assay

The approach to evaluation is syndromic.

Pulmonary infection: The most common presentation is of a pulmonary syndrome. The presentation is usually an illness over a few weeks with variable symptoms which could include cough, fever, breathing difficulty and haemoptysis. In one retrospective study assessing the role of bronchoscopy, 73 patients with pulmonary infections in SOT recipients were noted; 6 cases of invasive candidiasis and 4 of aspergillosis were identified [31]. In another prospective study of 54 pulmonary infections in SOT recipients, 6.4% of them had IFI, with *Aspergillus* as commonest agent [32]. As can be seen in the studies discussed earlier, the importance of PJP has reduced possibly due to the widespread use of prophylaxis. In fact, it is more often seen as a late infection at present.

The management approach in this situation should start with a radiological assessment to suspect fungal disease. Diffuse lung disease is better approached by bronchoscopic route—especially if PJP is considered; nodular masses are best biopsied under imaging guidance. For nodular masses, bronchoscopic assessment may be of limited value, except for galactomannan estimation—the causative organism may not be seen on cultures. Serological testing by galactomannan has a sensitivity of 22% and specificity of 84% in this population [33]. The consideration for nodular lesions should include Aspergillosis, other mould infections, endemic mycoses and Cryptococcosis.

Central nervous system infections: This carries a significant morbidity and mortality in the transplant setting. Neurological complications after transplant are commonly seen in 30–60% of SOT transplant recipients [34]. The presentations are of a meningitis due to cryptococcosis, a focal mass lesion due to haematogenous spread of moulds, or direct extension to base of brain and frontal lobe from sinus mould infection.

Fungal meningitis usually presents as a subacute or chronic illness with evolving headache and mental status change. The most common fungal cause is *Cryptococcus*; endemic/dimorphic fungi like *Histoplasma* could also present as meningitis.

Focal mass lesion/abscess is usually due to bacterial infection. Fungal infections tend to cause larger single masses. Although *Aspergillus* is the most common cause; *Mucorales*, dimorphic fungi and dermataceous fungi also need to be considered. *Candida* produces multiple small abscesses [23].

Sinus disease extending to the brain is usually due to mucormycosis [35]; other agents like *Aspergillus, Fusarium* and *Scedosporium* should also be considered. The role of uncontrolled diabetes, renal failure and prior voriconazole use as risk factors is well established.

Skin manifestations of fungal infections: Superficial fungal infections are more likely to be found in this population in view of the immune suppression and steroid use, but the approach to management is no different from a normal host. Cutaneous fungal infections may present as localized skin disease, which could disseminate. Cutaneous cryptococcosis may present as a variety of lesions including necrotizing fasciitis [36]. Cutaneous aspergillosis and mucormycosis results from trivial trauma like infected intravenous catheters. Lesions start as papules and can evolve into an eschar. Rarely, this route of inoculation can cause infection with dematiaceous or pigmented fungi.

Cutaneous skin infection could be a marker- forget window infection like cryptococcosis. Patients with cryptococcal meningitis may present with umbilicated skin lesion, hence biopsy from skin lesion showing *Cryptococcus* warrants evaluation for dissemination.

Sometimes IFI can present as a sepsis syndrome, and the most common cause being *Candida*. This is most common in patients with intra-abdominal transplants. This is often noted in the setting of an ICU patient who is on parenteral nutrition, graft dysfunction, requiring re-exploration, after CMV disease, and with renal dysfunction requiring dialysis. Blood culture is ideal, and beta-D glucan as a biomarker may be used.

Among the non-Candida yeast that can be isolated from blood culture, *Cryptococcus* and *Histoplasma* are important; others like *Trichosporon* species are emerging as important pathogens [37]. Though yeast like organisms are the fungi most commonly seen in blood culture, moulds such as *Fusarium* and *Scedosporium* could also be isolated from blood in disseminated infections.

8.7 Diagnosis of IFI

- High index of suspicion is required
- Cultures from sterile sites are diagnostic
- Isolation of fungus should trigger systemic search
- Biomarker BD glucan and galactomannan can be used
- Newer technology gene sequencing and MALDI improve identification

The diagnosis starts with a high index of suspicion of disease. Early identification is key to initiate appropriate therapy and better outcomes. The presence of fungus at non-sterile sites is not diagnostic of IFI, but increases the likelihood of the same. All isolation of fungus should trigger a systematic search for the possibility of an IFI.

The use of cultures is ideal for diagnosis *of Candida* infections, and speciation is required to identify the agent and optimize therapy. However, with the emergence of drug resistance, in vitro antifungal susceptibility testing may also be mandatory.

The use of cryptococcal antigen assay has made the approach to diagnosis of cryptococcosis easier and quicker. Cultures from sterile sites are diagnostic.

Non-*Candida* yeast infections are sometimes seen in this population, and some of it may be the effect of local epidemiology.

Dimorphic fungi represent an ever-present threat—as reactivational disease, as donor-derived infection or as new acquisition. Diagnosis is made by cultures from sterile sites. In the case of *Histoplasma*, the availability of urine antigen could help.

Early diagnosis of mould infections represents a significant challenge. Early diagnosis of mould infections represents a significant challenge, as this often presents as deep infections in the most debilitated recipient. There may be reluctance in doing a full workup which includes imaging and invasive procedures like biopsy and then may lead to unnecessary empirical therapy. Histopathology is essential for diagnosis and cultures for speciation. The newer technologies like gene sequencing and MALDI improve identification. The rise of drug resistance appears to be concern, and this is based on local epidemiology; the lack of standardized testing techniques makes this a significant challenge. The use of galactomannan estimation for pulmonary aspergillosis is best validated for broncho-alveolar lavage (BAL) samples in lung transplant recipients, and using a cut-off of 1.5 could reduce false positivity [38], but there is inadequate data in other solid organ transplants. A lateral flow device appears to show promise for diagnosis of aspergillosis in one study [39].

8.8 Treatment of IFI

- Candidemia, preferred drug is echinocandins
- Mould infection
  - Surgical resection
  - Amphotericin B (liposomal preferred)
- Aspergillus
  - Voriconazole
  - Posaconazole if vori is not tolerated
- Check for drug interactions
- Duration of therapy depends on clinical response, radiological clearance and improvement of biomarker
- PET scan can help assess activity of IFI

Both empiric and targeted therapy of IFI are no different from normal hosts but are more challenging in view of the drug interactions.

For treatment of candidemia, echinocandins are preferred. Although all of them are equally effective, caspofungin has significant interactions with the immune suppressive drugs, which need attention. Caspofungin may also need dose adjustment in patients with significant liver dysfunction. Micafungin and anidulafungin have the advantage of ease of use.

Treatment of mould infections remains a challenge. Surgical resection remains cornerstone of therapy. Empiric therapy is usually with amphotericin B, preferably with a liposomal preparation in view of its tolerability. Patients intolerant to amphotericin B may be switched to posaconazole.

Definitive therapy depends on the identification of the pathogen. Voriconazole is the preferred agent for aspergillosis, but the interactions with the agents of immune suppression can be challenging. Posaconazole is an alternative in such patients. For other moulds like Mucorales, amphotericin B remains the agent of choice. The role of isavuconazole in this population remains to be determined.

The duration of therapy is difficult to determine in such patients. A combination of clinical response, radiological clearance and stability with possible improvement in biomarkers is often considered before stopping therapy. Increasingly, PET scan is being used to assess activity of fungal infections [40]. However, given the continued immune suppression, these patients will need continued long-term monitoring.

8.9 Prophylaxis Against IFI

- Renal transplant recipient does not require prophylaxis
- Prophylaxis for liver transplant recipients is based on risk factors; fluconazole for candidiasis, liposomal amphotericin B for mould infection risk. Echinocandin is an alternative
- Posaconazole not used due to drug interaction with immunosuppression
- Lung transplant use of nebulized amphotericin B lipid formulation is favoured
- Use of voriconazole is a challenge due to drug interaction

Transplant organ	Agent	Duration
Kidney	None	
Liver	None in low risk Fluconazole in intermediate risk Liposomal amphotericin B or echinocandin in high risk	2–4 weeks
Lung	Oral voriconazole and/or inhaled amphotericin B	3–12 months
Heart	Itraconazole/voriconazole in high risk	2–6 months

Kidney transplant recipients do not require prophylaxis routinely.

Most liver transplant recipients do not require prophylaxis. However, those with additional risk factors benefit from prophylaxis. The approach is often tiered, based on whether the risk is for invasive candidiasis or mould infection. For those with only risk of candidiasis, fluconazole is considered appropriate, although the rising risk of fluconazole resistance represents a challenge. In those with risk of mould infection, the use of liposomal amphotericin B or echinocandin could be considered. The choice has to be based on the local epidemiology. Caspofungin has the least published data in this area. A study with micafungin did not show a benefit, probably because the recipients had much less severe liver disease [41]. Anidulafungin showed a trend towards benefit in this situation, and was superior in those exposed to fluconazole pre-transplant [42]. Liposomal amphotericin B would be considered appropriate in centres with non-*Aspergillus* mould infection and may even be administered as a once weekly option, but the concern of renal toxicity remains a concern [43]. The newer azoles like posaconazole have not been tried in this situation due to the significant interaction with the agents of immunosuppression.

Patients undergoing lung transplant are at highest risk of invasive fungal infection, and the relative importance of mould infection is highest in this population. There is very little trial data in this setting, but the consensus favours the use of nebulized amphotericin B, especially lipid formulations to prevent IFI [44]. Oral voriconazole has replaced itraconazole as the oral agent of choice but its use is a challenge in view of the drug interactions and significant toxicity from long-term use.

The role of prophylaxis in heart transplant is less well understood. Inhaled amphotericin B is an option, in view of the risk of mould infection [45].

8.10 Fungal Infections in Stem Cell Transplant (SCT)

- IFI in SCT depends on type of transplant, indication of transplant, regimen used, neutropenia duration and GVHD
- Low platelet makes diagnosis through biopsy difficult
- Aspergillosis and candidiasis are leading fungal infections

The risk of IFI is significantly higher in the stem cell transplant recipients than the solid organ recipients. The risk is determined by multiple factors, including the type of transplant, the underlying indication for transplant, regimen used, the duration of neutropenia, incidence and severity of graft-versus-host disease (GVHD), among others. There is considerable difference in the worldwide epidemiology of the IFI that occur in this population, and the distinction is difficult to quantify in view of the limited workup of such patients in developing countries. In general, the workup of patients with suspected IFI is very challenging given the low platelet count which makes biopsy near impossible. In addition, the limited availability of biomarkers like galactomannan forces the clinician to empiricism. Finally, the poor outcome even with aggressive case management discourages attempts at a definitive diagnosis when the financial burden can be a major challenge.

Country	Japan [46]	China [47]	China [48]	Taiwan [49]	India [50]
Prophylaxis	Fluconazole/ micafungin	Fluconazole	Fluconazole	Fluconazole/ micafungin	Fluconazole
Incidence	10.2%	13.4%	22.5%	7.4%	15.9%
Organisms	Aspergillus	Aspergillus	Candida	Candida	Aspergillus
	Trichosporon	Mucorales	Aspergillus	Aspergillus	Candida
		Candida			Mucorales
Mortality	86%	75.6%	58.9%	35.1%	

The risk of IFI in the developed world is primarily accounted for by *Aspergillus* and *Candida*. Based on autopsy study, the identification of IFI has not changed much but the relative importance of mould, primarily *Aspergillus*, has risen at the cost of reduction in *Candida* infection [51]. Recent data have shown a drop in the incidence of aspergillosis in autopsy studies, possibly due to use of mould active prophylaxis. It is interesting to note that infections apart from *Candida* and *Aspergillus* were quite rare [52]. Based on the TRANSNET data, the rate of IFI was between 5.8 and 8.1% [53], depending on the match. Aspergillosis and candidiasis were the leading infections and mucormycosis accounted for 8% only. The mortality for fusariosis was more than 90%; for the others, it was about 65–75%.

In comparison, studies from Asia have shown a much higher incidence of fungal infection. This is in spite of the data being from more recent cohorts, and with appropriate prophylaxis. The other striking feature was the different epidemiology, with more candidiasis in some cohorts, and a relative higher incidence of mucormycosis, as has been noted in renal transplant recipients. The relative lack of data from many countries makes interpretation and generalizations difficult. Overall it appears that the mortality is comparable to the West when adjusted for epidemiology.

8.11 Presentation of IFI in HSCT

- Fluconazole prophylaxis resulted in reduction of *Candida* infection with increase in azole resistant *Candida*
- Candidiasis presents as candidemia and hepatosplenic candidiasis
- Mucositis and IVC increases risk of candidemia
- Seeds to eye, skin or viscera as abscess
- Mould infection occurs via inhalation, invasion through skin breaks and GIT
- It involves sinus or lung and disseminates to organ like brain and skin

Candida was a major pathogen in the pre-prophylaxis era, being associated with significant mortality. With the widespread use of fluconazole prophylaxis, there is a reduction in overall incidence, but with a relative increase in azole resistant *Candida* species [54].

Invasive candidiasis presents in two ways—as Candidemia or as a tissue disease, as in hepatosplenic candidiasis.

Candidemia usually starts from the gastrointestinal tract due to mucositis or from intravenous catheters. Patients present as a sepsis syndrome, and can have seeding of other locations like the eye, skin or viscera as abscesses.

Hepatosplenic candidiasis starts from the gastrointestinal tract and spread to the liver and spleen by the portal system. Although this occurs during the neutropenic phase, it becomes evident only during engraftment. The patients present with fever, pain and elevated liver enzymes.

Mould infections usually present as respiratory disease, involving the sinus or the lung. Following tissue invasion, dissemination can occur to other organs, with preference to the brain and skin. Invasion through skin breaks and the gastrointestinal tract have also been documented.

8.12 Diagnosis of IFI

- Candidemia
  - Blood culture gold standard
  - Repeat culture until clearance
  - Eye exam after neutrophil engrafted
  - BD glucan pan-fungal biomarker. High false positive
- Hepatosplenic candidiasis
  - Imaging
  - Biopsy
- Moulds
  - Radiologically presents as cavitary nodule with halo sign, infiltrate, tracheobronchitis and bronchopneumonia
  - Engraftment changes radiological picture
- Galactomannan assay in BAL for invasive aspergillosis

The gold standard for diagnosis of candidemia is a blood culture. This is required for diagnosis, speciation and susceptibility testing. Follow-up cultures are also required for documentation of clearance. Furthermore, a dilated eye examination should be performed after the return of neutrophils to exclude eye involvement [55]. Beta-D glucan testing is an alternative to culture methods but suffers from a high false positivity rate in less than optimum laboratory services of developing countries. Since beta-D glucan test is pan-fungal biomarker, the identification of fungal pathogen may be difficult in absence of culture. Hepatosplenic candidiasis requires clinical suspicion, and imaging can show lesions which may even be necrotic. Biopsy may show granulomatous disease as well, but the organism may not be apparent.

Identification of mould infection requires a high degree of suspicion, and the use of radiology for early diagnosis. Although the typical presentation is of a cavitating nodular lesion with a halo sign, mould infection can present in many different radiological forms. The other well recognized forms include lobar infiltrates, tracheobronchitis and bronchopneumonia. The return of neutrophils usually changes the radiological picture significantly. The yield of aetiological agent by BAL culture may be poor, but the use of the galactomannan test has revolutionized the ability to diagnose invasive aspergillosis.

8.13 Treatment of IFI

- Candidemia
  - Echinocandin drug of choice
  - Line removal decision advisable though can be deferred
  - Treat till 14 days after negative culture
  - Eye examination once neutrophils engrafted
- Moulds
  - Amphotericin B lipid formulation, gold standard initial empiric therapy

- Aspergillus
  - Voriconazole
- Echinocandin considered for salvage therapy
- Combination of voriconazole and echinocandin may help in serious cases

Guidelines recommend the use of echinocandins as the agents of choice for candidemia [55]. The duration is for 14 days after negative cultures; regular blood cultures are required for documentation. Screening for eye involvement needs to be delayed till the return of neutrophils. Although it is advisable to remove lines, this may be difficult in neutropenic hosts, and with the increased activity of echinocandins in biofilms, it may be possible to defer this decision [56].

Amphotericin B, especially its lipid formulations, has been the gold standard in the initial empiric therapy of mould infections. Voriconazole has been accepted as the best therapy for proven aspergillosis following a large head to head trial [57]. Echinocandins also have activity and are considered for salvage in treatment for those intolerant to other options. A more recent trial has suggested the superiority of combination therapy of voriconazole with anidulafungin in aspergillosis when probable group is included in comparison [58].

Treatment of other infections like mucormycosis is less well studied. Liposomal amphotericin B remains the agent of choice for treatment. The availability of newer options like posaconazole and isavuconazole is likely to influence these decisions in the future.

The role of surgery, the use of immune modulators, and iron chelators is unclear, as is the required duration of treatment in such situations.

8.14 Prophylaxis Against IFI

- Fluconazole used as standard of care
- Posaconazole
  - AML undergoing induction therapy
  - GVHD in post-allogenic transplant
- Echinocandin popularly used due to less toxicity and activity against invasive aspergillosis
- Amphotericin B lipid formulation can be also used as once weekly option

The awareness of the risk of fungal infections has led to numerous studies to assess the role of prophylaxis in this setting. The earliest study demonstrated the efficacy of fluconazole in reducing IFI in this population [59]. This had established fluconazole as standard of care in this population, especially with survival benefit. Subsequent studies with itraconazole have not clearly demonstrated an overall superiority over fluconazole in terms of survival [60].

Since the publication of the landmark trial demonstrating the superiority of posaconazole in prophylaxis against IFI in patients with AML undergoing induction therapy, it has become the standard of care [61]. It is also strongly indicated in patients post-allogenic transplant with graft-versus-host disease (GVHD) [62]. This benefit has subsequently been confirmed by numerous real-life experiences.

Echinocandins have become popular given their relative lack of toxicity, and minimal potential for interactions. Micafungin is the one best studied for this indication, and a major trial showed superiority in comparison with fluconazole [63]. Given its intrinsic activity against *Aspergillus*, there is also trend towards fewer invasive aspergillosis after echinocandin use.

Studies involving amphotericin B, especially its lipid formulations, are fewer in number, and the results seemed encouraging in a study with the use of a higher dose as a once weekly option [64].

Fungal infections represent a dreaded complication after transplant, and the approach is different in different parts of the world. A good understanding of the epidemiology, risk factors, presentation and availability of testing can help better guide a logical and effective approach to prophylaxis and therapy in this setting.

References

1. Pappas PG, Alexander BD, Andes DR, et al. Invasive fungal infections among organ transplant recipients: results of the Transplant-Associated Infection Surveillance Network (TRANSNET). Clin Infect Dis. 2010;50(8):1101–11.
2. Andes DR, Safdar N, Baddley JW, et al. The epidemiology and outcomes of invasive Candida infections among organ transplant recipients in the United States: results of the Transplant-Associated Infection Surveillance Network (TRANSNET). Transpl Infect Dis. 2016;18(6):921–31.
3. Husain S, Tollemar J, Dominguez EA, et al. Changes in the spectrum and risk factors for invasive candidiasis in liver transplant recipients: prospective, multicenter, case-controlled study. Transplantation. 2003;75(12):2023–9.
4. Raghuram A, Restrepo A, Safadjou S, et al. Invasive fungal infections following liver transplantation: incidence, risk factors, survival, and impact of fluconazole resistant Candida parapsilosis (2003-2007). Liver Transpl. 2012;18(9):1100–9.
5. Saliba F, Delvart V, Ichai P, et al. Fungal infections after liver transplantation: outcomes and risk factors revisited in the MELD era. Clin Transpl. 2013;27(4):E454–61.
6. Rifkind D, Marchioro TL, Schneck SA, Hill RB Jr. Systemic fungal infections complicating renal transplantation and immunosuppressive therapy. Clinical, microbiologic, neurologic and pathologic features. Am J Med. 1967;43:28–38.
7. Echenique IA, Angarone MP, Gordon RA, et al. Invasive fungal infection after heart transplantation: a 7-year, single-center experience. Transpl Infect Dis. 2017;19(1).
8. Tissot F, Pascual M, Hullin R, Yerly P, Tozzi P, Meylan P, Manuel O. Impact of targeted antifungal prophylaxis in heart transplant recipients at high risk for early invasive fungal infection. Transplantation. 2014;97(11):1192–7.
9. Einollahi B, Lessan-Pezeshki M, Pourfarziani V, et al. Invasive fungal infections following renal transplantation: a review of 2410 recipients. Ann Transplant. 2008;13:55–8.
10. Patel MH, Patel RD, Vanikar AV, et al. Invasive fungal infections in renal transplant recipients: a single center study. Ren Fail. 2017;39(1):294–8.
11. Mangini S, Alves BR, Silvestre OM, et al. Heart transplantation: review. Einstein (Sao Paulo). 2015;13(2):310–8.
12. Afonso Júnior JE, Werebe Ede C, Carraro RM, et al. Lung transplantation. Einstein (Sao Paulo). 2015;13(2):297–304.

13. Ezzatzedegan S, Chen S, Chapman JR. Invasive fungal infections and renal transplantation. Int J Organ Transplant Med. 2012;3(1):18–25.
14. John GT, Shankar V, Talaulikar G, et al. Epidemiology of systemic mycoses among renal-transplant recipients in India. Transplantation. 2003;75(9):1544–51.
15. Haridasan S, Parameswaran S, Beemanathi SH, et al. Subcutaneous phaeohypomycosis in kidney transplant recipients: a series of seven cases. Tranplant Infect Dis. 2017;19.
16. Patel HV, Kute VB, Vanikar AV, Shah PR, Gumber MR, Trivedi HL. Blastomyces dermatitidis in a renal transplant recipient. Saudi J Kidney Dis Transplant. 2014;25(5):1042–5.
17. Ben Salem M, Hamouda M, Mohamed M, et al. Blastomyces dermatitidis in a renal transplant recipient: a case report. Transplant Proc. 2017;49(7):1583–6.
18. Guimarães LF, Halpern M, de Lemos AS, et al. Invasive fungal infection in renal transplant recipients in a Brazilian center: local epidemiology matters. Transplant Proc. 2016;48(7):2306–9.
19. Trabelsi H, Neji S, Sellami H, et al. Invasive fungal infections in renal transplant recipients: about 11 cases. J Mycol Med. 2013;23(4):255–60.
20. Al Salmi I, Metry AM, Al Ismaili F, et al. Transplant tourism and invasive fungal infection. Int J Infect Dis. 2018;69:120–9.
21. Altiparmak MR, Apavdin S, Trablus S, et al. Systemic fungal infections after renal transplant. Scand J Infect Dis. 2002;34(4):284–8.
22. Olivari D, Mainradi V, Rando K, et al. Risk factors of mortality after liver transplantation in Uruguay. Transplant Proc. 2018;50(2):499–502.
23. Zicker M, Colombo AL, Ferraz-Neto BH, Camargo LF. Epidemiology of fungal infections in liver transplant recipients: a six year study of a large Brazilian liver transplantation center. Mem Inst Oswaldo Cruz. 2011;106(3):339–45.
24. Khillan V, Kale P, Pamecha V, Rathor N, Sarin SK. Infections in liver donor liver transplant recipients: a study of time line, aetiology, and antimicrobial resistance of bacterial and fungal infections from the developing world. Indian J Med Microbiol. 2017;35(4):604–6.
25. Bassetti M, Peghin M, Carnelutti A, et al. Invasive candida infections in liver transplant recipients: clinical features and risk factors for mortality. Transplant Direct. 2017;3(5):e156.
26. Yang CH, He XS, Chen J, et al. Fungal infection in patients after liver transplantation in years 2003 to 2012. Ann Transplant. 2012;17(4):59–63.
27. Shi XJ, Lü SC, He L, et al. Diagnosis and treatment of fungal infection after liver transplantation. Chin Med J. 2011;124(7):1015–7.
28. Ohkubo T, Sugawara Y, Takayama T, Kokudo N, Makuuchi MJ. The risk factors of fungal infection in living-donor liver transplantations. Hepatobiliary Pancreat Sci. 2012;19(4):382–8.
29. Nampoory MR, Khan ZU, Johny KV, et al. Invasive fungal infections in renal transplant recipients. J Infect. 1996;33(2):95–101.
30. Nagao M, Fujimoto Y, Yamamoto M, et al. Epidemiology of invasive fungal infections after liver transplantation and the risk factors of late-onset invasive aspergillosis. J Infect Chemother. 2016;22(2):84–9.
31. Eyüboğlu FÖ, Küpeli E, Bozbaş SS, et al. Evaluation of pulmonary infections in solid organ transplant patients: 12 years of experience. Transplant Proc. 2013;45(10):3458–61.
32. Giannella M, Muñoz P, Alarcon JM, Mularoni A, Grossi P, Bouza E, PISOT study group. Pneumonia in solid organ transplant recipients: a prospective multicenter study. Transpl Infect Dis. 2014;16(2):232–41.
33. Pfeiffer CD, Fine JP, Safdar N. Diagnosis of invasive aspergillosis using a galactomannan assay: a meta-analysis. Clin Infect Dis. 2006;42:1417–27.
34. Zunt JR. Central nervous system infection during immunosuppression. Neurol Clin. 2002;20(1):1–22.
35. Singh N, Aguado JM, Bonatti H, et al. Zygomycosis in solid organ transplant recipients: a prospective, matched case-control study to assess risks for disease and outcome. J Infect Dis. 2009;200:1002–11.
36. Yoneda T, Itami Y, Hirayama A, et al. Cryptococcal necrotizing fasciitis in a patient after renal transplantation—a case report. Transplant Proc. 2014;46:620–2.

37. De Almeida JN, Hennequin C. Invasive Trichosporon infection: a systematic review on a re-emerging fungal pathogen. Front Microbiol. 2016;7:1629.
38. Pasqualotto AC, Xavier MO, Sánchez LB, de Oliveira Costa CD, Schio SM, Camargo SM, Camargo JJ, Sukiennik TC, Severo LC. Diagnosis of invasive aspergillosis in lung transplant recipients by detection of galactomannan in the bronchoalveolar lavage fluid. Transplantation. 2010;90(3):306–11.
39. Miceli MH, Goggins MI, Chander P, Sekaran AK, Kizy AE, Samuel L, Jiang H, Thornton CR, Ramesh M, Alangaden G. Performance of lateral flow device and galactomannan for the detection of Aspergillus species in bronchoalveolar fluid of patients at risk for invasive pulmonary aspergillosis. Mycoses. 2015;58:368–37.
40. Hot A, Maunoury C, Poiree S, et al. Diagnostic contribution of positron emission tomography with [^{18}F]fluorodeoxyglucose for invasive fungal infections. Clin Microbiol Infect. 2011;17:409–17.
41. Saliba F, Pascher A, Cointault O, et al. Randomized trial of micafungin for the prevention of invasive fungal infection in high-risk liver transplant recipients. Clin Infect Dis. 2015;60(7):997–1006.
42. Winston DJ, Limaye AP, Pelletier S, Safdar N, Morris MI, Meneses K, Busuttil RW, Singh N. Randomized, double-blind trial of anidulafungin versus fluconazole for prophylaxis of invasive fungal infections in high-risk liver transplant recipients. Am J Transplant. 2014;14(12):2758–64.
43. Giannella M, Ercolani G, Cristini F, et al. High-dose weekly liposomal amphotericin b antifungal prophylaxis in patients undergoing liver transplantation: a prospective phase II trial. Transplantation. 2015;99(4):848–54.
44. Bhaskaran A, Mumtaz K, Husain S. Anti-Aspergillus prophylaxis in lung transplantation: a systematic review and meta-analysis. Curr Infect Dis Rep. 2013;15:514–25.
45. Husain S, Sole A, Alexander BA, Aslam S, Avery R, Benden C, et al. The 2015 International Society for Heart and Lung Transplantation guidelines for the management of fungal infections in mechanical circulatory support and cardiothoracic organ transplant recipients: executive summary. J Heart Lung Transplant. 2016;35:261–82.
46. Miyakoshi S, Kusumi E, Matsumura T, et al. Invasive fungal infection following reduced-intensity cord blood transplantation for adult patients with hematologic diseases. Biol Blood Marrow Transplant. 2007;13(7):771–7.
47. Sun YQ, Xu LP, Liu DH, et al. The incidence and risk factors of invasive fungal infection after haploidentical haematopoietic stem cell transplantation without in vitro T-cell depletion. Clin Microbiol Infect. 2012;18(10):997–1003.
48. Shi JM, Pei XY, Luo Y, et al. Invasive fungal infection in allogeneic hematopoietic stem cell transplant recipients: single center experiences of 12 years. J Zhejiang Univ Sci B. 2015;16(9):796–804.
49. Liu YC, Chien SH, Fan NW, et al. Incidence and risk factors of probable and proven invasive fungal infection in adult patients receiving allogeneic hematopoietic stem cell transplantation. J Microbiol Immunol Infect. 2016;49(4):567–74.
50. George B, Mathews V, Srivastava A, Chandy M. Infections among allogeneic bone marrow transplant recipients in India. Bone Marrow Transplant. 2004;33:311–5.
51. Chamilos G, Luna M, Lewis RE, et al. Invasive fungal infections in patients with hematologic malignancies in a tertiary care cancer center: an autopsy study over a 15-year period (1989-2003). Haematologica. 2006;91:986–9.
52. Lewis RE, Cahyame-Zuniga L, Leventakos K, et al. Epidemiology and sites of involvement of invasive fungal infections in patients with haematological malignancies: a 20-year autopsy study. Mycoses. 2013;56:638–45.
53. Kontoyiannis DP, Marr KA, Park BJ, et al. Prospective surveillance for invasive fungal infections in hematopoietic stem cell transplant recipients, 2001–2006: overview of the Transplant-Associated Infection Surveillance Network (TRANSNET) database. Clin Infect Dis. 2010;50(8):1091–100.

54. Marr KA, Seidel K, White TC, Bowden RA. Candidemia in allogeneic blood and marrow transplant recipients: evolution of risk factors after the adoption of prophylactic fluconazole. J Infect Dis. 2000;181:309–16.
55. Pappas PG, Kaufman CA, Andes DR, et al. Clinical practice guideline for the management of candidiasis: 2016 update by the Infectious Diseases Society of America. Clin Infect Dis. 2016;62:e1–50.
56. Swaminathan S, Kamat S, Pinto NA. Antifungal agent activity in biofilms. Ind J Med Microbiol. 2018;36(1):87–92.
57. Herbrecht R, Denning DW, Patterson TF, et al. Voriconazole versus amphotericin B for primary therapy of invasive aspergillosis. N Engl J Med. 2002;347:408–15.
58. Marr KA, Schlamm HT, Herbrecht R, et al. Combination antifungal therapy for invasive aspergillosis: a randomized trial. Ann Intern Med. 2015;162(2):81–9.
59. Goodman JL, Winston DJ, Greenfield RA, et al. A controlled trial of fluconazole to prevent fungal infections in patients undergoing bone marrow transplantation. N Engl J Med. 1992;326:845–51.
60. Sharpe MD, Ghent C, Grant D, Horbay GL, McDougal J, David Colby W. Efficacy and safety of itraconazole prophylaxis for fungal infections after orthotopic liver transplantation: a prospective, randomized, double-blind study. Transplantation. 2003;76(6):977–83.
61. Cornely OA, Maertens J, Winston DJ, et al. Posaconazole vs. fluconazole or itraconazole prophylaxis in patients with neutropenia. N Engl J Med. 2007;356:348–59.
62. Ullmann AJ, Lipton JH, Vesole DH, et al. Posaconazole or fluconazole for prophylaxis in severe graft-versus-host disease. N Engl J Med. 2007;356(4):335–47.
63. van Burik JA, Ratanatharathorn V, Stepan DE, et al. National Institute of Allergy and Infectious Diseases Mycoses Study Group. Micafungin versus fluconazole for prophylaxis against invasive fungal infections during neutropenia in patients undergoing hematopoietic stem cell transplantation. Clin Infect Dis. 2004;39:1407–16.
64. El Cheikh J, Castagna L, Wang L, et al. Once-weekly liposomal amphotericin B for prophylaxis of invasive fungal infection after graft-versus-host disease in allogeneic hematopoietic stem cell transplantation: a comparative retrospective single-center study. Hematol Oncol Stem Cell Ther. 2010;3:167–73.

Mycoses in Hematological Malignancies

9

Pankaj Malhotra

Key Points

- The patients with hematological malignancies constitute one of the important risk groups for invasive fungal diseases.
- The prevalence of invasive fungal diseases is higher in acute leukemia than lymphomas and myeloma.
- The highest incidence of fungal infections is seen in acute myeloid leukemia receiving intensive chemotherapy.
- Out of all fungal diseases, mold infections are acquired from the environment, whereas candidiasis is mostly endogenous in origin.
- Once acquired, the invasive fungal diseases are difficult to treat and are important cause of morbidity and mortality.
- Every effort should be made for the prevention of these infections by control of environment (treatment of patients in HEPA filter rooms) and/or use of prophylaxis in an appropriate setting.
- Fortunately we have a variety of antifungal drugs (azoles, echinocandins, and amphotericin) that can be used both as prophylaxis and for treatment in an appropriate clinical setting.

9.1 Introduction

9.1.1 Magnitude of Problem

There has been a rising incidence of invasive fungal diseases (IFD) among patients with hematological malignancies in recent times [1]. The predominant reasons for the increased incidence are related to the use of intensive chemotherapy and highly immunosuppressive

P. Malhotra (✉)
Department of Internal Medicine, Postgraduate Institute of Medical Education and Research (PGIMER), Chandigarh, India

A. Chakrabarti (ed.), *Clinical Practice of Medical Mycology in Asia*,
https://doi.org/10.1007/978-981-13-9459-1_9

medications along with increasing environmental pollution. The fungal infections are also increasingly diagnosed because of increased awareness as well as availability of newer diagnostic techniques [1]. Patients who develop IFD have multiple underlying risk factors and therefore they are also more prone to develop co-infections with bacterial/viral or other fungal pathogens [2] (Table 9.1). This is illustrated by a study looking at concurrent lung infections in patients with hematological malignancies and invasive

Table 9.1 Risk factors for invasive fungal infections in non-transplant hematological disorders

Therapy and hospital care related
Type of chemotherapy
Type of immunosuppressive therapy (specifically T-cell immune suppressants and purine analogues in the past 90 days)
Central venous catheters
Mucositis (chemotherapy or radiotherapy induced)
Multiple cycles of chemotherapy
Corticosteroids (a mean dose of >0.3 mg/kg/day equivalent of prednisone for >3 weeks)
Use of total parenteral nutrition
Prolonged hospitalization[a]
Hyperglycemia (especially plasma glucose >250 mg/dL)[a]
Non-removal of tapes/ECG leads from the patient
Disease related
Prolonged and persistent neutropenia
Neutrophil functional impairment
Lymphopenia
Hypogammaglobulinemia
Hyperglycemia (especially plasma glucose >250 mg/dL)[a]
Hypoalbuminemia (serum albumin <3.0 gm/dL)
Iron overload
Mucositis (chemotherapy or radiotherapy induced)
Past history of treated invasive fungal infection
Disease status (newly diagnosed, in remission, relapsed, refractory)
Type of malignancy
Increasing age
Co-morbidities and organ dysfunction
Fungal colonization
Prolonged hospitalization[a]
Affordability of appropriate antifungal agents
Compliance of antifungal medication
Environment related
Dusty environment (ongoing construction/destruction)
Overall microbial exposure (colonization, environment, prior infection)
Use of contaminated intravenous fluids/sets
Intensive chemotherapy in non-HEPA filter rooms

Some of the factors may be interlinked with each other (high-dose chemotherapy with development of mucositis and neutropenia)

Generally patients who develop IFD have multiple risk factors

[a]Common risk factors

pulmonary aspergillosis, wherein out of 126 patients of invasive aspergillosis (IA), 62 (49%) patients had evidence of dual infections either with bacterial, viral, or another fungal infection [2]. One of the important risk factors for development of IFD is fungal colonization in patients receiving intensive chemotherapy (Table 9.1). The rates of fungal colonization vary widely and are highest for acute myeloid leukemia (AML, 78.8%), non-Hodgkin lymphoma (NHL, 69.2%) followed by acute lymphoblastic leukemia (ALL, 64%) [3]. IFD can either be yeasts (mostly candidiasis) or mold infections (aspergillosis and mucormycosis). Candidiasis is mostly endogenous that gains entry through breached mucosal surfaces of the body due to the use of intensive chemotherapy. Molds (filamentous) are ubiquitous soil inhabitants whose conidia gain entry through inhalation and are mostly responsible for sino-pulmonary infections. Even though there have been great improvements in the investigative techniques for early diagnosis of IFD, they are still far from being termed as "satisfactory." The uncertainty in making a definitive diagnosis and the need for stratification of such patients have led to the use of terms "possible," "probable," and "proven" fungal infections in patients with hematological disorders [4]. The incidence and prevalence of IFD are calculated based on "probable" and "proven" fungal infections. However, in clinic, much higher numbers of patients with "possible" fungal infections are seen than "probable" or "proven" infections. This point is illustrated by the largest series of autopsied patients with underlying hematological malignancies where proven IFD were identified only in 31% of patients [5]. However, 75% of these infections were not identified pre-mortem signifying the weakness of current methods of diagnosis of these infections. This series of autopsied patients also showed increase in the incidence of invasive mold infections over a 15-year period from 19 to 25% [5]. According to another large study SEIFEM-2004 (Sorveglianza Epidemiologica Infezioni Fungine Emopatie Maligne) carried out among 11,802 patients with hematologic malignancies, there were 4.6% proven or probable IFD and 69% of these infections occurred in patients with acute myeloid leukemia (AML) [6]. More than 50% IFD were caused by mold infections and IFD attributable mortality rates were 39% in this series [6]. **The highest attributable mortality was due to mucormycosis (64%) followed by fusariosis (53%) and aspergillosis (42%)** [6]. The incidence of mucormycosis has gone up in recent times especially among patients with acute leukemia. The overall prevalence of mucormycosis was 78% and significantly found to be more common in patients of AML (51%) than ALL (27%) [7, 8]. Similarly, out of 59 patients of proven or probable invasive aspergillosis (IA) in a large hospital in Korea, 25 patients (46.3%) had underlying AML and 10 (18.5%) patients had underlying ALL. Overall mortality at 12 weeks was 40% [9]. In the SAIF ("Surveillance des Aspergilloses Invasivesen France") network, out of 393 adult patients with IA, 77.6% patients had underlying hematological malignancies [10]. However, with the availability of newer antifungal agents and use of prophylaxis, the risk of IA appears to be decreasing. In a recently conducted meta-analysis, the risk of IA was estimated to range from 4 to 11% and case fatality rates of 29% [11].

This data suggests that IFD pose a significant burden among patients with hematological malignancies and their prevalence has significantly increased in recent years (Table 9.2). The detailed discussion on fungal infections in AML, ALL, and chronic leukemia is discussed below. Fungal infections in bone marrow transplantation are discussed in a separate chapter.

Table 9.2 Prevalence and risk factors for IFD in hematological disorders in Asian countries

Type of malignancy	Prevalence of fungal infection (range)%	Risk factors and confounding factors	When fungal infections were common Early/late After specific drug therapy? Immune modulators	Common fungal agents	Any interesting or unique epidemiology in Asian countries	Personal comments
AML	37–48% IA 4–15% Candidiasis 8–18% Mucormycosis 1–1.9%	Prolonged and persistent neutropenia	During induction phase	Molds	*A.flavus* common than *A. fumigatus*, infection-related mortality generally high.	Treatment should be preferably in HEPA filtered rooms. Antifungal prophylaxis strongly recommended.
ALL	Overall 6.5% Yeasts infections 1.88% Aspergillosis 3.75%, Mucormycosis 0.34%, Fusariosis 0.08%	Corticosteroids, neutropenia	Induction, consolidation	Candida	Non-albicans Candida species common	Azoles increase the neurotoxicity of vincristine
Lymphomas	Overall 1.4% Aspergillosis 0.7%, yeasts infections 0.6%	Corticosteroids, purine analogues, neutropenia	High-dose chemotherapy or use of purine analogues	Molds	–	PJI common in HL
CLL	Molds 0.4% Yeasts 0.1%	Use of purine analogues, alemtuzumab, corticosteroids	FCR regimen (fludarabine, cyclophosphamide, rituximab), Hypogammaglobulinemia	Molds	–	Antifungal prophylaxis must if patient receiving purine analogues or alemtuzumab
CML	Mold 2.3%, Yeasts 0.2%	Common in accelerated phase or blast crisis	High-dose chemotherapy akin to treatment of acute leukemia	Molds	–	Fungal infections uncommon in chronic phase
MM	Molds 0.3% Yeasts 0.2%	Corticosteroids	Hypogammaglobulinemia	Candida	–	Antifungal prophylaxis is used if patients are on high-dose dexamethasone regimens

AML acute myeloid leukemia, *ALL* Acute lymphoblastic leukemia, *CLL* chronic lymphocytic leukemia, *CML* chronic myeloid leukemia, *MM* multiple myeloma, *IA* invasive aspergillosis, *PJI* Pneumocystis jirovecii infection, *HL* Hodgkin lymphoma

9.2 IFD in AML

AML is one of the aggressive leukemia that requires the use of intensive chemotherapy for its cure. The incidence of neutropenia following intensive chemotherapy is universal and persists for an average of 10 days to 3 weeks depending upon various factors. Thus, prolonged and persistent neutropenia following intensive chemotherapy used for curative treatment of AML is the most important risk factor for IFD in AML. Studies conducted in 1960–1980 suggested candidiasis as the commonest IFD in these patients. The frequency of IFD was noted to be between 13 and 28% [12]. **After the results of landmark study on the use of fluconazole as prophylaxis in these patients, the risk of invasive candidiasis declined but paradoxically led to increase in mold infections** [13]. The studies conducted in the last decade suggest that IA is the commonest IFD in these patients followed by candidiasis. The prevalence of proven and probable IFD is to the tune of 37–48% [4]. However, the prevalence rates of IFD vary depending upon various factors. Invasive candidiasis was reported to have an incidence of 8–18% and mortality of 30–40%, whereas IA had an incidence of 4–15% and mortality rate of 60–85% [14]. **The universal use of fluconazole prophylaxis has also led to increase in the prevalence of non-albicans Candida species in these patients.** In the SEIFEM-2008 study conducted between 2004 and 2007 in Italy, 140 patients with proven or probable IA cases among AML patients were analyzed [15]. In this series, the incidence of IA was 10% during post-induction or following consolidation therapy in AML. The aspergillosis-attributable mortality rate was between 30 and 40%. In a series of patients with AML and MDS from The Netherlands treated in HOVON treatment protocol (Hemato-Oncologie voor Volwassenen Nederland), the prevalence of probable and proven IA was 30% and mortality rate at 12 weeks after starting antifungal therapy was 22% [16]. The data on IFD in children is scarce. However, in one of the largest series of 1047 children hospitalized in hematology/oncology department, 80% had mold infections (non-Aspergillus 55%) and 20% had candidemia (60% had non-albicans Candida species) [17]. In all patients of IFD occurring in hematological malignancies, 35% had AML as underlying hematological disorder [17]. **Along with the increased incidence of IA, there is parallel rise in the incidence of mucormycosis among patients with AML** undergoing intensive chemotherapy. In the autopsy series spanning over 15-year period (1989–2003), the rate of mucormycosis was noted to have gone up from 0.9% to nearly 4% [4]. The reported incidence of mucormycosis in AML varies between 1 and 1.9% [18]. AML patients are also predisposed to get other fungal infections like fusariosis, *Pneumocystis jirovecii* infection (PJI), *Scedosporium*, and *Trichosporon* infections. PJI occurred in 12 out of 2171 new cases of adult acute leukemia (0.5%) [19]. Invasive fusariosis was reported in 46% patients of AML in a series on 177 patients of invasive fusariosis occurring in hematological disorders [20]. *Out of 52 cases of Trichosporon* species and *Geotrichum capitatum*, 64.5% patients had underlying AML [21]. Similarly out of 39 patients of *Scedosporium* infection described in literature, 64% patients had underlying AML [22]. Cryptococcosis is an uncommon infection; however, out of 17 cases reported in patients with hematological disorders, 35% patients had underlying AML [23].

It is clear from the abovementioned literature that AML patients constitute as one of the commonest underlying condition for the development of IFD. **In fact, the risk of IFD is considered much higher in AML patients than the patients undergoing stem cell transplantation (SCT).** In a series reported from Italy, the incidence of IFD was 16.9% in AML vs 8.2% of patients undergoing SCT. The attributable mortality rates, however, were more in SCT patients (69.6%) as compared to patients with AML (34.8%) [24]. Because of the high mortality associated by IFD in AML, the available guidelines advocate the routine use of antifungal prophylaxis in all AML patients undergoing intensive chemotherapy (Table 9.3). In one series of 322 AML patients undergoing standard chemotherapy, use of prophylactic fluconazole was able to reduce the incidence of IFD [25]. **Posaconazole is considered superior to fluconazole and itraconazole for prophylaxis in AML and myelodysplastic syndrome patients**. In the landmark trial comparing posaconazole vs fluconazole vs. itraconazole in patients undergoing chemotherapy for AML and myelodysplastic syndrome, posaconazole was more effective than fluconazole or itraconazole in preventing IFD and also improved overall survival in these patients [26]. Hence ECIL 3 guidelines recommend routine use of posaconazole as antifungal prophylaxis in AML patients undergoing standard chemotherapy [27]. **Other antifungal agents viz. voriconazole, echinocandins, and amphotericin B have been recommended as prophylaxis with equivalent results by NCCN guidelines**. Retrospective analysis of use of voriconazole as antifungal prophylaxis in AML does suggest that it is an effective prophylactic agent [28, 29]. **In developing countries, amphotericin B deoxycholate is a cheaper alternative as antifungal prophylaxis in AML patients undergoing intensive chemotherapy**. Nevertheless, physicians in Asia have wider choice of using these agents as prophylaxis in their patients based on several parameters (Table 9.3).

9.3 IFD in ALL

The intensity of chemotherapy and immunosuppressive medication in ALL is generally lower as compared to AML and hence **ALL patients have a reduced risk than AML patients for developing IFD during chemotherapy**. However, the risk of IFD has gone up in recent years. In the autopsy series spanning over a time interval from 1989 to 2003, the prevalence of IFD in ALL patients was noted to have gone up from 16 to 21% over this period of time [4]. One of the largest retrospective study of IFD in hematological disorders reported incidence of **IFD (molds and yeasts) to the tune of 6.5% in ALL** [5]. The incidence of yeast infections was 1.88%, aspergillosis 3.75%, mucormycosis 0.34%, and fusariosis 0.08%. Most infections occurred during induction phase of chemotherapy. **The attributable mortality rates were highest in mucormycosis 50%, followed by aspergillosis 43%, and least for candidiasis of 36%.** ALL is generally a disease of childhood. Among 2021 children of ALL, one fifth deaths were attributable to IFD [30]. The risk factors for IFD in ALL are prolonged neutropenia, use of corticosteroids and broad-spectrum antibiotics besides many other risk factors as listed in Table 9.1.

Table 9.3 Types of antifungal therapy used in hematology oncology setting

Type of therapy	Explanation	Initiation of therapy	Termination of therapy	Drugs used
Prophylactic	Prevention of fungal infection	Started on the day the induction therapy	Continued until the risk factor disappears (myeloid constitution in case of neutropenia)	Posaconazole (200 mg TDS), Voriconazole (200 mg BD), liposomal amphotericin B, Fluconazole 400 mg OD, Itraconazole 200 mg BD, Caspofungin 50 mg OD, micafungin 50 mg OD
Empiric	Clinical suspicion	Day 3 to day 7 of febrile neutropenia	Continued until the recovery of neutropenia	Amphotericin B, Caspofungin, Voriconazole
Preemptive	Surrogate markers positive (Galactomannan +ve)	Started as soon as surrogate markers become positive	Continued until recovery of neutropenia	Amphotericin B, Caspofungin, Voriconazole
Directed	Fungal species on histopathology or culture	Started as soon as result come as positive	Continued until 2-weeks of culture becoming negative (e.g., continued for two more weeks when blood fungal culture become sterile after initial positivity with *Candida* spp.)	Voriconazole for Aspergillus, Amphotericin B and Posaconazole for Mucormycosis, Echinocandins for Candida and Aspergillus

Lungs are the commonest organs affected by IFD. However, unlike AML, there is no consensus on the routine use of antifungal prophylaxis in ALL. **A word of caution when using itraconazole, voriconazole, and posaconazole as prophylaxis in ALL patients. These azoles are potent inhibitors of P450 3A4 enzyme system and can increase the neurotoxicity of vincristine which is an important chemotherapy drug in the treatment of ALL.**

9.4 Lymphomas

The incidence of **IFD is generally lower in both non-Hodgkin lymphoma (NHL) and Hodgkin lymphoma (HL)** and they are discussed together. In the SEIFEM-2004 study, the incidence of mold and yeast infections together was 1.4% among NHL and HL patients [5]. Among the mold infections, aspergillosis was the commonest infection with an incidence of 0.7% and attributable mortality rate of 52–67% in NHL and

HL, respectively. The incidence of yeast infections was 0.6%. In the autopsy series on lymphoma in the decade spanning 1989–2003, IFD were found in 10–11% of lymphoma patients [4]. The major risk factors for IFD in lymphoma patients again are prolonged neutropenia, mucositis, and use of immunosuppressive medications (corticosteroids, purine analogues, alemtuzumab). Abnormalities of T-cell function are common in patients with HL. These patients thus are at highest risk of infections by PJI and cryptococcosis [31]. However, the **routine use of antifungal prophylaxis is not recommended in lymphoma patients based on abovementioned factors**.

9.5 Chronic Lymphocytic Leukemia (CLL)

In the SEIFEM-2004 study, the incidence of mold infections was 0.4% and yeast infections was 0.1% among 1104 CLL patients [5]. In the autopsy study spanning over a 15-year period, the incidence of IFD in CLL had gone up from 5 to 11% [4]. The major risk factors in CLL are use of T-cell immunosuppressive therapy in the form of corticosteroids, purine analogues and alemtuzumab.

9.6 Chronic Myeloid Leukemia (CML)

The incidence of mold infections was 2.3% and yeasts 0.2% in 596 patients of CML studied in the SEIFEM study [5]. However in the autopsy study conducted over a 15-year period, the incidence of IFD had shown a decline from 17 to 6% in patients with CML [4]. CML has got two phases of disease—chronic and advanced. **It is the advanced phase of the disease (accelerated and blastic) where IFD occur frequently because of use of intensive chemotherapy**. With the availability of targeted therapies since 2000 onwards, the number of CML patients transforming into advanced phase have declined leading to decline in the incidence of IFD in CML.

9.7 Multiple Myeloma (MM)

The incidence of mold infections was 0.3% and of yeasts 0.2% in 1616 patients of MM [4]. The attributable mortality rate due to *Aspergillus* infection was close to 75% though the number of patients were small in this series. The predisposing factors for fungal infections are presence of immune dysfunction and use of corticosteroids in patients with MM.

9.8 Diagnosis of IFD

9.8.1 When to Suspect?

The diagnosis of IFD is suspected when the clinical signs and symptoms of patients are generally not explained by usual bacterial infections and the

clinical condition of patient is deteriorating on appropriate broad-spectrum antibiotics. World-over, the most common underlying conditions among patients with IFD are malignant hematological disorders. However, even among patients with hematological disorders, IFD are more common among patients who receive either high-dose chemotherapy that results in prolonged neutropenia (e.g., induction therapy in AML), or highly immunosuppressive therapy (e.g., fludarabine in CLL). Ongoing construction and destruction in the hospital are other risk factors for the increasing incidence of mold infections [28]. Generally multiple risk factors are present in patients who are diagnosed with IFD and hence the **index of suspicion for IFD should be kept high in an appropriate clinical setting** (Table 9.1). Superficial candidiasis (oral candidiasis) and skin infections (Tinea) are generally diagnosed on general physical examination. Candidemia is diagnosed on blood culture positivity. Mold infections are difficult to diagnose. In patients with prolonged neutropenia (>7 days), persistent fever beyond 3 days of appropriate antibiotics generally raise the suspicion of IFD. A high resolution of the CT scan of the chest (HRCT) is strongly recommended before the initiation of antifungal treatment. **HRCT chest can show plethora of findings but presence of cavitation, halo sign, and air-crescent signs are hallmarks of mold infections.** The involvement of nasal sinuses also suggests presence of mold infection. Biopsy of the involved area and histopathology should be performed whenever possible as they form the gold standard tests for "proven" IFD. However, biopsy may not always be possible as patients are generally ill and have severe neutropenia and thrombocytopenia precluding any invasive investigation in them. Broncho-alveolar lavage (BAL), however, can still be carried out in a few patients and analysis of BAL fluid is helpful to some extent. Attempt should always be made for tissue diagnosis by CT/ultrasound guided aspiration/biopsy and endobronchial ultrasound technique (EBUS). In thrombocytopenic patients, such procedure can be attempted after infusion of platelets. In the last decade, testing for two fungal wall antigens galactomannan (GM) and 1,3-b-d-glucan (BG) have been added in the armamentarium of diagnosis of IFD. Instead of one single value, rising titers of GM favor diagnosis of aspergillosis [32]. β-D-glucan is a major cell wall component of most fungal species (with exception of *Mucorales* and *Cryptococcus* spp.), and is released in blood and tissues of patients in the course of IFD [33]. Though there is no uniformity on the cutoff values of both GM and BG and on the number of tests to be carried out before confirming these tests as positive, the tests are useful to screen out IFD. The positive test in an immunocompromised host will put patients into the "probable" category of IFD, whereas "possible" fungal infections are diagnosed based only on host and clinical criteria for IFD.

There are various guidelines available for diagnosis and management of Aspergillosis mainly from The European Society for Clinical Microbiology and Infectious Diseases, the European Confederation of Medical Mycology, and the European Respiratory Society [34]. These guidelines recommend computed tomography, bronchoscopy, and bronchoalveolar lavage for suspected invasive pulmonary aspergillosis. The diagnosis should be confirmed by direct microscopy, preferably with optical brighteners, histopathology, and cultures of the tissue. Biomarkers like serum and BAL galactomannan aid in the diagnosis of invasive aspergillosis. The guidelines also put emphasis on identification of species as well as antifungal drug susceptibility testing [34].

9.9 Treatment Approach

The treatment of IFD is carried out by risk-categorizing the patients based on underlying hematological condition, type of chemotherapy or immunosuppressive therapy, and multiple other risk factors (Table 9.1), e.g., febrile neutropenia in AML constitutes the highest-risk category for IFD (even higher risk than patients with stem cell transplantation) [35–38]. **Thus, the antifungal treatment is divided into prophylactic, empiric, pre-emptive, or directed** (Table 9.3). Patients in the highest-risk category (AML, ALL on high-dose chemotherapy protocol) are generally candidates for prophylactic antifungal treatment [39]. The choice of antifungal drugs is based on anticipated risk of infection (yeast, mold, etc). The prophylaxis treatment is generally continued until the risk factors for IFD are under control (e.g., absolute neutrophil count more than 500/μL). Empiric antifungal treatment is considered in the clinical setting of neutropenia and persistent fever despite use of broad-spectrum antibiotics [40]. This is usually initiated on day 4 to day 7 of persistent neutropenic fever though there is some evidence that early empiric antifungal therapy is better [41]. Pre-emptive antifungal treatment approach is carried out in patients who have evidence of IFD on surrogate marker such as an antigen or genomic detection test, but without evidence of clinical disease [37]. Directed antifungal treatment therapy applies to patients with evidence of fungal infection and clinical manifestations [42, 43].

There are also guidelines from various societies (e.g., European, German) available on primary prophylaxis of invasive fungal infections in patients with hematological malignancies [44, 45]. Posaconazole delayed-release tablets are recommended as primary prophylaxis for AML and MDS patients undergoing intensive induction therapy. Intravenous posaconazole is recommended only if oral route is contraindicated. If the incidence of IFD is less than 8%, fluconazole can be considered as prophylaxis [13]. There are no clear recommendations for any particular drug as prophylaxis in ALL or other hematological disorders. Fluconazole probably remains the best choice as prophylactic agent in ALL. If voriconazole is used as prophylaxis, therapeutic drug monitoring is strongly recommended [44, 45].

9.10 Prevention of IFD

Candidiasis mostly arises from endogenous flora whenever there is breach of mucosal barrier (mucositis) due to chemotherapy. Hence prophylactic use of fluconazole has been shown to be effective in reducing the rate of invasive candidiasis in patients with mucositis due to chemotherapy. Mold infections on the other hand arise because of inhalation of spores from the environment. Thus control of environment with use of high-efficiency particulate air (HEPA) filters and protective isolation is the key to prevent mold infections [43]. The ongoing construction activities near the hospital are well-known risk factors for the occurrence of mold infections [28]. Thus it is preferable to treat acute leukemia patients in HEPA filter room and they should keep themselves in some form of protective environment after discharge from hospital.

9.11 Asian Data [46–64]

There are a few review articles [46–49] and published studies [50–64] from Asian countries on the prevalence of IFD. Based on the available literature, **it is believed that prevalence of IFD is equal or higher than the reported prevalence from the western countries**. However, there are countries in Asia, which are more developed than others, and the prevalence of IFD in these countries is similar to what is generally seen in the west.

9.11.1 Major Studies from India

In an autopsy study of 72 patients with underlying hematological malignancy, 29% patients had systemic IFD [50]. Ten patients each had aspergillosis and invasive candidiasis. All *Aspergillus* infections were pulmonary while 90% of candidiasis was involving the gastrointestinal tract. The other infections in this series were mucormycosis, cryptococcosis, and trichosporonosis.

An analysis of 382 febrile episodes [51] occurring in patients with AML found the prevalence of IFD as 15.7% (17.9% in neutropenic patients). Empiric antifungal therapy was used in 37.5% of patients. An earlier study conducted in the same institute in the year 2000 [52] showed usage of empiric amphotericin B in 54 (22.5%) patients of acute leukemia who had 240 episodes of fever (both neutropenic and non-neutropenic). The proven IFD was documented in nine patients. Another analysis [53] from the same group in the year 2012 showed 30% patients having IFD (possible 20.5, probable 8.5%, and proven 1%) in 200 episodes of febrile neutropenia following chemotherapy. Interestingly, no patient was documented to have candidemia or invasive candidiasis. All patients received antifungal prophylaxis in the form of either itraconazole or amphotericin B.

In 222 patients of AML undergoing intensive therapy at a tertiary care center in South India, the incidence of IFD was found to be 38.7% with proven fungal infection rates of 5.4%. Use of posaconazole prophylaxis led to decrease in the incidence of IFD [54].

The incidence of fungal infections was also found to be high (18.3%) in acute promyelocytic leukemia treated with non-chemotherapy agents indirectly implicating environment as one of the risk factors for invasive fungal infections in the developing countries [55].

9.11.2 Other Studies from Asia

An analysis of autopsied patients in Japan showed increase in the incidence of mycoses from 1.6 to 4.66% in 1990 [56]. While *Aspergillus* was the commonest fungal pathogen found among acute leukemia patients (37.5%), *Candida* spp. were common among patients with solid tumors.

There are a few published studies on mycoses from Taiwan [57–59]. In the evaluation of children with 82 episodes of febrile neutropenia [57], IFD were found in 35.4% of febrile episodes. The most common presentation of IFD was pneumonia (69%). The overall mortality was 51.7%. A study on candidemia in hematological malignancies showed that it was more common in patients with ALL [58]. *Candida tropicalis* was the most common *Candida* spp. followed by *Candida albicans*. All *Candida* spp. were sensitive to caspofungin while among azoles, the sensitivity was 99%, 91.3%, and 51.5% with voriconazole, fluconazole, and itraconazole, respectively. In another study of 46 patients with underlying hematological malignancy and with fungal sinusitis, AML was found to be the commonest underlying hematological disorder [59]. *A. flavus* was the commonest pathogen isolated. The overall mortality at 6 weeks was 41.3%.

In a study from Korea on 54 patients with IA, the most common underlying hematological disorder was again found to be AML [9]. The overall mortality at 12 weeks was 38.9% and IA attributable mortality was 33.3%. Uncontrolled disease state and hypoalbuminemia were the commonest risk factors for mortality in this study.

In another study done in a large tertiary care hospital of Singapore, the prevalence of IFD was 10.7% among patients of ALL, AML, and SCT who were receiving antifungal prophylaxis either with fluconazole or itrazonazole [60]. The most common fungal pathogen isolated was *Aspergillus*. The prevalence of IFD during induction chemotherapy was 8.9% for AML and 1.0% for ALL. The in-hospital mortality was 28.2% and IFD attributable mortality was 12.8%.

The common drugs to treat aspergillosis are voriconazole, itraconazole, posaconazole, echinocandins, and amphotericin B. Experience of voriconazole in the treatment of IA in patients with hematological malignancies in a study from China suggests that it was safe and effective in 81.6% patients [61].

GM is an important test for making a probable diagnosis of IA. A study conducted in Thailand [62] evaluated GM in patients with febrile neutropenia and found that the cutoff GM index of more than 0.75 had sensitivity of 94.1% and a specificity of 78.8%.

In another study on 94 patients with IA in a tertiary care hospital in Thailand, acute leukemia was the commonest underlying condition (30%) [63]. The most common organ affected was lungs in 68% of patients. Contrary to other reports from Asia, *A. fumigatus* was the commonest *Aspergillus* spp. in this series. The mortality in this series was 47%.

From the abovementioned studies, it is clear that there are a few differences in the epidemiology of IFD in Asia compared to West in the form of higher incidence of fungal infections in the developing countries of Asian region. However, much more work is required to be done and published from these countries to comment on the epidemiology and novel risk factors for IFD [46–49].

9.12 Conclusions

It is clear from the above data that patients with hematological disorders have the highest risk of developing IFD. Out of all hematological disorders, AML has the highest risk followed by ALL (risks of IFD in stem cell transplantation are discussed in a separate chapter). Most IFD happens during the induction phase of chemotherapy. The IFD carries a high risk of attributable mortality and hence varied antifungal treatment strategies are used to decrease this risk. Antifungal prophylaxis in high-risk setting, use of empiric and pre-emptive antifungal therapy in appropriate clinical setting are important strategies. However, we are still far away from effectively preventing, diagnosing and carrying definitive treatment of IFD in patients with hematological disorders.

References

1. Ruhnke M, Böhme A, Buchheidt D, et al. Infectious Diseases Working Party in Haematology and Oncology of the German Society for Haematology and Oncology. Diagnosis of invasive fungal infections in hematology and oncology—guidelines from the Infectious Diseases Working Party in Haematology and Oncology of the German Society for Haematology and Oncology (AGIHO). Ann Oncol. 2012;23:823–33.
2. Georgiadou SP, Kontoyiannis DP. Concurrent lung infections in patients with hematological malignancies and invasive pulmonary aspergillosis: how firm is the Aspergillus diagnosis? J Infect. 2012;65:262–8.
3. Gözdaşoğlu S, Ertem M, Büyükkeçeci Z, et al. Fungal colonization and infection in children with acute leukemia and lymphoma during induction therapy. Med Pediatr Oncol. 1999;32: 344–8.
4. De Pauw B, Walsh TJ, Donnelly JP, et al. European Organization for Research and Treatment of Cancer/Invasive Fungal Infections Cooperative Group; National Institute of Allergy and Infectious Diseases Mycoses Study Group (EORTC/MSG) Consensus Group. Revised definitions of invasive fungal disease from the European Organization for Research and Treatment of Cancer/Invasive Fungal Infections Cooperative Group and the National Institute of Allergy and Infectious Diseases Mycoses Study Group (EORTC/MSG) Consensus Group. Clin Infect Dis. 2008;46:1813–21.
5. Chamilos G, Luna M, Lewis RE, et al. Invasive fungal infections in patients with hematologic malignancies in a tertiary care cancer center: an autopsy study over a 15-year period (1989–2003). Haematologica. 2006;91:986–9.
6. Pagano L, Caira M, Candoni A, et al. The epidemiology of fungal infections in patients with hematologic malignancies: the SEIFEM-2004 study. Haematologica. 2006;91:1068–75.
7. Karthaus M, Cornely OA. Recent developments in the management of invasive fungal infections in patients with hematological malignancies. Ann Hematol. 2005;84:207–16.
8. Pagano L, Offidani M, Fianchi L, et al. GIMEMA (Gruppo Italiano Malattie EMatologiche dell'Adulto) Infection Program. Mucormycosis in hematologic patients. Haematologica. 2004;89:207–14.
9. Kwon JC, Kim SH, Park SH, et al. Prognosis of invasive pulmonary aspergillosis in patients with hematologic diseases in Korea. Tuberc Respir Dis (Seoul). 2012;72:284–92.

10. Lortholary O, Gangneux JP, Sitbon K, et al. French Mycosis Study Group. Epidemiological trends in invasive aspergillosis in France: the SAIF network (2005–2007). Clin Microbiol Infect. 2011;17:1882–9.
11. van de Peppel RJ, Visser LG, Dekkers OM, de Boer MGJ. The burden of invasive aspergillosis in patients with haematological malignancy: a meta-analysis and systematic review. J Infect. 2018;76:550–62.
12. Bennett JE. The changing face of febrile neutropenia-from monotherapy to moulds to mucositis. Management of mycoses in neutropenic patients: a brief history, 1960–2008. J Antimicrob Chemother. 2009;63(Suppl 1):i23–6.
13. Goodman JL, Winston DJ, Greenfield RA, et al. A controlled trial of fluconazole to prevent fungal infections in patients undergoing bone marrow transplantation. N Engl J Med. 1992;326:845–51.
14. Wirk B, Wingard JR. Current approaches in antifungal prophylaxis in high risk hematologic malignancy and hematopoietic stem cell transplant patients. Mycopathologia. 2009;168:299–311.
15. Pagano L, Caira M, Candoni A, et al. Invasive aspergillosis in patients with acute myeloid leukemia: a SEIFEM-2008 registry study. Haematologica. 2010;95:644–50.
16. Slobbe L, Polinder S, Doorduijn JK, et al. Outcome and medical costs of patients with invasive aspergillosis and acute myelogenous leukemia-myelodysplastic syndrome treated with intensive chemotherapy: an observational study. Clin Infect Dis. 2008;15(47):1507–12.
17. Mor M, Gilad G, Kornreich L, Fisher S, Yaniv I, Levy I. Invasive fungal infections in pediatric oncology. Pediatr Blood Cancer. 2011;56:1092–7.
18. Skiada A, Lanternier F, Groll AH, et al. European Conference on Infections in Leukemia. Diagnosis and treatment of mucormycosis in patients with hematological malignancies: guidelines from the 3rd European Conference on Infections in Leukemia (ECIL 3). Haematologica. 2013;98:492–504.
19. Pagano L, Fianchi L, Mele L, et al. Pneumocystis carinii pneumonia in patients with malignant haematological diseases: 10 years' experience of infection in GIMEMA centres. Br J Haematol. 2002;117:379–86.
20. Girmenia C, Pagano L, Corvatta L, Mele L, del Favero A, Martino P. The epidemiology of fusariosis in patients with haematological diseases. Gimema Infection Programme. Br J Haematol. 2000;111:272–6.
21. Girmenia C, Pagano L, Martino B, et al. GIMEMA Infection Program. Invasive infections caused by Trichosporon species and Geotrichum capitatum in patients with hematological malignancies: a retrospective multicenter study from Italy and review of the literature. J Clin Microbiol. 2005;43:1818–28.
22. Caira M, Girmenia C, Valentini CG, et al. Scedosporiosis in patients with acute leukemia: a retrospective multicenter report. Haematologica. 2008;93:104–10.
23. Pagano L, Fianchi L, Caramatti C, et al. Gruppo Italiano Malattie EMatologiche dell'Adulto Infection Program. Cryptococcosis in patients with hematologic malignancies. A report from GIMEMA-infection. Haematologica. 2004;89:852–6.
24. Caira M, Girmenia C, Fadda RM, et al. Invasive fungal infections in patients with acute myeloid leukemia and in those submitted to allogeneic hemopoietic stem cell transplant: who is at highest risk? Eur J Haematol. 2008;81:242–3.
25. Rex JH, Anaissie EJ, Boutati E, Estey E, Kantarjian H. Systemic antifungal prophylaxis reduces invasive fungal in acute myelogenous leukemia: a retrospective review of 833 episodes of neutropenia in 322 adults. Leukemia. 2002;16:1197–9.
26. Cornely OA, Maertens J, Winston DJ, et al. Posaconazole vs. fluconazole or itraconazole prophylaxis in patients with neutropenia. N Engl J Med. 2007;356:348–59.
27. Maertens J, Marchetti O, Herbrecht R, et al. Third European Conference on Infections in Leukemia. European guidelines for antifungal management in leukemia and hematopoietic stem cell transplant recipients: summary of the ECIL 3—2009 update. Bone Marrow Transplant. 2011;46:709–18.

28. Chabrol A, Cuzin L, Huguet F, et al. Prophylaxis of invasive aspergillosis with voriconazole or caspofungin during building work in patients with acute leukemia. Haematologica. 2010;95:996–1003.
29. Barreto JN, Beach CL, Wolf RC, et al. The incidence of invasive fungal infections in neutropenic patients with acute leukemia and myelodysplastic syndromes receiving primary antifungal prophylaxis with voriconazole. Am J Hematol. 2013;88:283–8.
30. Grigull L, Beier R, Schrauder A, et al. Invasive fungal infections are responsible for one-fifth of the infectious deaths in children with ALL. Mycoses. 2003;46:441–6.
31. Fisher RI, DeVita VT Jr, Bostick F, et al. Persistent immunologic abnormalities in long-term survivors of advanced Hodgkin's disease. Ann Intern Med. 1980;92:595–9.
32. Hoenigl M, Salzer HJ, Raggam RB, et al. Impact of galactomannan testing on the prevalence of invasive aspergillosis in patients with hematological malignancies. Med Mycol. 2012;50:266–9.
33. Lamoth F, Cruciani M, Mengoli C, et al. Third European Conference on Infections in Leukemia (ECIL-3). β-Glucan antigenemia assay for the diagnosis of invasive fungal infections in patients with hematological malignancies: a systematic review and meta-analysis of cohort studies from the Third European Conference on Infections in Leukemia (ECIL-3). Clin Infect Dis. 2012;54:633–43.
34. Ullmann AJ, Aguado JM, Arikan-Akdagli S, et al. Diagnosis and management of Aspergillus diseases: executive summary of the 2017 ESCMID-ECMM-ERS guideline. Clin Microbiol Infect. 2018;24(Suppl 1):e1–e38.
35. Girmenia C, Aversa F, Busca A, et al. Sorveglianza Epidemiologica delle Infezioni Fungine nelle Emopatie Maligne; Invasive Fungal Infections Cooperative Group of the European Organization for Research and Treatment of Cancer; Gruppo Italiano Malattie Ematologiche dell'Adulto; Associazione Italiana Ematologia ed Oncologia Pediatrica; Gruppo ItalianoTrapianto di Midollo Osseo. A hematology consensus agreement on antifungal strategies for neutropenic patients with hematological malignancies and stem cell transplant recipients. Gruppo Italiano Malattie Ematologiche dell'Adulto, Gruppo Italiano Trapianto di Midollo Osseo, Associazione Italiana Ematologia ed Oncologia Pediatrica, Invasive Fungal Infections Cooperative Group of the European Organization for Research and Treatment of Cancer and Sorveglianza Epidemiologica delle Infezioni Fungine nelle Emopatie Maligne. Hematol Oncol. 2013;31:117–26.
36. Bow EJ. Of yeasts and hyphae: a hematologist's approach to antifungal therapy. Hematology Am Soc Hematol Educ Program. 2006:361–7.
37. Mikolajewska A, Schwartz S, Ruhnke M. Antifungal treatment strategies in patients with haematological diseases or cancer: from prophylaxis to empirical, pre-emptive and targeted therapy. Mycoses. 2012;55:2–16.
38. Hicheri Y, Toma A, Maury S, et al. Updated guidelines for managing fungal diseases in hematology patients. Expert Rev Anti Infect Ther. 2010;8:1049–60.
39. Almyroudis NG, Segal BH. Antifungal prophylaxis and therapy in patients with hematological malignancies and hematopoietic stem cell transplant recipients. Expert Rev Anti Infect Ther. 2010;8:1451–66.
40. Ferrara JJ, MacDougall C, Gallagher JC. Empiric antifungal therapy in patients with febrile neutropenia. Pharmacotherapy. 2011;31:369–85.
41. Malhotra P, Makkar A, Guru Murthy GS, Varma N, Varma S, Chakrabarti A. Empirical amphotericin B therapy on day 4 or day 8 of febrile neutropenia. Mycoses. 2014;57:110–5.
42. Maschmeyer G. The changing face of febrile neutropenia-from monotherapy to moulds to mucositis. Prevention of mould infections. J Antimicrob Chemother. 2009;63(Suppl 1):i27–30.
43. Lee LD, Hachem RY, Berkheiser M, Hackett B, Jiang Y, Raad II. Hospital environment and invasive aspergillosis in patients with hematologic malignancy. Am J Infect Control. 2012;40:247–9.
44. Primary prophylaxis of invasive fungal infections in patients with haematological malignancies: 2017 update of the recommendations of the Infectious Diseases Working Party (AGIHO)

of the German Society for Haematology and MedicalOncology (DGHO). Ann Hematol. 2018;97:197–207.
45. European guidelines for primary antifungal prophylaxis in adult haematology patients: summary of the updated recommendations from the European Conference on Infections in Leukaemia. J Antimicrob Chemother. 2018;73:3221–30.
46. Slavin MA, Chakrabarti A. Opportunistic fungal infections in the Asia-Pacific region. Med Mycol. 2012;50:18–25.
47. Chakrabarti A, Slavin MA. Endemic fungal infections in the Asia-Pacific region. Med Mycol. 2011;49:337–44.
48. Chakrabarti A, Singh R. The emerging epidemiology of mould infections in developing countries. Curr Opin Infect Dis. 2011;24:521–6.
49. Chakrabarti A, Chatterjee SS, Das A, Shivaprakash MR. Invasive aspergillosisin developing countries. Med Mycol. 2011;49(Suppl 1):S35–47.
50. Srivastava VM, Krishnaswami H, Srivastava A, Dennison D, Chandy M. Infections in haematological malignancies: an autopsy study of 72 cases. Trans R Soc Trop Med Hyg. 1996;90:406–8.
51. Gupta A, Singh M, Singh H, Kumar L, Sharma A, Bakhshi S, Raina V, Thulkar S. Infections in acute myeloid leukemia: an analysis of 382 febrile episodes. Med Oncol. 2010;27:1037–45.
52. Jagarlamudi R, Kumar L, Kochupillai V, Kapil A, Banerjee U, Thulkar S. Infections in acute leukemia: an analysis of 240 febrile episodes. Med Oncol. 2000;17:111–6.
53. Ghosh I, Raina V, Kumar L, Sharma A, Bakhshi S, Thulkar S, Kapil A. Profile of infections and outcome in high-risk febrile neutropenia: experience from a tertiary care cancer center in India. Med Oncol. 2012;29:1354–60.
54. Korula A, Abraham A, Abubacker FN, et al. Invasive fungal infection following chemotherapy for acute myeloid leukaemia—experience from a developing country. Mycoses. 2017;60:686–91.
55. Yanamandra U, Karunakaran P, Khandwal A, et al. Invasive fungal infections in acute promyelocytic leukemia on dual differentiating agents: real world data. Indian J Hematol Blood Transfus. 2018;34:466–8.
56. Yamazaki T, Kume H, Murase S, Yamashita E, Arisawa M. Epidemiology of visceral mycoses: analysis of data in annual of the pathological autopsy cases in Japan. J Clin Microbiol. 1999;37:1732–8.
57. Lai HP, Chen YC, Chang LY, et al. Invasive fungal infection in children with persistent febrile neutropenia. J Formos Med Assoc. 2005;104:174–9.
58. Chen CY, Huang SY, Tsay W, et al. Clinical characteristics of candidaemia in adults with haematological malignancy,and antimicrobial susceptibilities of the isolates at a medical centre in Taiwan,2001–2010. Int J Antimicrob Agents. 2012;40:533–8.
59. Chen CY, Sheng WH, Cheng A, et al. Invasive fungal sinusitis in patients with hematological malignancy: 15 years experience in a single university hospital in Taiwan. BMC Infect Dis. 2011;11:250.
60. Lee SY, Yeo CL, Lee WH, et al. Prevalence of invasive fungal disease in hematological patients at a tertiary university hospital in Singapore. BMC Res Notes. 2011;4:42.
61. Zhang XZ, Huang XE, Xu YL, Zhang XQ, Su AL, Shen ZS. Phase II study on voriconazole for treatment of Chinese patients with malignant hematological disorders and invasive aspergillosis. Asian Pac J Cancer Prev. 2012;13:2415–8.
62. Suankratay C, Kanitcharaskul P, Arunyingmongkol K. Galactomannan antigenemia for the diagnosis of invasive aspergillosis in neutropenic patients with hematological disorders. J Med Assoc Thai. 2006;89:1851–8.
63. Kiertiburanakul S, Thibbadee C, Santanirand P. Invasive aspergillosis in a tertiary-care hospital in Thailand. J Med Assoc Thai. 2007;90:895–902.
64. Malhotra P, Chauhan S, Bhatt P, et al. Cryptococcal meningitis in acute lymphoblastic leukemia. J Assoc Physicians India. 2004;52:831–2.

Part III

Fungal Allergy

Allergic Bronchopulmonary Aspergillosis

10

Valliappan Muthu and Ritesh Agarwal

Key Points

- Allergic bronchopulmonary aspergillosis (ABPA) can complicate asthma and cystic fibrosis. The burden of ABPA complicating asthma is substantial, especially in the Indian subcontinent.
- All patients with asthma, irrespective of the severity, should be routinely investigated for ABPA.
- Specific IgE against *A. fumigatus* is the best investigation to screen asthmatic patients for ABPA.
- ABPA is currently diagnosed on the basis of a constellation of clinical, radiological, and immunological findings.
- The ABPA working group of the International Society for Human and Animal Mycology (ISHAM) has proposed new diagnostic and staging criteria with precise definitions.
- Glucocorticoids (to suppress the immune hyperactivity), and antifungal azoles (to reduce the fungal burden in the airways), are the primary treatment modalities employed in the management of ABPA.
- Glucocorticoids are the preferred therapy for acute stage of ABPA. Itraconazole and voriconazole may be used as alternative agents.

10.1 Introduction

Aspergillus spp. cause several diseases in humans, the nature and severity of which depends on the interaction between the virulence of the *Aspergillus* spp. and the immunity of the host [1]. The spectrum of pulmonary diseases caused by *Aspergillus fumigatus* includes aspergilloma, allergic *Aspergillus* sinusitis, hypersensitivity

V. Muthu · R. Agarwal (✉)
Department of Pulmonary Medicine, Post Graduate Institute of Medical Education and Research (PGIMER), Chandigarh, India

A. Chakrabarti (ed.), *Clinical Practice of Medical Mycology in Asia*,
https://doi.org/10.1007/978-981-13-9459-1_10

Table 10.1 Spectrum of pulmonary disorders caused by *Aspergillus*

Saprophytic
Aspergillus colonization
Aspergilloma
Inflammatory
Hypersensitivity pneumonitis
Allergic
Asthma with *Aspergillus* sensitization
Allergic *Aspergillus* sinusitis
Allergic bronchopulmonary aspergillosis
Semi-invasive
Chronic pulmonary aspergillosis
Chronic cavitary pulmonary aspergillosis
Chronic fibrosing pulmonary aspergillosis
Chronic necrotizing pulmonary aspergillosis
Invasive
Airway invasive aspergillosis
Invasive pulmonary aspergillosis

pneumonitis, allergic bronchopulmonary aspergillosis (ABPA), chronic pulmonary aspergillosis (CPA), and invasive pulmonary aspergillosis (Table 10.1) [2]. Of these, ABPA is a complex pulmonary disorder caused by immunological reactions against the fungal products released from *A. fumigatus* colonizing the airways of individuals with bronchial asthma or cystic fibrosis (CF) [3]. When fungi other than *A. fumigatus* cause an ABPA-like syndrome, the entity is termed as allergic bronchopulmonary mycosis (ABPM) [4, 5].

ABPA clinically manifests as poorly controlled asthma, expectoration of mucus plugs, hemoptysis, recurrent pulmonary opacities, and bronchiectasis. Despite its description seven decades back by Hinson et al. [6], the diagnosis of ABPA continues to remain elusive. A diagnostic delay of several years between the first symptom and the final diagnosis is not uncommon [7]. In fact, ABPA continues to be mistaken for pulmonary tuberculosis, especially in the developing countries [8]. Currently, ABPA is diagnosed on the basis of a composite criteria including clinical, radiological, and immunological findings. A working group of "ABPA in asthmatics" has been constituted by the International Society of Human and Animal Mycology (ISHAM). This group has laid down new criteria for the diagnosis and staging of ABPA, so as to enable easy recognition and treatment of ABPA [5]. The current chapter summarizes the recent advances made in the identification and management of this enigmatic entity.

10.2 Burden of the Disease

Aspergillus sensitization (AS) is defined by either an elevated level of IgE against *A. fumigatus* or the presence of immediate cutaneous hyperreactivity to *Aspergillus* antigen. The community prevalence of AS and/or ABPA remains unknown. The only community-based data on AS using IgE against *A. fumigatus*, is from the

National Health and Nutrition Examination Survey (United States), where the prevalence was found to be 6.4% among apparently healthy adults [9].

Denning et al. has estimated the global asthma and ABPA burden to be 193 and 4.8 million, respectively, assuming the prevalence of ABPA in asthma of about 2.5% [10]. Intuitively, the burden of ABPA would vary according to the estimates of the prevalence of ABPA in asthma. Using the same model, the burden of adult asthmatics and ABPA patients in India are estimated at 23.7 million and 592,719, respectively. However, if the prevalence rates of ABPA in asthma are changed to 5%, 7%, and 20%, the population of ABPA patients in India rises to 1.2, 1.7, and 4.7 million, respectively [11]. Similarly, the estimates available from other Asian countries including Nepal, Thailand, Philippines, Malaysia, Qatar, and others suggest a significant burden of ABPA (ranging from 35 to 123 cases per 100,000 population) [12–17].

The prevalence of AS and/or ABPA from asthma clinics is substantially higher. In a systematic review, the pooled prevalence of AS and ABPA in asthmatics was shown to be 28% [95% confidence intervals (CI), 24–34] and 13% [95% CI, 8–19], respectively [18]. AS and ABPA may be even more prevalent in patients with severe asthma. In patients with severe acute asthma admitted to the ICU, we found the prevalence of AS and ABPA to be about 51% and 39%, respectively [19]. Although this high prevalence could represent referral bias, other centers from India have also reported a high prevalence of AS (25–32%) and ABPA (7–8%) in asthmatics [20, 21]. The prevalence of AS and ABPA in subjects with CF was found to be 39% [95% CI, 33–45] and 9% [95% CI, 7–11], respectively [22]. However, reliable data on CF from the Asian population are lacking [23].

The true prevalence of ABPM is unknown. Several thermotolerant fungi including *Candia*, *Bipolaris*, *Schizophyllum*, and others have been shown to cause ABPM [24]. However, most reports are in the form of brief cases and case series [4]. However, the burden may be significant. In one study, a high prevalence (96.2%) of sensitization to *A. flavus* was noted, and possibly 30.2% of the subjects had ABPM [25].

10.3 Pathogenesis

Exposure to high concentrations of *Aspergillus* conidia may have an association with ABPA [26, 27]. Environmental factors are however not the primary determinants of disease susceptibility, as not all subjects with bronchial asthma develop ABPA, despite being exposed to the same environment. Fungal spores themselves cannot trigger immune reactions due to the presence of surface hydrophobin, which prevents immune recognition [28]. It is hypothesized that in patients with asthma or CF, the presence of viscid mucus leads to defective clearance of conidia, allowing them to germinate into hyphae. Recently, other risk factors with mucus hypersecretion including chronic obstructive pulmonary disease and pulmonary tuberculosis-related fibrocavitary disease have also been suggested as predisposing factors for ABPA [29, 30]. Certain genetic polymorphisms can cause persistence of *A. fumigatus*, leading to hyphal growth (Table 10.2) [5, 31, 32]. There is emerging evidence that mutations in

Table 10.2 Genetic factors involved in the pathogenesis of allergic bronchopulmonary aspergillosis

HLA associations
Interleukin 10 polymorphisms
Surfactant protein A2 gene polymorphisms
CFTR gene mutations
Transforming growth factor-β polymorphisms
Mannose-binding lectin polymorphisms
Interleukin 4 receptor alpha polymorphisms
CHIT-1 gene polymorphisms
Toll-like receptor 9 gene polymorphisms

HLA human leukocyte antigen, *CFTR* cystic fibrosis transmembrane regulator, *CHIT1* chitinase gene
Refer to references [5, 31] for further details

cystic fibrosis transmembrane regulator (CFTR), which are usually implicated in CF, might also predispose to the development of ABPA in individuals with bronchial asthma [33, 34]. In susceptible asthmatics, several single-nucleotide polymorphisms have recently been identified, which could possibly contribute to the development of ABPA [35]. During fungal growth, several proteins and proteases are released, which are then recognized by the immune effector cells [36], triggering the secretion of several proinflammatory cytokines [37–40]. Murine models have demonstrated that *A. fumigatus* proteases Asp f5 and Asp f13 are important mediators of recruiting inflammatory cells and airway remodeling [41].

On exposure to *A. fumigatus*, the pulmonary dendritic cells prime the naïve Th-cells, transforming them into *Aspergillus*-specific T cells. The latter is usually a Th1 type of response. On the contrary, in hosts susceptible to develop ABPA, a Th2 type of response is triggered with a subsequent secretion of IL-4, IL-5, and IL-13 cytokines [42–46]. A recent study showed that the *Aspergillus* conidia had a unique property of stimulating the human peripheral blood mononuclear cells by a complement receptor-3-dependent pathway, to produce a Th2 skewed response in susceptible individuals [47]. This initiates a profound immune response with the influx of neutrophils, eosinophils, and other inflammatory cells [48, 49], resulting in IgE (total as well as *A. fumigatus*-specific) synthesis (Fig. 10.1) [50]. Understanding the immunopathogenesis of ABPA can pave way for the development of newer treatment options. For instance, the role of vitamin D in suppressing Th2 inflammation and its potential utility in ABPA has been recently explored [51–53].

10.4 Clinical Presentation

ABPA commonly presents as poorly controlled asthma. Expectoration of mucus plugs, fever, hemoptysis, malaise, weight loss, and fleeting pulmonary opacities are the other common manifestations. However, the sensitivity and specificity of these clinical signs and symptoms to diagnose ABPA is poor. For instance, the expectoration of brownish black mucus plugs, believed to be the most characteristic symptom

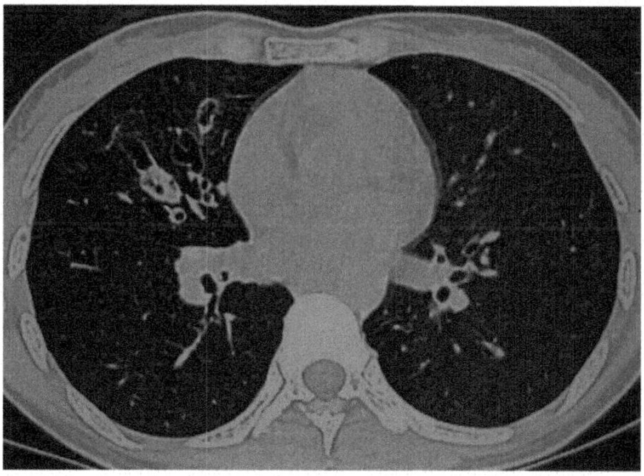

Fig. 10.1 High-resolution computed tomography of the thorax (lung windows) showing bronchiectasis in the medial segment of the right middle lobe extending to the periphery

of ABPA, is seen in only 31–69% of patients [54–56]. Though the classic manifestation of ABPA is with poorly controlled asthma, it is not uncommon in individuals with well-controlled asthma. In fact, several cases are diagnosed only on routine screening performed for the diagnosis of ABPA [8, 56, 57]. In our series of 155 cases, 19% of ABPA had well-controlled asthma [56]. Rarely, ABPA may be detected after the development of complications such as cor pulmonale, type 2 respiratory failure, or secondary amyloidosis [58].

10.5 Investigations for Diagnosing ABPA

The investigations employed in the diagnosis of ABPA include cutaneous testing with *Aspergillus* antigen, IgE levels (total and *A. fumigatus*-specific), eosinophil count, *A. fumigatus*-specific IgG (or *Aspergillus* precipitins), chest radiograph, and high-resolution computed tomography (HRCT) of the chest. Recently, *A. fumigatus*-specific IgE and IgG (detected using fluorescent enzyme immunoassay) have been shown to be more sensitive than skin test against *Aspergillus* and serum precipitins, respectively [59, 60]. HRCT chest findings in ABPA include bronchiectasis (arbitrarily classified as central, if confined to the medial two thirds of the lung), mucoid impaction (hypodense or hyperdense), centrilobular nodules, tree-in-bud opacities, mosaic attenuation, and pleuropulmonary fibrosis [61, 62]. Central bronchiectasis (CB) has been considered the most characteristic imaging feature of ABPA (Fig. 10.1). However, bronchiectasis can extend to the periphery in about 26–39% of the ABPA patients [62, 63]. Moreover, the sensitivity of CB to diagnose ABPA was only 37% in one study [64]. Since bronchiectasis can also occur in asthmatic patients without ABPA, its specificity is also questionable [65]. On the contrary, high-attenuation mucus (HAM, defined as mucus that appears visually denser than the paraspinal skeletal muscle) is a pathognomonic finding (Fig. 10.2) [56, 66–68] and has the highest specificity in diagnosis of ABPA [59]. In fact, the presence of HAM confirms ABPA as the etiology of bronchiectasis [69]. In the later stages,

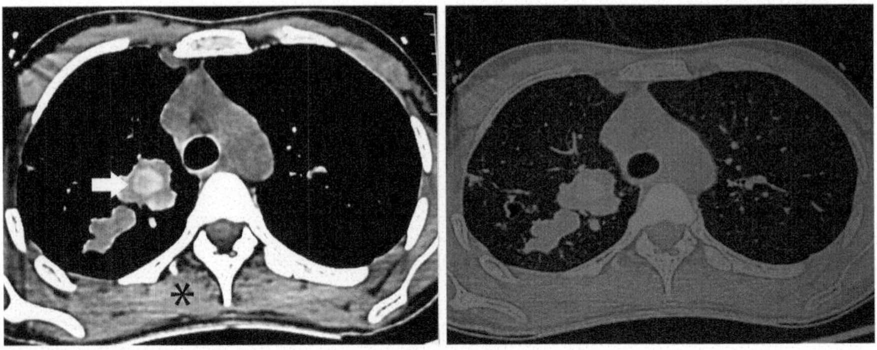

Fig. 10.2 High-resolution computed tomography of the thorax (mediastinal window, right panel) showing high-attenuation mucus (arrow) within a bronchocele (mucus filled bronchiectatic cavity). The mucus is visually denser than the paraspinal skeletal muscle (asterisk). The corresponding lung window is shown in the left panel

pleuropulmonary fibrosis and aspergilloma could represent another complication, namely CPA [70]. In situations where radiation due to CT thorax is to be avoided, MRI may be considered as an alternative [71]. Bronchiectasis with impacted mucous can be demonstrated on MRI [72]. Corresponding to the HAM on CT, an MRI T2 turbo spin can show nodules with hypointense foci [73].

The immunological investigations for diagnosing ABPA utilize the crude antigens of *A. fumigatus*, against which antibodies (IgE and IgG) are detected. The commercial availability of recombinant technology has enabled *A. fumigatus* antigens to be isolated in its pure form. A number of recombinant *Aspergillus* proteins (rAsp) have been evaluated in ABPA (rAsp f1, rAsp f2, rAsp f3, rAsp f4, and rAsp f6) [74–76]. A recent meta-analysis suggested that combination of specific IgE against rAsp antigens may be more useful than IgE against individual rAsp antigens [77]. Other immunological investigation which is in the experimental phase is the basophil activation test, which measures the upregulation of CD203c on the basophils after stimulation by *Aspergillus* antigen [78–80]. Galactomannan (a component of *Aspergillus* cell wall) estimation in serum has been approved for use in the diagnosis of invasive aspergillosis. However, serum galactomannan has a sensitivity and specificity of 26% and 82%, respectively, in ABPA [81]. Thus, the utility of serum galactomannan in ABPA seems to be limited [82].

10.6 Diagnostic Criteria

The Patterson criteria (eight major and three minor) were the most widely used criteria for diagnosing ABPA complicating asthma. However, there were several problems with the Patterson criteria. There was a lack of consensus on the number of criteria required for a diagnosis, with different centers using different number of criteria [83]. Also, the criteria offered equal weightage to all the individual components, while in reality, certain components appear more important than others.

Table 10.3 Diagnostic criteria for allergic bronchopulmonary aspergillosis (Adapted from references [5, 84])

ISHAM-ABPA working group criteria
A. *Predisposing conditions*
Bronchial asthma, cystic fibrosis
B. *Essential criteria (both must be met)*
• Serum *Aspergillus fumigatus*-specific IgE levels >0.35 kUA/L or positive type I *Aspergillus* skin test
• Elevated serum total IgE levels >1000 IU/mL[a]
C. *Additional criteria (at least two of three)*
• Presence of precipitating (or IgG) antibodies against *A. fumigatus* in serum
• Thoracic imaging findings consistent with ABPA[b]
• Peripheral blood eosinophil count >500 cells/μL (may be historical)
Proposed modifications to ISHAM-ABPA working group criteria[c]
A. *Predisposing conditions*
Bronchial asthma, cystic fibrosis, chronic obstructive pulmonary disease, post-tuberculous fibrocavitary disease
B. *Essential criteria (both must be met)*
• Serum *Aspergillus fumigatus*-specific IgE levels >0.35 kUA/L
• Elevated serum total IgE levels >1000 IU/mL[a]
C. *Additional criteria (at least two of three)*
• Presence of IgG antibodies against *A. fumigatus* in serum (Phadia, Immulite, and others)
• Thoracic imaging findings consistent with ABPA[b]
• Peripheral blood eosinophil count >500 cells/μL (may be historical)

[a]If all other criteria are present, an IgE value <1000 IU/mL is also acceptable

[b]Chest radiographic features consistent with ABPA include transitory findings such as consolidation, nodules, tram-track opacities, toothpaste/finger-in-glove opacities, fleeting opacities or findings of permanent lung destruction including parallel line and ring shadows, bronchiectasis, and pleuropulmonary fibrosis

[c]The newly proposed criteria might have a few modifications: (1) addition of other risk factors predisposing to ABPA, (2) *Aspergillus* skin test positivity to be completely replaced by *A. fumigatus*-specific IgE >0.35 kUA/L, (3) serum precipitins to be replaced by serum *A. fumigatus*-specific IgG

Finally, there was no cut-off for the IgE levels and eosinophil count. The criteria suggested by the ISHAM-ABPA working group have addressed the limitations of the previous criteria (Table 10.3). The ISHAM-ABPA criteria continues to evolve, and in our opinion, certain modifications will further improve its diagnostic performance (Table 10.3) [84]. The diagnostic criteria for ABPM are similar to ABPA, except that the sensitization to the specific fungi should be documented [3, 4, 85].

10.7 Diagnostic Algorithm

In the past, cutaneous testing was the preferred method of screening asthmatic patients for ABPA [8, 19, 29, 56, 62, 68, 86–91]. However, *A. fumigatus*-specific IgE (>0.35 kUA/L) should be the preferred modality to screen asthmatic patients for

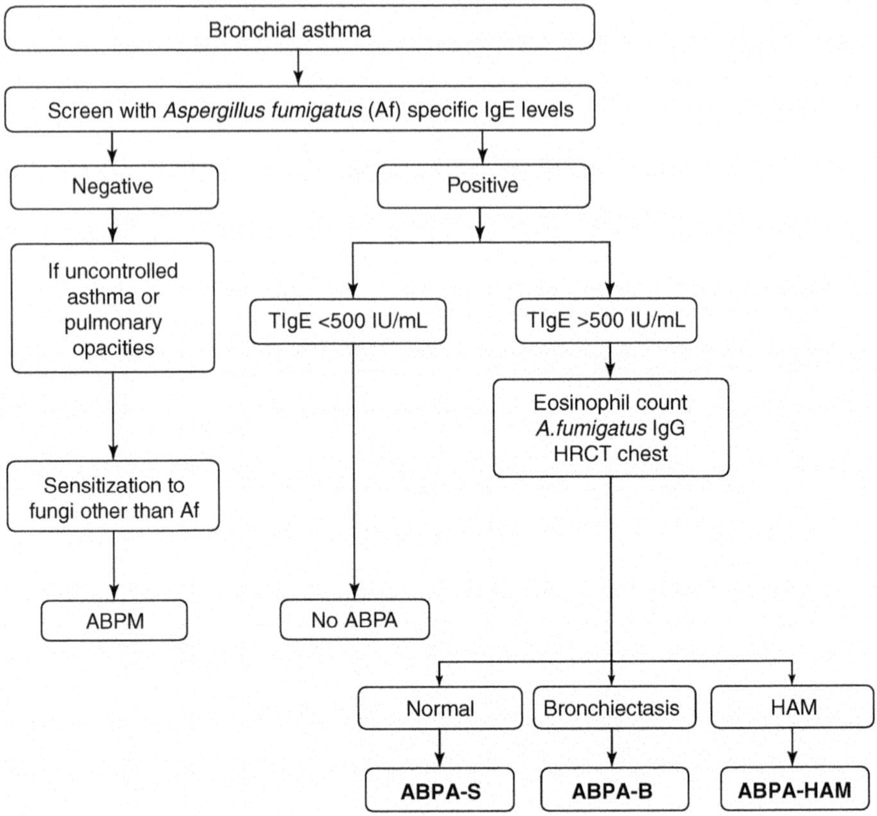

Fig. 10.3 A simple algorithm for the diagnosis of ABPA

ABPA, as it is the most sensitive test available for the diagnosis of ABPA. Using latent class analysis, the sensitivity of *Aspergillus* skin test (type 1 reaction) and *A. fumigatus*-specific IgE level (>0.35 kUA/L) was 88–94% and 100%, respectively [59]. Thus, skin testing can potentially miss 6–12% of ABPA cases. Hence, all subjects with asthma should be screened for ABPA using *A. fumigatus*-specific IgE (Fig. 10.3). If it is negative (<0.35 kUA/L), further investigations for ABPA are generally not required. Routine diagnostic testing for ABPM is not required given the rarity of the disorder. In those with *A. fumigatus*-specific IgE >0.35 kUA/L, the next step is to obtain serum total IgE. A total IgE <500 IU/mL excludes ABPA in the vast majority. In subjects with serum total IgE >500 IU/mL, other investigations including *A. fumigatus*-specific IgG, peripheral blood eosinophil count, and HRCT of the thorax are required to both confirm the diagnosis and determine the radiological stage and the extent of the disease.

10.8 Staging

Once the diagnosis of ABPA is confirmed, the disease needs to be staged clinically and radiologically. Besides enabling prognostication, staging also helps in defining response to therapy and early identification of exacerbations. Initially, ABPA was classified into five stages [92], but due to the lack of precise definitions, there was considerable ambiguity in this classification [8]. The ISHAM-ABPA working group now classifies ABPA into seven stages (stage 0–6) with accurate definitions (Table 10.4). However, a patient need not pass through the stages in a sequential manner.

Table 10.4 Clinical staging of ABPA in asthma [5]

Stage	Definition	Features
0	Asymptomatic	• No previous diagnosis of ABPA • Controlled asthma (as per the GINA/EPR-3 guidelines) • Satisfying the diagnostic criteria of ABPA (Table 10.1)
1	Acute	• No previous diagnosis of ABPA • Uncontrolled asthma/symptoms consistent with ABPA • Meeting the diagnostic criteria of ABPA
1a	With mucoid impaction	Mucoid impaction observed on thoracic imaging or bronchoscopy
1b	Without mucoid impaction	Absence of mucoid impaction on thoracic imaging or bronchoscopy
2	Response	• Clinical and/or radiological improvement AND • Decline in IgE by ≥25% of baseline at 8 weeks
3	Exacerbation	• Clinical and/or radiological worsening AND • Increase in IgE by ≥50% from the baseline established during remission/response
4	Remission	• Sustained clinicoradiological improvement AND • IgE levels persisting at or below baseline (or increase by <50%) for ≥6 months off treatment
5a	Treatment-dependent ABPA	• ≥2 exacerbations within 6 months of discontinuing therapy OR • Worsening of clinical and/or radiological condition, accompanied by immunological worsening (rise in IgE levels) on tapering oral steroids/azoles
5b	Glucocorticoid-dependent asthma	Systemic glucocorticoids are required for asthma control, while the ABPA activity is controlled (as indicated by IgE levels and thoracic imaging)
6	Advanced ABPA	• Extensive bronchiectasis due to ABPA on chest imaging AND • Complications (such as cor pulmonale and/or chronic type II respiratory failure)

EPR 3 third expert panel report, *GINA* global initiative against asthma

Stage 0 includes patients with well-controlled asthma where ABPA is detected on routine screening. On the other hand, symptomatic patients fulfilling all the diagnostic criteria for ABPA (Table 10.3) are classified as **stage 1**. Patients in stage 1 are further subclassified as Ia or Ib depending on the presence or absence of mucoid impaction. Stages 2 through 5 are encountered during therapy of ABPA. Once treatment is initiated, there is improvement in symptoms, pulmonary function, and chest radiograph with a decline in IgE levels by at least 25% in 8 weeks; this is labeled as response (**stage 2**). Total IgE levels are measured periodically to determine the "new" baseline value of an individual patient. Thereafter, a 50% increase in serum IgE levels over the new baseline, along with clinical or radiological worsening, is defined as an ABPA exacerbation (**stage 3**). Patients with only clinical worsening and no increase in total IgE (by >50%) or radiological worsening are classified as asthma exacerbation. Patients with HRCT chest findings of fungal ball and/or HAM are likely to experience frequent exacerbations [68, 90]. ABPA is said to be in remission (**stage 4**), if there is no exacerbation over the next 6 months of stopping therapy. Patients in remission should be followed up every 3 months during the first year and then annually. Further monitoring may be tailored depending on the patient's clinical status. Patients in **stage 5** are those with either "treatment-dependent ABPA" wherein the disease requires repeated courses of glucocorticoids (or azoles) to prevent ABPA exacerbations or the "glucocorticoid-dependent asthma" group, which requires prolonged use of steroids for asthma control. Patients with widespread bronchiectasis and/or fibrosis who develop either type II respiratory failure or cor pulmonale are classified as **stage 6**. It is important to remember that even in advanced stages, ABPA can be active, both clinically and immunologically, and may require treatment [93, 94].

ABPA was previously classified as ABPA with central bronchiectasis (ABPA-CB) or serological ABPA (ABPA-S) depending on whether bronchiectasis was present or absent, respectively [91, 95, 96]. Another stage of ABPA namely ABPA-CB with other radiological findings (ABPA-CB-ORF) has also been proposed [97]. Our group had proposed classifying ABPA into ABPA-S, ABPA-CB, and ABPA-CB with HAM (ABPA-CB-HAM) as this classification scheme was most consistently associated with immunological severity [68]. The ISHAM-ABPA working group has laid down a classification incorporating all the radiological findings of ABPA. ABPA is now classified into four major radiological categories (Table 10.5), namely serological ABPA (ABPA-S), ABPA with bronchiectasis (ABPA-B), ABPA with high-attenuation mucus (ABPA-HAM), and ABPA with chronic pleuropulmonary fibrosis (ABPA-CPF). The radiological staging is not only helpful in predicting disease severity but also has prognostic value [61].

Table 10.5 Radiological classification of ABPA based on CT chest findings [5]

ABPA-S: Serological ABPA
ABPA-B: ABPA with bronchiectasis
ABPA-HAM: ABPA with high-attenuation mucus
ABPA-CPF: ABPA with chronic pleuropulmonary fibrosis

10.9 Natural History

The natural history of ABPA remains unknown. However, most experts believe that sensitization to the fungus is the first step in its development [85]. It is also not clear whether ABPA-S is the earliest stage in the pathogenesis of ABPA or represents a subgroup of patients who are genetically predisposed not to develop bronchiectasis. The course of ABPA is characterized by recurrent episodes of remission and relapse, either spontaneously or despite treatment. The disease is a non-acute, low-grade respiratory syndrome of varying severity that may lurk for several years without diagnosis. There is a persistent airway inflammation with tissue damage and airway remodeling. Untreated ABPA can progress relentlessly, resulting in bronchiectasis and/or pulmonary fibrosis. Hence it is prudent to screen all asthmatic patients for ABPA [83].

10.10 Complications

The complications of ABPA include worsening of asthma control manifested by recurrent asthma and ABPA exacerbations, and the development of bronchiectasis. Some patients with ABPA, especially those with delayed diagnosis or suboptimal treatment, can develop extensive bronchiectasis and pleuropulmonary fibrosis culminating in the development of type 2 respiratory failure and cor pulmonale. An occasional patient with ABPA has presented with pulmonary hypertension [98]. Another important complication of ABPA is the development of chronic pulmonary aspergillosis [99]. Other complications include large airway collapse, which may necessitate therapeutic bronchoscopy [100].

10.11 Pharmacotherapy of ABPA

The management strategy for ABPA includes the use of glucocorticoids to suppress the immune hyperactivity and antifungals (azoles) to decrease the fungal burden in the airways. The goals of therapy are asthma control, maintenance of normal activity, control of pulmonary inflammation, prevention of acute exacerbations of ABPA and preventing or arresting the progression of bronchiectasis (and pulmonary fibrosis). Three randomized controlled trials performed in the last decade have clarified the uncertainties surrounding the treatment of ABPA, to a certain extent [101–103].

10.11.1 Glucocorticoids

Oral glucocorticoids: are the current treatment of choice in ABPA [8, 56, 68, 86, 90]. However, the dose and duration has varied from center to center. The two commonly used regimens were the high-dose (prednisolone, 0.75 mg/kg for 6 weeks, 0.5 mg/kg for 6 weeks, then tapered every 6 weeks by 5 mg, and discontinued after

8–10 months) [8, 104], and the medium-dose protocol (prednisolone 0.5 mg/kg/day for 2 weeks, then alternate days for 6–8 weeks, and finally tapered every 2 weeks by 5–10 mg and discontinued after 3–5 months) [105]. A head-to-head comparison of these two regimens found them to be equally efficacious, in terms of reducing the exacerbation at 1 year and the proportion of subjects remaining glucocorticoid-dependent at 2 years [101]. Although a composite response (clinical, radiological, and immunological outcome) at 6 weeks was significantly better in the high-dose arm, this was also associated with a significantly higher adverse effects. Thus, medium-dose glucocorticoids should be the preferred initial therapy for ABPA complicating asthma and high-dose steroids reserved for those not responding to the former.

Inhaled corticosteroids: have no role in the primary treatment of ABPA, even though inhaled steroids achieve high airway concentrations. The level of evidence on the use of inhaled steroids in ABPA is very poor, and in most of these studies, the patients continued to receive oral steroids [106–111]. In one study, inhaled steroids failed to control the immunological activity in patients with ABPA, while the use of oral steroids led to a clinical as well as immunological response [87]. Inhaled steroids should therefore be used only for asthma control.

Intravenous glucocorticoids: Pulse doses of intravenous methylprednisolone (15 mg/kg, maximum of 1 g) are useful in ABPA exacerbations, refractory to other therapies [112]. Anecdotal reports describe its usefulness in both CF and asthma patients with ABPA [112–114]. Long-term steroid usage in ABPA may result in the downregulation of steroid receptors, thereby producing a steroid-resistant state and rendering the usual oral dose ineffective (0.5 mg/kg of prednisolone). Pulse doses of glucocorticoids are believed to overcome this steroid resistance by its non-genomic actions that are independent of the glucocorticoid receptors [115]. Pulse doses of methylprednisolone have also been used in pediatric ABPA to avoid the side effects associated with daily glucocorticoid use [116].

10.11.2 Antifungal agents

Antifungal agents with activity against *A. fumigatus* would diminish fungal load in the airways and thus attenuate the immune responses in ABPA. Although systemic corticosteroids are highly effective in ABPA, there are two major issues with the use of steroids. First, almost 50% of patients experience an exacerbation once steroids are tapered, and almost 20–45% can become glucocorticoid-dependent [8, 95]. Moreover, the use of steroids on a prolonged basis is associated with increased risk of adverse events, including serious ones [117, 118]. Natamycin, fluconazole, and ketoconazole are not effective in ABPA as they have limited efficacy against *A. fumigatus* [119–121].

Triazoles: The currently available triazoles have an acceptable side effect profile and can be used in ABPA. Two RCTs have also evaluated itraconazole in glucocorticoid-dependent ABPA [122, 123]. In one study, 55 subjects with "steroid-dependent" ABPA were randomized to receive either 400 mg/day of oral itraconazole or placebo for 4 months. The overall composite response criteria (reduction in corticosteroid dose by ≥50%;a decline in total IgE by 25% or more; and at least one of the following [increase in exercise capacity by ≥25%, improvement in pulmonary function test values by 25% or more, radiographic resolution]) were better with itraconazole. However, the study failed to demonstrate statistical significance when each outcome was examined separately [122]. In another study, 29 "clinically stable" ABPA patients (50% were already on steroids) were randomized to either itraconazole therapy (400 mg/day orally) or placebo. Itraconazole resulted in a significant decline in total IgE levels and sputum inflammatory markers. The authors also noted a decrease in the number of exacerbations requiring glucocorticoid therapy, though the study was not designed to evaluate exacerbations [123]. Pooled analysis showed that itraconazole could significantly decrease IgE levels by ≥25% compared to placebo, but with no significant improvement in lung function [124].

Until recently, the role of azole monotherapy vis-à-vis glucocorticoids in acute stage of ABPA remained unclear. Two RCTs are now available in acute-stage ABPA complicating asthma where azole monotherapy has been compared with glucocorticoids. The first RCT compared medium doses of glucocorticoid ($n = 63$) with itraconazole ($n = 68$) and showed a significantly better composite response at 6 weeks with glucocorticoids (100% vs. 88% respectively, $p = 0.007$) [102]. Nevertheless, considering the safety profile and the fact that majority of patients with ABPA did show a response, it was concluded that itraconazole could still be considered as the initial therapy for acute-stage ABPA. This is especially pertinent in those cases where adverse effects of glucocorticoids are a concern. The second RCT was an exploratory study comparing voriconazole monotherapy ($n = 25$) and medium-dose glucocorticoids ($n = 25$) in subjects with acute-stage ABPA [103]. The primary outcomes (composite response criteria and ABPA exacerbations till 2 years) were similar in both the groups. Voriconazole was as effective as glucocorticoids and had fewer side effects (transient derangements in liver function, photosensitivity, and visual disturbance). Newer azoles such as posaconazole are also possibly efficacious in ABPA [125]. All the existing evidence is in ABPA complicating asthma, and the role of azoles in CF-ABPA has not been evaluated in randomized trials.

Nebulized amphotericin B: Amphotericin B binds to the fungal cell membrane, leading to pore formation, increased cell permeability, and cell death. Inhaled amphotericin B achieves concentration in bronchoalveolar lavage fluid well above the minimal inhibitory concentration of *A. fumigatus* (0.5 mg/L), while the corresponding serum concentration of amphotericin is negligible. Though several case reports and case series describe its usefulness, the efficacy of nebulized amphotericin B in ABPA exacerbation seems to be limited [126]. It may be considered in subjects where other options are either unavailable or not tolerated. Nebulized amphotericin B along with nebulized budesonide has also been used in the treatment of ABPA complicating CF [127–130]. In a pilot study, we randomized ABPA (complicating asthma) subjects with recurrent exacerbations (≥2) to receive either nebulized budesonide ($n = 9$) or nebulized amphotericin B (conventional) along with nebulized budesonide ($n = 12$), after inducing response with either prednisolone or itraconazole [131]. The amphotericin B arm had a significantly lesser number of patients experiencing exacerbation (8% vs. 66.7% in the budesonide arm, $p = 0.016$), though the time to first exacerbation was similar in both the study groups. Thus, in selected patients with recurrent ABPA exacerbations, nebulized amphotericin B may have a role. However, larger trials are required. Alteration in the pulmonary surfactant due to the deoxycholate component of conventional amphotericin B and the resultant bronchospasm may be averted with the use of lipid formulations of amphotericin [132].

10.11.3 Monoclonal Antibodies

Omalizumab, a humanized monoclonal antibody against IgE, has been evaluated in ABPA. Data from small case series suggest marginal improvement in symptoms, lung function, and a decline in the requirement of oral steroids [133–136]. However, there are conflicting reports, with some suggesting improvement, while no significant benefit was observed in few other studies [137–139]. A small randomized double-blind placebo-controlled trial ($n = 13$) with a cross-over design showed that omalizumab was superior to placebo in chronic ABPA complicating asthma. There was a reduction in the exacerbation frequency during the treatment phase (with omalizumab) and a decline in fractional exhaled nitric oxide [140].

Mepolizumab and benralizumab (monoclonal antibodies against interleukin-5) either alone or in combination with omalizumab has also been tried in few cases of refractory ABPA [141–144]. The role of these monoclonal antibodies in the initial management of ABPA currently remains unknown, and further trials are required.

10.11.4 Supportive Therapies

Nebulized hypertonic saline (3%, 3–5 mL) benefits by reducing the viscosity of sputum [145]. Hypertonic saline may precipitate bronchospasm; hence, the first dose of nebulization should be supervised and preceded by inhaled salbutamol. Hypertonic saline is not recommended for patients with poor lung function (FEV1 < 1 L), thereby restricting its utility where it is most useful. *Pneumococcal and influenza vaccines* are recommended in subjects with ABPA, though disease-specific guidelines are lacking. Poor response to vaccination (with 23-valent polysaccharide vaccine) as compared to healthy adults suggests that an alternative vaccination strategy may be superior in ABPA patients, such as delaying vaccination till the patient is off glucocorticoids or combining a polysaccharide and 13-valent conjugate vaccine [146]. When ABPA progresses to end-stage lung disease, lung transplantation is the only available option; ABPA can rarely recur in donor lungs [147, 148]. Long-term antibiotic therapy may be required in patients who have recurrent bacterial colonization, while azithromycin therapy may be required in those experiencing recurrent exacerbations of bronchiectasis unrelated to ABPA [149].

10.12 Treatment Protocol

Not all patients with ABPA require treatment (Table 10.6). Patients with ABPA-S and well-controlled asthma (stage 0) require only treatment for asthma control and close monitoring to ensure that the disease is not progressing. However, patients in stage 0 with organ damage such as bronchiectasis (or fleeting pulmonary opacities) generally require treatment as outlined below. Symptomatic patients with ABPA (stage 1 or stage 3) should be initially treated with steroids (or antifungal azoles). Table 10.7 summarizes the various treatment options available and their dosages. The endpoint of therapy in ABPA is a 25–50% decline in total IgE, which is usually associated with clinical, spirometric, and radiological improvements [86, 150]. Patients presenting with large airway collapse should be reassessed after 3–4 weeks of steroid therapy. If the collapse is persistent, therapeutic bronchoscopy should be performed. Steroid treatment is initially continued for at least 4–6 months. For the first exacerbation, we prefer a combination of glucocorticoids and itraconazole. In those with recurrent exacerbations, one may consider prolonged therapy with any one or more of the following: itraconazole, low-dose corticosteroids, omalizumab, monthly pulses of methyl prednisolone, or nebulized amphotericin B. High doses of inhaled steroids should not be used as a sole therapy in the treatment of ABPA. While instituting the combination of inhaled steroids (especially budesonide, occasionally fluticasone) and itraconazole, the minimum required dose of inhaled steroid should be used. Otherwise, some patients can develop cushingoid effects and secondary adrenal insufficiency [151–155].

10.13 Monitoring of Patients

Patients should be closely monitored, initially every 6–8 weeks with serum IgE (total) values, chest radiograph, and spirometry. The clinical response is reflected by symptomatic and radiologic improvement along with decline in the total serum IgE

Table 10.6 Stage-wise treatment of patients with ABPA

Stage	Treatment
0	ABPA-S may not require any treatment, close follow-up ABPA-B and other stages: as for stage 1
1	Prednisolone (or itraconazole or voriconazole) for at least 4–6 months
2	Close observation with follow-up every 6–8 weeks
3	Prednisolone plus itraconazole (200 mg twice daily for at least 4–6 months)
4	Close observation with follow-up every 3–6 months
5	Initial exacerbation to be controlled with steroids followed by any of the following (itraconazole, low-dose glucocorticoids, omalizumab, monthly pulses of methyl prednisolone or nebulized amphotericin B)
6	Pharmacological control of asthma, steroids, or azoles depending on the disease activity, oxygen therapy, domiciliary noninvasive ventilation

Table 10.7 Summary of treatment options for ABPA and their dosages

Oral glucocorticoids
Prednisolone (or equivalent) 0.5 mg/kg/day for 4 weeks, 0.25 mg/kg/day for 4 weeks, 0.125 mg/kg/day for 4 weeks, taper over the next month; total duration: 4 months
Oral azoles (therapeutic drug monitoring to titrate drug doses are recommended)
Oral itraconazole 200 mg twice a day, for 16–24 weeks
Oral voriconazole 200 mg twice a day, for 16–24 weeks
Nebulized amphotericin B
Amphotericin B deoxycholate Daily: 5–40 mg twice daily Intermittent: 20 mg (10 mg twice daily) thrice weekly
Liposomal amphotericin B Intermittent: 25 mg twice weekly
Amphotericin B lipid complex Intermittent: 50 mg twice weekly
Pulse methylprednisolone
15 mg/kg/day (maximum 1 g) given as intravenous infusion for three consecutive days
Omalizumab
375 mg subcutaneous injection every 2 weeks for a period of 4–6 months
Inhaled corticosteroids
Single-agent inhaled corticosteroid therapy should not be used for controlling immunological activity of ABPA. However, they are useful agents in the management of asthma
Follow-up and monitoring
• Patients are followed up with monitoring of clinical symptoms (cough, dyspnea), chest radiograph, and total IgE levels, every 8 weeks • Monitor for adverse effects of treatment • Satisfactory response to therapy is suggested when there is clinical and/or radiological improvement along with at least 25% decline in IgE levels • Monitor IgE frequently to establish the "new" baseline level for an individual patient • Clinical and/or radiological worsening along with 50% increase in IgE levels suggests an ABPA exacerbation

values. Once remission is achieved, patients should be followed up initially every 3–6 months and then at least annually. Although some patients may enter into prolonged period of remission, exacerbations are known to occur several years after remission [156]. Patients should be counseled regarding the side effects of therapy, especially that of glucocorticoids.

10.14 ABPA in Special Situations

ABPA complicating cystic fibrosis: The association of CF and ABPA was first reported in 1965 [157]. Allergic aspergillosis is now recognized as a potential and catastrophic complication of CF [158]. The prevalence of AS and ABPA in CF ranges from 27% to 41% and 6% to 10%, respectively [3]. The differentiation of CF-lung disease from ABPA can be challenging, as they share common features including wheeze, fleeting opacities, mucous plugging, and bronchiectasis. The development of ABPA in CF (occurs in 8–10% of CF patients) [159] has been associated with higher rates of microbial colonization, deterioration of lung functions, poor nutritional status, and complications (such as pneumothorax and hemoptysis) [160–162]. Further, the immunological parameters may improve spontaneously, causing difficulties in diagnosis [163]. In this context, the finding of HAM in patients with CF confirms ABPA as the cause of pulmonary manifestations [69]. The CF foundation criteria is used for the diagnosis and management of ABPA complicating CF, and the treatment strategy is similar to that of ABPA complicating asthma [164].

ABPA without underlying risk factors—"ABPA de novo": ABPA most commonly develops in subjects with asthma or CF. The occurrence of ABPA has also been occasionally demonstrated in other disorders including chronic obstructive pulmonary disease [29, 165, 166], bronchiectasis (idiopathic [167], post-tubercular [30, 168], ciliary dyskinesia [169], Swyer-James-MacLeod's syndrome [170], and chronic granulomatous disease [171]). Occasionally, ABPA can occur without any underlying disease, the so-called de novo ABPA [172]. The de novo presentation is often mistaken for other pulmonary disorders because of the absence of asthma [173].

ABPA and chronic pulmonary aspergillosis: Chronic pulmonary aspergillosis (CPA) represents a chronic infection of the lung parenchyma, in contrast to ABPA which is an allergic response to *A. fumigatus* [174]. However, differentiating ABPA from CPA may be difficult, as the clinical features are nonspecific and several investigations (radiological and immunological) are common to both the diseases. In fact, a recent study showed that 5% CPA patients satisfy all the criteria of ABPA, and 22% met the obligatory criteria for ABPA [175]. Also, some patients of ABPA may go on to develop CPA [99]. The treatments of these two diseases are different (glucocorticoids for ABPA and antifungal triazoles for CPA), and hence, it is important that they are classified correctly. Currently, the management of patients with overlap of ABPA and CPA is not clear.

The simultaneous occurrence of ABPA and aspergilloma during the initial stages of the disease probably represents a severe form of ABPA with increased propensity for recurrent relapses [90]. In this circumstance, oral glucocorticoids are beneficial as their administration alleviates asthma, thus decreasing sputum production [176]. In fact, we have shown disappearance of aspergilloma after treatment with oral steroids alone [90]. In the later stages, aspergilloma and pleuropulmonary fibrosis could represent a manifestation of CPA [70]. Azoles may be warranted in this situation, and glucocorticoids are reserved for those with demonstrable disease activity due to ABPA. Occasionally, aspergilloma can antedate the diagnosis of ABPA. It is believed that some of these patients may harbor the genetic mutations listed in Table 10.2, and *Aspergillus* antigens trigger immunologic activation leading to ABPA [176–178].

Sinobronchial allergic mycosis (SAM) syndrome: Allergic *Aspergillus* rhinosinusitis (AARS) represents an allergic response to *A. fumigatus* within the sinus cavity [179]. It may coexist with ABPA [180] and is then referred to as the SAM syndrome [181]. Patients present with epistaxis, nasal obstruction, rhinorrhea, and headache. The diagnosis of AARS is suspected radiologically if there is presence of

HAM and/or bony erosion visualized on paranasal CT scan and is confirmed by histopathological demonstration of fungal elements, allergic mucin, and Charcot–Leyden crystals [182]. The mycological and immunological features of allergic fungal sinusitis resemble ABPA. The treatment of allergic fungal rhinosinusitis in contrast to ABPA is primarily surgical [183].

ABPA in children: Data from children with ABPA are sparse [184]. The prevalence of ABPA in children ranges from 2% of asthmatic children in Russia to 18.2% of CF patients in India [23, 185, 186]. Treatment protocols are extrapolated from studies in adults, and the principles are similar. However, since growth retardation is a concern, the lowest possible dose of glucocorticoid is used and for the shortest duration possible. Steroid sparing agents such as antifungals, omalizumab, and nebulized amphotericin may be considered for the maintenance of remission [187, 188].

ABPA during pregnancy and lactation: Glucocorticoids are the treatment of choice during pregnancy. Though the use of itraconazole has not been associated with increased congenital anomalies in two studies, higher rates of miscarriage were observed in the itraconazole exposed subjects [189, 190]. Nebulized amphotericin may be safe in pregnancy [191]. Anecdotal reports suggest that omalizumab has not been associated with congenital anomalies, prematurity, or low birth weight [192]. However, we prefer using glucocorticoids, and in those with contraindications, we use inhaled amphotericin B.

References

1. Geiser DM, Klich MA, Frisvad JC, Peterson SW, Varga J, Samson RA. The current status of species recognition and identification in Aspergillus. Stud Mycol. 2007;59:1–10. https://doi.org/10.3114/sim.2007.59.01.
2. Agarwal R, Chakrabarti A. Epidemiology of allergic bronchopulmonary aspergillosis. In: Pasqualotto AC, editor. Aspergillosis: from diagnosis to prevention. New York: Springer; 2010. p. 671–88.
3. Agarwal R. Allergic bronchopulmonary aspergillosis. Chest. 2009;135(3):805–26. https://doi.org/10.1378/chest.08-2586.
4. Chowdhary A, Agarwal K, Kathuria S, Gaur SN, Randhawa HS, Meis JF. Allergic bronchopulmonary mycosis due to fungi other than Aspergillus: a global overview. Crit Rev Microbiol. 2014;40(1):30–48. https://doi.org/10.3109/1040841x.2012.754401.
5. Agarwal R, Chakrabarti A, Shah A, Gupta D, Meis JF, Guleria R, et al. Allergic bronchopulmonary aspergillosis: review of literature and proposal of new diagnostic and classification criteria. Clin Exp Allergy. 2013;43(8):850–73. https://doi.org/10.1111/cea.12141.
6. Hinson KF, Moon AJ, Plummer NS. Broncho-pulmonary aspergillosis; a review and a report of eight new cases. Thorax. 1952;7(4):317–33.
7. Kirsten D, Nowak D, Rabe KF, Magnussen H. Diagnosis of bronchopulmonary aspergillosis is often made too late. Med Klin (Munich). 1993;88(6):353–6.
8. Agarwal R, Gupta D, Aggarwal AN, Behera D, Jindal SK. Allergic bronchopulmonary aspergillosis: lessons from 126 patients attending a chest clinic in North India. Chest. 2006;130(2):442–8. https://doi.org/10.1378/chest.130.2.442.
9. Gergen PJ, Arbes SJ Jr, Calatroni A, Mitchell HE, Zeldin DC. Total IgE levels and asthma prevalence in the US population: results from the national health and nutrition examination survey 2005-2006. J Allergy Clin Immunol. 2009;124(3):447–53. https://doi.org/10.1016/j.jaci.2009.06.011.

10. Denning DW, Pleuvry A, Cole DC. Global burden of allergic bronchopulmonary aspergillosis with asthma and its complication chronic pulmonary aspergillosis in adults. Med Mycol. 2013;51(4):361–70. https://doi.org/10.3109/13693786.2012.738312.
11. Agarwal R, Denning DW, Chakrabarti A. Estimation of the burden of chronic and allergic pulmonary aspergillosis in India. PLoS One. 2014;9(12):e114745. https://doi.org/10.1371/journal.pone.0114745.
12. Gugnani HC, Denning DW, Rahim R, Sadat A, Belal M, Mahbub MS. Burden of serious fungal infections in Bangladesh. Eur J Clin Microbiol Infect Dis. 2017;36(6):993–7. https://doi.org/10.1007/s10096-017-2921-z.
13. Khwakhali US, Denning DW. Burden of serious fungal infections in Nepal. Mycoses. 2015;58(Suppl 5):45–50. https://doi.org/10.1111/myc.12393.
14. Taj-Aldeen SJ, Chandra P, Denning DW. Burden of fungal infections in Qatar. Mycoses. 2015;58(Suppl 5):51–7. https://doi.org/10.1111/myc.12386.
15. Velayuthan RD, Samudi C, Lakhbeer Singh HK, Ng KP, Shankar EM, Denning DW. Estimation of the burden of serious human fungal infections in Malaysia. J Fungi (Basel). 2018;4(1):38. https://doi.org/10.3390/jof4010038.
16. Batac MCR, Denning D. Serious fungal infections in the Philippines. Eur J Clin Microbiol Infect Dis. 2017;36(6):937–41. https://doi.org/10.1007/s10096-017-2918-7.
17. Chayakulkeeree M, Denning DW. Serious fungal infections in Thailand. Eur J Clin Microbiol Infect Dis. 2017;36(6):931–5. https://doi.org/10.1007/s10096-017-2927-6.
18. Agarwal R, Aggarwal AN, Gupta D, Jindal SK. *Aspergillus* hypersensitivity and allergic bronchopulmonary aspergillosis in patients with bronchial asthma: systematic review and meta-analysis. Int J Tuberc Lung Dis. 2009;13(8):936–44.
19. Agarwal R, Nath A, Aggarwal AN, Gupta D, Chakrabarti A. Aspergillus hypersensitivity and allergic bronchopulmonary aspergillosis in patients with acute severe asthma in a respiratory intensive care unit in North India. Mycoses. 2010;53(2):138–43. https://doi.org/10.1111/j.1439-0507.2008.01680.x.
20. Ghosh T, Dey A, Biswas D, Chatterjee S, Haldar N, Maiti PK. Aspergillus hypersensitivity and allergic bronchopulmonary aspergillosis among asthma patients in eastern India. J Indian Med Assoc. 2010;108(12):863–5.
21. Sarkar A, Mukherjee A, Ghoshal AG, Kundu S, Mitra S. Occurrence of allergic bronchopulmonary mycosis in patients with asthma: an Eastern India experience. Lung India. 2010;27(4):212–6. https://doi.org/10.4103/0970-2113.71949.
22. Maturu VN, Agarwal R. Prevalence of Aspergillus sensitization and allergic bronchopulmonary aspergillosis in cystic fibrosis: systematic review and meta-analysis. Clin Exp Allergy. 2015;45(12):1765–78. https://doi.org/10.1111/cea.12595.
23. Sharma VK, Raj D, Xess I, Lodha R, Kabra SK. Prevalence and risk factors for allergic bronchopulmonary aspergillosis in Indian children with cystic fibrosis. Indian Pediatr. 2014;51(4):295–7.
24. Woolnough K, Fairs A, Pashley CH, Wardlaw AJ. Allergic fungal airway disease: pathophysiologic and diagnostic considerations. Curr Opin Pulm Med. 2015;21(1):39–47. https://doi.org/10.1097/mcp.0000000000000129.
25. Sehgal IS, Choudhary H, Dhooria S, Aggarwal AN, Bansal S, Garg M, et al. Prevalence of sensitization to Aspergillus flavus in patients with allergic bronchopulmonary aspergillosis. Med Mycol. 2019;57(3):270–6. https://doi.org/10.1093/mmy/myy012.
26. Kramer MN, Kurup VP, Fink JN. Allergic bronchopulmonary aspergillosis from a contaminated dump site. Am Rev Respir Dis. 1989;140(4):1086–8.
27. Allmers H, Huber H, Baur X. Two year follow-up of a garbage collector with allergic broncho pulmonary aspergillosis (ABPA). Am J Ind Med. 2000;37(4):438–42. https://doi.org/10.1002/(SICI)1097-0274(200004)37:4<438::AID-AJIM14>3.0.CO;2-A.
28. Aimanianda V, Bayry J, Bozza S, Kniemeyer O, Perruccio K, Elluru SR, et al. Surface hydrophobin prevents immune recognition of airborne fungal spores. Nature. 2009;460(7259):1117–21. https://doi.org/10.1038/nature08264.

29. Agarwal R, Hazarika B, Gupta D, Aggarwal AN, Chakrabarti A, Jindal SK. Aspergillus hypersensitivity in patients with chronic obstructive pulmonary disease: COPD as a risk factor for ABPA? Med Mycol. 2010;48(7):988–94.
30. Dhooria S, Kumar P, Saikia B, Aggarwal AN, Gupta D, Behera D, et al. Prevalence of Aspergillus sensitisation in pulmonary tuberculosis-related fibrocavitary disease. Int J Tuberc Lung Dis. 2014;18(7):850–5. https://doi.org/10.5588/ijtld.13.0838.
31. Agarwal R. Allergic bronchopulmonary aspergillosis: lessons learnt from genetics. Indian J Chest Dis Allied Sci. 2011;53(3):137–40.
32. Gago S, Overton NLD, Ben-Ghazzi N, Novak-Frazer L, Read ND, Denning DW, et al. Lung colonization by Aspergillus fumigatus is controlled by ZNF77. Nat Commun. 2018;9(1):3835. https://doi.org/10.1038/s41467-018-06148-7.
33. Agarwal R, Khan A, Aggarwal AN, Gupta D. Link between CFTR mutations and ABPA: a systematic review and meta-analysis. Mycoses. 2012;55(4):357–65. https://doi.org/10.1111/j.1439-0507.2011.02130.x.
34. Gamaletsou MN, Hayes G, Harris C, Brock J, Muldoon EG, Denning DW. F508del CFTR gene mutation in patients with allergic bronchopulmonary aspergillosis. J Asthma. 2018;55(8):837–43. https://doi.org/10.1080/02770903.2017.1373808.
35. Overton NL, Denning DW, Bowyer P, Simpson A. Genetic susceptibility to allergic bronchopulmonary aspergillosis in asthma: a genetic association study. Allergy Asthma Clin Immunol. 2016;12:47. https://doi.org/10.1186/s13223-016-0152-y.
36. Park SJ, Mehrad B. Innate immunity to Aspergillus species. Clin Microbiol Rev. 2009;22(4):535–51. https://doi.org/10.1128/CMR.00014-09.
37. Tomee JF, Wierenga AT, Hiemstra PS, Kauffman HK. Proteases from Aspergillus fumigatus induce release of proinflammatory cytokines and cell detachment in airway epithelial cell lines. J Infect Dis. 1997;176(1):300–3.
38. Tomee JF, Kauffman HF, Klimp AH, de Monchy JG, Koeter GH, Dubois AE. Immunologic significance of a collagen-derived culture filtrate containing proteolytic activity in Aspergillus-related diseases. J Allergy Clin Immunol. 1994;93(4):768–78. https://doi.org/10.1016/009/0091-6749(94)90257-7.
39. Hogaboam CM, Blease K, Schuh JM. Cytokines and chemokines in allergic bronchopulmonary aspergillosis (ABPA) and experimental Aspergillus-induced allergic airway or asthmatic disease. Front Biosci. 2003;8:e147–56.
40. Kauffman HF. Immunopathogenesis of allergic bronchopulmonary aspergillosis and airway remodeling. Front Biosci. 2003;8:e190–6.
41. Namvar S, Warn P, Farnell E, Bromley M, Fraczek M, Bowyer P, et al. Aspergillus fumigatus proteases, Asp f 5 and Asp f 13, are essential for airway inflammation and remodelling in a murine inhalation model. Clin Exp Allergy. 2015;45(5):982–93. https://doi.org/10.1111/cea.12426.
42. Knutsen AP, Mueller KR, Levine AD, Chouhan B, Hutcheson PS, Slavin RG. Asp f I CD4+ TH2-like T-cell lines in allergic bronchopulmonary aspergillosis. J Allergy Clin Immunol. 1994;94(2 Pt 1):215–21.
43. Chauhan B, Knutsen A, Hutcheson PS, Slavin RG, Bellone CJ. T cell subsets, epitope mapping, and HLA-restriction in patients with allergic bronchopulmonary aspergillosis. J Clin Invest. 1996;97(10):2324–31.
44. Chauhan B, Santiago L, Kirschmann DA, Hauptfeld V, Knutsen AP, Hutcheson PS, et al. The association of HLA-DR alleles and T cell activation with allergic bronchopulmonary aspergillosis. J Immunol. 1997;159(8):4072–6.
45. Schuyler M. The Th1/Th2 paradigm in allergic bronchopulmonary aspergillosis. J Lab Clin Med. 1998;131(3):194–6. https://doi.org/10.1016/S0022-2143(98)90089-0.
46. Knutsen AP, Bellone C, Kauffman H. Immunopathogenesis of allergic bronchopulmonary aspergillosis in cystic fibrosis. J Cyst Fibros. 2002;1(2):76–89. https://doi.org/10.1016/S1569-1993(02)00033-4.
47. Becker KL, Gresnigt MS, Smeekens SP, Jacobs CW, Magis-Escurra C, Jaeger M, et al. Pattern recognition pathways leading to a Th2 cytokine bias in allergic bronchopulmonary aspergillosis patients. Clin Exp Allergy. 2015;45(2):423–37. https://doi.org/10.1111/cea.12354.

48. Kauffman HK, Tomee JFC. Inflammatory cells and airway defense against Aspergillus fumigatus. Immunol Allergy Clin N Am. 1998;18(3):619–40.
49. Kauffman HF, Tomee JF, van de Riet MA, Timmerman AJ, Borger P. Protease-dependent activation of epithelial cells by fungal allergens leads to morphologic changes and cytokine production. J Allergy Clin Immunol. 2000;105(6 Pt 1):1185–93. https://doi.org/10.1016/S0091674900380599.
50. Moss RB. Pathophysiology and immunology of allergic bronchopulmonary aspergillosis. Med Mycol. 2005;43(Suppl 1):S203–6.
51. Nguyen NL, Chen K, McAleer J, Kolls JK. Vitamin D regulation of OX40 ligand in immune responses to Aspergillus fumigatus. Infect Immun. 2013;81(5):1510–9. https://doi.org/10.1128/iai.01345-12.
52. Nguyen NL, Pilewski JM, Celedon JC, Mandalapu S, Blanchard ML, DeRicco A, et al. Vitamin D supplementation decreases Aspergillus fumigatus specific Th2 responses in CF patients with aspergillus sensitization: a phase one open-label study. Asthma Res Pract. 2015;1:3. https://doi.org/10.1186/s40733-015-0003-5.
53. Dodamani MH, Muthu V, Thakur R, Pal A, Sehgal IS, Dhooria S, et al. A randomized trial of vitamin D in acute-stage allergic bronchopulmonary aspergillosis complicating asthma. Mycoses. 2019;62(4):320–7. https://doi.org/10.1111/myc.12879.
54. Kumar R, Gaur SN. Prevalence of allergic bronchopulmonary aspergillosis in patients with bronchial asthma. Asian Pac J Allergy Immunol. 2000;18(4):181–5.
55. Chakrabarti A, Sethi S, Raman DS, Behera D. Eight-year study of allergic bronchopulmonary aspergillosis in an Indian teaching hospital. Mycoses. 2002;45(8):295–9.
56. Agarwal R, Gupta D, Aggarwal AN, Saxena AK, Chakrabarti A, Jindal SK. Clinical significance of hyperattenuating mucoid impaction in allergic bronchopulmonary aspergillosis: an analysis of 155 patients. Chest. 2007;132(4):1183–90. https://doi.org/10.1378/chest.07-0808.
57. Eaton T, Garrett J, Milne D, Frankel A, Wells AU. Allergic bronchopulmonary aspergillosis in the asthma clinic. A prospective evaluation of CT in the diagnostic algorithm. Chest. 2000;118(1):66–72.
58. Muthu V, Sehgal IS, Dhooria S, Bal A, Agarwal R. Allergic bronchopulmonary aspergillosis presenting as nephrotic syndrome due to secondary amyloidosis: case report and systematic review of the literature. Lung India. 2018;35(4):332–5. https://doi.org/10.4103/lungindia.lungindia_180_17.
59. Agarwal R, Maskey D, Aggarwal AN, Saikia B, Garg M, Gupta D, et al. Diagnostic performance of various tests and criteria employed in allergic bronchopulmonary aspergillosis: a latent class analysis. PLoS One. 2013;8(4):e61105. https://doi.org/10.1371/journal.pone.0061105.
60. Agarwal R, Dua D, Choudhary H, Aggarwal AN, Sehgal IS, Dhooria S, et al. Role of Aspergillus fumigatus-specific IgG in diagnosis and monitoring treatment response in allergic bronchopulmonary aspergillosis. Mycoses. 2017;60(1):33–9. https://doi.org/10.1111/myc.12541.
61. Agarwal R, Khan A, Garg M, Aggarwal AN, Gupta D. Pictorial essay: allergic bronchopulmonary aspergillosis. Indian J Radiol Imaging. 2011;21(4):242–52. https://doi.org/10.4103/0971-3026.90680.
62. Agarwal R, Khan A, Garg M, Aggarwal AN, Gupta D. Chest radiographic and computed tomographic manifestations in allergic bronchopulmonary aspergillosis. World J Radiol. 2012;4(4):141–50. https://doi.org/10.4329/wjr.v4.i4.141.
63. Agarwal R. Allergic bronchopulmonary aspergillosis: lessons for the busy radiologist. World J Radiol. 2011;3(7):178–81.
64. Reiff DB, Wells AU, Carr DH, Cole PJ, Hansell DM. CT findings in bronchiectasis: limited value in distinguishing between idiopathic and specific types. Am J Roentgenol. 1995;165(2):261–7.
65. Fairs A, Agbetile J, Hargadon B, Bourne M, Monteiro WR, Brightling CE, et al. IgE sensitisation to Aspergillus fumigatus is sssociated with reduced lung function in asthma. Am J Respir Crit Care Med. 2010;182(11):1362–8. https://doi.org/10.1164/rccm.201001-0087OC.

66. Agarwal R, Aggarwal AN, Gupta D. High-attenuation mucus in allergic bronchopulmonary aspergillosis: another cause of diffuse high-attenuation pulmonary abnormality. Am J Roentgenol. 2006;186(3):904. https://doi.org/10.2214/AJR.05.0125.
67. Phuyal S, Garg MK, Agarwal R, Gupta P, Chakrabarti A, Sandhu MS, et al. High-attenuation mucus impaction in patients with allergic bronchopulmonary Aspergillosis: objective criteria on high-resolution computed tomography and correlation with serologic parameters. Curr Probl Diagn Radiol. 2016;45(3):168–73. https://doi.org/10.1067/j.cpradiol.2015.07.006.
68. Agarwal R, Khan A, Gupta D, Aggarwal AN, Saxena AK, Chakrabarti A. An alternate method of classifying allergic bronchopulmonary aspergillosis based on high-attenuation mucus. PLoS One. 2010;5(12):e15346. https://doi.org/10.1371/journal.pone.0015346.
69. Agarwal R. High attenuation mucoid impaction in allergic bronchopulmonary aspergillosis. World J Radiol. 2010;2(1):41–3. https://doi.org/10.4329/wjr.v2.i1.41.
70. Smith NL, Denning DW. Underlying conditions in chronic pulmonary aspergillosis including simple aspergilloma. Eur Respir J. 2011;37(4):865–72. https://doi.org/10.1183/09031936.00054810.
71. Sodhi KS, Gupta P, Shrivastav A, Saxena AK, Mathew JL, Singh M, et al. Evaluation of 3 T lung magnetic resonance imaging in children with allergic bronchopulmonary aspergillosis: pilot study. Eur J Radiol. 2019;111:88–92. https://doi.org/10.1016/j.ejrad.2018.12.021.
72. Dournes G, Berger P, Refait J, Macey J, Bui S, Delhaes L, et al. Allergic bronchopulmonary aspergillosis in cystic fibrosis: MR imaging of airway mucus contrasts as a tool for diagnosis. Radiology. 2017;285(1):261–9. https://doi.org/10.1148/radiol.2017162350.
73. Garg MK, Gupta P, Agarwal R, Sodhi KS, Khandelwal N. MRI: a new paradigm in imaging evaluation of allergic bronchopulmonary aspergillosis? Chest. 2015;147(2):e58–9. https://doi.org/10.1378/chest.14-2347.
74. Crameri R, Hemmann S, Ismail C, Menz G, Blaser K. Disease-specific recombinant allergens for the diagnosis of allergic bronchopulmonary aspergillosis. Int Immunol. 1998;10(8):1211–6.
75. Hemmann S, Menz G, Ismail C, Blaser K, Crameri R. Skin test reactivity to 2 recombinant Aspergillus fumigatus allergens in a fumigatus-sensitized asthmatic subjects allows diagnostic separation of allergic bronchopulmonary aspergillosis from fungal sensitization. J Allergy Clin Immunol. 1999;104(3 Pt 1):601–7. https://doi.org/10.1016/S0091674999005321.
76. Kurup VP, Banerjee B, Hemmann S, Greenberger PA, Blaser K, Crameri R. Selected recombinant Aspergillus fumigatus allergens bind specifically to IgE in ABPA. Clin Exp Allergy. 2000;30(7):988–93. https://doi.org/10.1016/cea837.
77. Muthu V, Sehgal IS, Dhooria S, Aggarwal AN, Agarwal R. Utility of recombinant Aspergillus fumigatus antigens in the diagnosis of allergic bronchopulmonary aspergillosis: a systematic review and diagnostic test accuracy meta-analysis. Clin Exp Allergy. 2018;48(9):1107–36. https://doi.org/10.1111/cea.13216.
78. Kozlova YI, Frolova EV, Uchevatkina AE, Bychkova NV, Filippova LV, Davydova NI, et al. Basophil activation test in the diagnosis of allergic bronchopulmonary aspergillosis. Mycoses. 2017;60:101. https://doi.org/10.1111/myc.12674.
79. Gernez Y, Waters J, Dunn C, Davies Z, Tirouvanziam R, Everson C, et al. Basophil activation is a reliable biomarker of allergic bronchopulmonary aspergillosis (ABPA) in CF: one year results of a longitudinal cohort study. J Allergy Clin Immunol. 2014;133(2):AB58.
80. Moss RB, Waters J, Dunn C, Davies Z, Everson C, Tirouvanziam R, et al. Basophil activation is a reliable biomarker of allergic bronchopulmonary aspergillosis (ABPA) in CF: interim results of a longitudinal cohort study. J Cyst Fibros. 2013;12:S46.
81. Agarwal R, Aggarwal AN, Sehgal IS, Dhooria S, Behera D, Chakrabarti A. Performance of serum galactomannan in patients with allergic bronchopulmonary aspergillosis. Mycoses. 2015;58(7):408–12. https://doi.org/10.1111/myc.12334.
82. Kono Y, Tsushima K, Yamaguchi K, Kurita N, Soeda S, Fujiwara A, et al. The utility of galactomannan antigen in the bronchial washing and serum for diagnosing pulmonary aspergillosis. Respir Med. 2013;107(7):1094–100. https://doi.org/10.1016/j.rmed.2013.04.007.
83. Agarwal R. Controversies in allergic bronchopulmonary aspergillosis. Int J Respir Care. 2010;6(2):53–4, 6-63.

84. Agarwal R, Sehgal IS, Dhooria S, Aggarwal AN. Developments in the diagnosis and treatment of allergic bronchopulmonary aspergillosis. Expert Rev Respir Med. 2016;10(12):1317–34. https://doi.org/10.1080/17476348.2016.1249853.
85. Agarwal R. Severe asthma with fungal sensitization. Curr Allergy Asthma Rep. 2011;11(5):403–13. https://doi.org/10.1007/s11882-011-0217-4.
86. Agarwal R, Gupta D, Aggarwal AN, Saxena AK, Saikia B, Chakrabarti A, et al. Clinical significance of decline in serum IgE levels in allergic bronchopulmonary aspergillosis. Respir Med. 2010;104(2):204–10.
87. Agarwal R, Khan A, Aggarwal AN, Saikia B, Gupta D, Chakrabarti A. Role of inhaled corticosteroids in the management of serological allergic bronchopulmonary aspergillosis (ABPA). Intern Med. 2011;50(8):855–60.
88. Agarwal R, Khan A, Aggarwal AN, Varma N, Garg M, Saikia B, et al. Clinical relevance of peripheral blood eosinophil count in allergic bronchopulmonary aspergillosis. J Infect Public Health. 2011;4(5–6):235–43. https://doi.org/10.1016/j.jiph.2011.08.006.
89. Agarwal R, Noel V, Aggarwal AN, Gupta D, Chakrabarti A. Clinical significance of Aspergillus sensitisation in bronchial asthma. Mycoses. 2011;54(5):e531–8. https://doi.org/10.1111/j.1439-0507.2010.01971.x.
90. Agarwal R, Aggarwal AN, Garg M, Saikia B, Gupta D, Chakrabarti A. Allergic bronchopulmonary aspergillosis with aspergilloma: an immunologically severe disease with poor outcome. Mycopathologia. 2012;174(3):193–201. https://doi.org/10.1007/s11046-012-9535-x.
91. Agarwal R, Garg M, Aggarwal AN, Saikia B, Gupta D, Chakrabarti A. Serologic allergic bronchopulmonary aspergillosis (ABPA-S): long-term outcomes. Respir Med. 2012;106(7):942–7. https://doi.org/10.1016/j.rmed.2012.03.001.
92. Patterson R, Greenberger PA, Radin RC, Roberts M. Allergic bronchopulmonary aspergillosis: staging as an aid to management. Ann Intern Med. 1982;96(3):286–91.
93. Lee TM, Greenberger PA, Patterson R, Roberts M, Liotta JL. Stage V (fibrotic) allergic bronchopulmonary aspergillosis. A review of 17 cases followed from diagnosis. Arch Intern Med. 1987;147(2):319–23.
94. Baur X, Weiss W, Jarosch B, Menz G, Schoch C, Schmitz-Schumann M, et al. Immunoprint pattern in patients with allergic bronchopulmonary aspergillosis in different stages. J Allergy Clin Immunol. 1989;83(4):839–44. https://doi.org/10.1016/0091-6749(89)90023-7.
95. Patterson R, Greenberger PA, Halwig JM, Liotta JL, Roberts M. Allergic bronchopulmonary aspergillosis. Natural history and classification of early disease by serologic and roentgenographic studies. Arch Intern Med. 1986;146(5):916–8.
96. Greenberger PA, Miller TP, Roberts M, Smith LL. Allergic bronchopulmonary aspergillosis in patients with and without evidence of bronchiectasis. Ann Allergy. 1993;70(4):333–8.
97. Kumar R. Mild, moderate, and severe forms of allergic bronchopulmonary aspergillosis: a clinical and serologic evaluation. Chest. 2003;124(3):890–2.
98. Agarwal R, Singh N, Gupta D. Pulmonary hypertension as a presenting manifestation of allergic bronchopulmonary aspergillosis. Indian J Chest Dis Allied Sci. 2009;51(1):37–40.
99. Lowes D, Chishimba L, Greaves M, Denning DW. Development of chronic pulmonary aspergillosis in adult asthmatics with ABPA. Respir Med. 2015;109(12):1509–15. https://doi.org/10.1016/j.rmed.2015.09.007.
100. Agarwal R, Aggarwal AN, Gupta N, Gupta D. A rare cause of acute respiratory failure—allergic bronchopulmonary aspergillosis. Mycoses. 2011;54(4):e223–7. https://doi.org/10.1111/j.1439-0507.2009.01830.x.
101. Agarwal R, Aggarwal AN, Dhooria S, Singh Sehgal I, Garg M, Saikia B, et al. A randomised trial of glucocorticoids in acute-stage allergic bronchopulmonary aspergillosis complicating asthma. Eur Respir J. 2016;47(2):490–8. https://doi.org/10.1183/13993003.01475-2015.
102. Agarwal R, Dhooria S, Singh Sehgal I, Aggarwal AN, Garg M, Saikia B, et al. A randomized trial of Itraconazole vs prednisolone in acute-stage allergic bronchopulmonary aspergillosis complicating asthma. Chest. 2018;153(3):656–64. https://doi.org/10.1016/j.chest.2018.01.005.

103. Agarwal R, Dhooria S, Sehgal IS, Aggarwal AN, Garg M, Saikia B, et al. A randomised trial of voriconazole and prednisolone monotherapy in acute-stage allergic bronchopulmonary aspergillosis complicating asthma. Eur Respir J. 2018;52(3):1801159. https://doi.org/10.1183/13993003.01159-2018.
104. Vlahakis NE, Aksamit TR. Diagnosis and treatment of allergic bronchopulmonary aspergillosis. Mayo Clin Proc. 2001;76(9):930–8.
105. Greenberger PA. Allergic bronchopulmonary aspergillosis. J Allergy Clin Immunol. 2002;110(5):685–92. https://doi.org/10.1016/S009167490201415X.
106. Hilton AM, Chatterjee SS. Bronchopulmonary aspergillosis—treatment with beclomethasone dipropionate. Postgrad Med J. 1975;51(Suppl 4):98–103.
107. Inhaled beclomethasone dipropionate in allergic bronchopulmonary aspergillosis. Report to the Research Committee of the British Thoracic Association. Br J Dis Chest. 1979;73(4):349–56.
108. Heinig JH, Weeke ER, Groth S, Schwartz B. High-dose local steroid treatment in broncho pulmonary aspergillosis. A pilot study. Allergy. 1988;43(1):24–31.
109. Balter MS, Rebuck AS. Treatment of allergic bronchopulmonary aspergillosis with inhaled corticosteroids. Respir Med. 1992;86(5):441–2.
110. Imbeault B, Cormier Y. Usefulness of inhaled high-dose corticosteroids in allergic bronchopulmonary aspergillosis. Chest. 1993;103(5):1614–7.
111. Seaton A, Seaton RA, Wightman AJ. Management of allergic bronchopulmonary aspergillosis without maintenance oral corticosteroids: a fifteen-year follow-up. QJM. 1994;87(9):529–37.
112. Singh Sehgal I, Agarwal R. Pulse methylprednisolone in allergic bronchopulmonary aspergillosis exacerbations. Eur Respir Rev. 2014;23(131):149–52. https://doi.org/10.1183/09059180.00004813.
113. Cohen-Cymberknoh M, Blau H, Shoseyov D, Mei-Zahav M, Efrati O, Armoni S, et al. Intravenous monthly pulse methylprednisolone treatment for ABPA in patients with cystic fibrosis. J Cyst Fibros. 2009;8(4):253–7. https://doi.org/10.1016/j.jcf.2009.04.008.
114. Thomson JM, Wesley A, Byrnes CA, Nixon GM. Pulse intravenous methylprednisolone for resistant allergic bronchopulmonary aspergillosis in cystic fibrosis. Pediatr Pulmonol. 2006;41(2):164–70. https://doi.org/10.1002/ppul.20333.
115. Groeneweg FL, Karst H, de Kloet ER, Joels M. Mineralocorticoid and glucocorticoid receptors at the neuronal membrane, regulators of nongenomic corticosteroid signalling. Mol Cell Endocrinol. 2012;350(2):299–309. https://doi.org/10.1016/j.mce.2011.06.020.
116. Ghdifan S, Couderc L, Michelet I, Leguillon C, Masseline B, Marguet C. Bolus methylprednisolone efficacy for uncontrolled exacerbation of cystic fibrosis in children. Pediatrics. 2010;125(5):e1259–64. https://doi.org/10.1542/peds.2009-2042.
117. Frauman AG. An overview of the adverse reactions to adrenal corticosteroids. Adverse Drug React Toxicol Rev. 1996;15(4):203–6.
118. Schacke H, Docke WD, Asadullah K. Mechanisms involved in the side effects of glucocorticoids. Pharmacol Ther. 2002;96(1):23–43.
119. Shale DJ, Faux JA, Lane DJ. Trial of ketoconazole in non-invasive pulmonary aspergillosis. Thorax. 1987;42(1):26–31.
120. Fournier EC. Trial of ketoconazole in allergic bronchopulmonary aspergillosis. Thorax. 1987;42(10):831.
121. Currie DC, Lueck C, Milburn HJ, Harvey C, Longbottom JL, Darbyshire JH, et al. Controlled trial of natamycin in the treatment of allergic bronchopulmonary aspergillosis. Thorax. 1990;45(6):447–50.
122. Stevens DA, Schwartz HJ, Lee JY, Moskovitz BL, Jerome DC, Catanzaro A, et al. A randomized trial of itraconazole in allergic bronchopulmonary aspergillosis. N Engl J Med. 2000;342(11):756–62. https://doi.org/10.1056/NEJM200003163421102.
123. Wark PA, Hensley MJ, Saltos N, Boyle MJ, Toneguzzi RC, Epid GD, et al. Anti-inflammatory effect of itraconazole in stable allergic bronchopulmonary aspergillosis: a randomized controlled trial. J Allergy Clin Immunol. 2003;111(5):952–7. https://doi.org/10.1016/S0091674903008509.

124. Wark PA, Gibson PG, Wilson AJ. Azoles for allergic glucocorticoids are the preferred first-line therapy with asthma. Cochrane Database Syst Rev. 2004;(3):CD001108. https://doi.org/10.1002/14651858.CD001108.pub2.
125. Chishimba L, Niven RM, Cooley J, Denning DW. Voriconazole and posaconazole improve asthma severity in allergic bronchopulmonary aspergillosis and severe asthma with fungal sensitization. J Asthma. 2012;49(4):423–33. https://doi.org/10.3109/02770903.2012.662568.
126. Chishimba L, Langridge P, Powell G, Niven RM, Denning DW. Efficacy and safety of nebulised amphotericin B (NAB) in severe asthma with fungal sensitisation (SAFS) and allergic bronchopulmonary aspergillosis (ABPA). J Asthma. 2015;52(3):289–95. https://doi.org/10.3109/02770903.2014.958853.
127. Laoudi Y, Paolini JB, Grimfed A, Just J. Nebulised corticosteroid and amphotericin B: an alternative treatment for ABPA? Eur Respir J. 2008;31(4):908–9. https://doi.org/10.1183/09031936.00146707.
128. Hayes D Jr, Murphy BS, Lynch JE, Feola DJ. Aerosolized amphotericin for the treatment of allergic bronchopulmonary aspergillosis. Pediatr Pulmonol. 2010;45(11):1145–8. https://doi.org/10.1002/ppul.21300.
129. Proesmans M, Vermeulen F, Vreys M, De Boeck K. Use of nebulized amphotericin B in the treatment of allergic bronchopulmonary aspergillosis in cystic fibrosis. Int J Pediatr. 2010;2010:376287. https://doi.org/10.1155/2010/376287.
130. Godet C, Meurice JC, Roblot F, Kauffmann-Lacroix C, Verdaguer M, Frat JP, et al. Efficacy of nebulised liposomal amphotericin B in the attack and maintenance treatment of ABPA. Eur Respir J. 2012;39(5):1261–3. https://doi.org/10.1183/09031936.00162311.
131. Ram B, Aggarwal AN, Dhooria S, Sehgal IS, Garg M, Behera D, et al. A pilot randomized trial of nebulized amphotericin in patients with allergic bronchopulmonary aspergillosis. J Asthma. 2016;53(5):517–24. https://doi.org/10.3109/02770903.2015.1127935.
132. Sehgal IS, Agarwal R. Role of inhaled amphotericin in allergic bronchopulmonary aspergillosis. J Postgrad Med. 2014;60(1):41–5. https://doi.org/10.4103/0022-3859.128806.
133. van der Ent CK, Hoekstra H, Rijkers GT. Successful treatment of allergic bronchopulmonary aspergillosis with recombinant anti-IgE antibody. Thorax. 2007;62(3):276–7. https://doi.org/10.1136/thx.2004.035519.
134. Perez-de-Llano LA, Vennera MC, Parra A, Guallar J, Marin M, Asensio O, et al. Effects of omalizumab in Aspergillus-associated airway disease. Thorax. 2011;66(6):539–40.
135. Tillie-Leblond I, Germaud P, Leroyer C, Tetu L, Girard F, Devouassoux G, et al. Allergic bronchopulmonary aspergillosis and omalizumab. Allergy. 2011;66(9):1254–6. https://doi.org/10.1111/j.1398-9995.2011.02599.x.
136. Wong R, Wong M, Robinson PD, Fitzgerald DA. Omalizumab in the management of steroid dependent allergic bronchopulmonary aspergillosis (ABPA) complicating cystic fibrosis. Paediatr Respir Rev. 2013;14(1):22–4. https://doi.org/10.1016/j.prrv.2012.11.004.
137. Nove-Josserand R, Grard S, Auzou L, Reix P, Murris-Espin M, Bremont F, et al. Case series of omalizumab for allergic bronchopulmonary aspergillosis in cystic fibrosis patients. Pediatr Pulmonol. 2017;52(2):190–7. https://doi.org/10.1002/ppul.23612.
138. Perisson C, Destruys L, Grenet D, Bassinet L, Derelle J, Sermet-Gaudelus I, et al. Omalizumab treatment for allergic bronchopulmonary aspergillosis in young patients with cystic fibrosis. Respir Med. 2017;133:12–5. https://doi.org/10.1016/j.rmed.2017.11.007.
139. Ashkenazi M, Sity S, Sarouk I, Bar Aluma BE, Dagan A, Bezalel Y, et al. Omalizumab in allergic bronchopulmonary aspergillosis in patients with cystic fibrosis. J Asthma Allergy. 2018;11:101–7. https://doi.org/10.2147/jaa.S156049.
140. Voskamp AL, Gillman A, Symons K, Sandrini A, Rolland JM, O'Hehir RE, et al. Clinical efficacy and immunologic effects of omalizumab in allergic bronchopulmonary aspergillosis. J Allergy Clin Immunol Pract. 2015;3(2):192–9. https://doi.org/10.1016/j.jaip.2014.12.008.
141. Altman MC, Lenington J, Bronson S, Ayars AG. Combination omalizumab and mepolizumab therapy for refractory allergic bronchopulmonary aspergillosis. J Allergy Clin Immunol Pract. 2017;5(4):1137–9. https://doi.org/10.1016/j.jaip.2017.01.013.

142. Terashima T, Shinozaki T, Iwami E, Nakajima T, Matsuzaki T. A case of allergic bronchopulmonary aspergillosis successfully treated with mepolizumab. BMC Pulm Med. 2018;18(1):53. https://doi.org/10.1186/s12890-018-0617-5.
143. Soeda S, Kono Y, Tsuzuki R, Yamawaki S, Katsube O, To M, et al. Allergic bronchopulmonary aspergillosis successfully treated with benralizumab. J Allergy Clin Immunol Pract. 2019;7(5):1633–5. https://doi.org/10.1016/j.jaip.2018.11.024.
144. Hirota S, Kobayashi Y, Ishiguro T, Nishida T, Kagiyama N, Shimizu Y, et al. Allergic bronchopulmonary aspergillosis successfully treated with mepolizumab: case report and review of the literature. Respir Med Case Rep. 2019;26:59–62. https://doi.org/10.1016/j.rmcr.2018.11.013.
145. Hogan C, Denning DW. Allergic bronchopulmonary aspergillosis and related allergic syndromes. Semin Respir Crit Care Med. 2011;32(6):682–92. https://doi.org/10.1055/s-0031-1295716.
146. Kosmidis C, Powell G, Borrow R, Morris J, Alachkar H, Denning DW. Response to pneumococcal polysaccharide vaccination in patients with chronic and allergic aspergillosis. Vaccine. 2015;33(51):7271–5. https://doi.org/10.1016/j.vaccine.2015.10.114.
147. Casey P, Garrett J, Eaton T. Allergic bronchopulmonary aspergillosis in a lung transplant patient successfully treated with nebulized amphotericin. J Heart Lung Transplant. 2002;21(11):1237–41. https://doi.org/10.1016/S1053249802004254.
148. Fitzsimons EJ, Aris R, Patterson R. Recurrence of allergic bronchopulmonary aspergillosis in the posttransplant lungs of a cystic fibrosis patient. Chest. 1997;112(1):281–2.
149. Polverino E, Goeminne PC, McDonnell MJ, Aliberti S, Marshall SE, Loebinger MR, et al. European Respiratory Society guidelines for the management of adult bronchiectasis. Eur Respir J. 2017;50(3). https://doi.org/10.1183/13993003.00629-2017.
150. Ricketti AJ, Greenberger PA, Patterson R. Serum IgE as an important aid in management of allergic bronchopulmonary aspergillosis. J Allergy Clin Immunol. 1984;74(1):68–71. https://doi.org/10.1016/0091-6749(84)90089-7.
151. Bolland MJ, Bagg W, Thomas MG, Lucas JA, Ticehurst R, Black PN. Cushing's syndrome due to interaction between inhaled corticosteroids and itraconazole. Ann Pharmacother. 2004;38(1):46–9. https://doi.org/10.1345/aph.1D222.
152. De Wachter E, Vanbesien J, De Schutter I, Malfroot A, De Schepper J. Rapidly developing Cushing syndrome in a 4-year-old patient during combined treatment with itraconazole and inhaled budesonide. Eur J Pediatr. 2003;162(7–8):488–9. https://doi.org/10.1007/s00431-003-1233-8.
153. Parmar JS, Howell T, Kelly J, Bilton D. Profound adrenal suppression secondary to treatment with low dose inhaled steroids and itraconazole in allergic bronchopulmonary aspergillosis in cystic fibrosis. Thorax. 2002;57(8):749–50.
154. Naef R, Schmid C, Hofer M, Minder S, Speich R, Boehler A. Itraconazole comedication increases systemic levels of inhaled fluticasone in lung transplant recipients. Respiration. 2007;74(4):418–22. https://doi.org/10.1159/000095941.
155. Gilchrist FJ, Cox KJ, Rowe R, Horsley A, Webb AK, Jones AM, et al. Itraconazole and inhaled fluticasone causing hypothalamic-pituitary-adrenal axis suppression in adults with cystic fibrosis. J Cyst Fibros. 2013;12(4):399–402. https://doi.org/10.1016/j.jcf.2012.10.007.
156. Halwig JM, Greenberger PA, Levine M, Patterson R. Recurrence of allergic bronchopulmonary aspergillosis after seven years of remission. J Allergy Clin Immunol. 1984;74(5):738–40. https://doi.org/10.1016/0091-6749(84)90238-0.
157. Mearns M, Young W, Batten J. Transient pulmonary infiltrations in cystic fibrosis due to allergic aspergillosis. Thorax. 1965;20(9):385–92.
158. Moss RB. Allergic bronchopulmonary aspergillosis and Aspergillus infection in cystic fibrosis. Curr Opin Pulm Med. 2010;16(6):598–603. https://doi.org/10.1097/MCP.0b013e32833e24a6.
159. Carsin A, Romain T, Ranque S, Reynaud-Gaubert M, Dubus JC, Mege JL, et al. Aspergillus fumigatus in cystic fibrosis: an update on immune interactions and molecular diagnostics

in allergic bronchopulmonary aspergillosis. Allergy. 2017;72(11):1632–42. https://doi.org/10.1111/all.13204.
160. Kraemer R, Delosea N, Ballinari P, Gallati S, Crameri R. Effect of allergic bronchopulmonary aspergillosis on lung function in children with cystic fibrosis. Am J Respir Crit Care Med. 2006;174(11):1211–20. https://doi.org/10.1164/rccm.200603-423OC.
161. Mastella G, Rainisio M, Harms HK, Hodson ME, Koch C, Navarro J, et al. Allergic bronchopulmonary aspergillosis in cystic fibrosis. A European epidemiological study. Epidemiologic registry of cystic fibrosis. Eur Respir J. 2000;16(3):464–71.
162. Nepomuceno IB, Esrig S, Moss RB. Allergic bronchopulmonary aspergillosis in cystic fibrosis: role of atopy and response to itraconazole. Chest. 1999;115(2):364–70.
163. Hutcheson PS, Rejent AJ, Slavin RG. Variability in parameters of allergic bronchopulmonary aspergillosis in patients with cystic fibrosis. J Allergy Clin Immunol. 1991;88(3 Pt 1): 390–4.
164. Stevens DA, Moss RB, Kurup VP, Knutsen AP, Greenberger P, Judson MA, et al. Allergic bronchopulmonary aspergillosis in cystic fibrosis—state of the art: cystic fibrosis foundation consensus conference. Clin Infect Dis. 2003;37(Suppl 3):S225–64. https://doi.org/10.1086/376525.
165. Agarwal R, Srinivas R, Jindal SK. Allergic bronchopulmonary aspergillosis complicating chronic obstructive pulmonary disease. Mycoses. 2008;51(1):83–5. https://doi.org/10.1111/j.1439-0507.2007.01432.x.
166. Mir E, Shah A. Allergic bronchopulmonary aspergillosis in a patient with chronic obstructive pulmonary disease. Prim Care Respir J. 2012;21(1):111–4. https://doi.org/10.4104/pcrj.2012.00001.
167. Bahous J, Malo JL, Paquin R, Cartier A, Vyas P, Longbottom JL. Allergic bronchopulmonary aspergillosis and sensitization to Aspergillus fumigatus in chronic bronchiectasis in adults. Clin Allergy. 1985;15(6):571–9.
168. Agarwal R, Singh N, Aggarwal AN. An unusual association between mycobacterium tuberculosis and Aspergillus fumigatus. Monaldi Arch Chest Dis. 2008;69(1):32–4.
169. Sharma B, Sharma M, Bondi E, Sharma M. Kartagener's syndrome associated with allergic bronchopulmonary aspergillosis. MedGenMed. 2005;7(2):25.
170. Sehgal IS, Dhooria S, Behera D, Agarwal R. Allergic bronchopulmonary aspergillosis complicating Swyer-James-Macleod's syndrome: case report and review of literature. Eur Ann Allergy Clin Immunol. 2016;48(3):99–102.
171. Eppinger TM, Greenberger PA, White DA, Brown AE, Cunningham-Rundles C. Sensitization to Aspergillus species in the congenital neutrophil disorders chronic granulomatous disease and hyper-IgE syndrome. J Allergy Clin Immunol. 1999;104(6):1265–72. https://doi.org/10.1016/S0091674999006788.
172. Glancy JJ, Elder JL, McAleer R. Allergic bronchopulmonary fungal disease without clinical asthma. Thorax. 1981;36(5):345–9.
173. Agarwal R, Aggarwal AN, Gupta D, Bal A, Das A. Case report: a rare cause of miliary nodules—allergic bronchopulmonary aspergillosis. Br J Radiol. 2009;82(980):e151–4. https://doi.org/10.1259/bjr/20940804.
174. Denning DW, Cadranel J, Beigelman-Aubry C, Ader F, Chakrabarti A, Blot S, et al. Chronic pulmonary aspergillosis: rationale and clinical guidelines for diagnosis and management. Eur Respir J. 2016;47(1):45–68. https://doi.org/10.1183/13993003.00583-2015.
175. Sehgal IS, Choudhary H, Dhooria S, Aggarwal AN, Garg M, Chakrabarti A, et al. Is there an overlap in immune response between allergic bronchopulmonary and chronic pulmonary aspergillosis? J Allergy Clin Immunol Pract. 2019;7(3):969–74. https://doi.org/10.1016/j.jaip.2018.08.034.
176. Ein ME, Wallace RJ Jr, Williams TW Jr. Allergic bronchopulmonary aspergillosis-like syndrome consequent to aspergilloma. Am Rev Respir Dis. 1979;119(5):811–20.
177. Safirstein BH. Aspergilloma consequent to allergic bronchopulmonary aspergillosis. Am Rev Respir Dis. 1973;108(4):940–3.

178. Rosenberg IL, Greenberger PA. Allergic bronchopulmonary aspergillosis and aspergilloma. Long-term follow-up without enlargement of a large multiloculated cavity. Chest. 1984;85(1):123–5.
179. Saravanan K, Panda NK, Chakrabarti A, Das A, Bapuraj RJ. Allergic fungal rhinosinusitis: an attempt to resolve the diagnostic dilemma. Arch Otolaryngol Head Neck Surg. 2006;132(2):173–8. https://doi.org/10.1001/archotol.132.2.173.
180. Shah A, Panchal N, Agarwal AK. Concomitant allergic bronchopulmonary aspergillosis and allergic Aspergillus sinusitis: a review of an uncommon association. Clin Exp Allergy. 2001;31(12):1896–905.
181. Venarske DL, deShazo RD. Sinobronchial allergic mycosis: the SAM syndrome. Chest. 2002;121(5):1670–6.
182. Agarwal R, Bansal S, Chakrabarti A. Are allergic fungal rhinosinusitis and allergic bronchopulmonary aspergillosis lifelong conditions? Med Mycol. 2017;55(1):87–95. https://doi.org/10.1093/mmy/myw071.
183. Braun JJ, Pauli G, Schultz P, Gentine A, Ebbo D, de Blay F. Allergic fungal sinusitis associated with allergic bronchopulmonary aspergillosis: an uncommon sinobronchial allergic mycosis. Am J Rhinol. 2007;21(4):412–6.
184. Jat KR, Vaidya PC, Mathew JL, Jondhale S, Singh M. Childhood allergic bronchopulmonary aspergillosis. Lung India. 2018;35(6):499–507. https://doi.org/10.4103/lungindia.lungindia_216_18.
185. Kozlova OP, Kozlova YI, Suslova IE, Aak OV, Ignatieva SM, Borzova UV, et al. Allergic bronchopulmonary aspergillosis in children with asthma in St. Petersburg, Russia. Mycoses. 2017;60:190. https://doi.org/10.1111/myc.12674.
186. Singh M, Das S, Chauhan A, Paul N, Sodhi KS, Mathew J, et al. The diagnostic criteria for allergic bronchopulmonary aspergillosis in children with poorly controlled asthma need to be re-evaluated. Acta Paediatr. 2015;104(5):e206–9. https://doi.org/10.1111/apa.12930.
187. Wright M, Cho E, Yang C. Omalizumab therapy for steroid-dependent ABPA in children with cystic fibrosis: a case series. J Cyst Fibros. 2016;15:S47.
188. Elmallah MK, Hendeles L, Hamilton RG, Capen C, Schuler PM. Management of patients with cystic fibrosis and allergic bronchopulmonary aspergillosis using anti-immunoglobulin e therapy (omalizumab). J Pediatr Pharmacol Ther. 2012;17(1):88–92. https://doi.org/10.5863/1551-6776-17.1.88.
189. De Santis M, Di Gianantonio E, Cesari E, Ambrosini G, Straface G, Clementi M. First-trimester itraconazole exposure and pregnancy outcome: a prospective cohort study of women contacting teratology information services in Italy. Drug Saf. 2009;32(3):239–44. https://doi.org/10.2165/00002018-200932030-00006.
190. Bar-Oz B, Moretti ME, Bishai R, Mareels G, Van Tittelboom T, Verspeelt J, et al. Pregnancy outcome after in utero exposure to itraconazole: a prospective cohort study. Am J Obstet Gynecol. 2000;183(3):617–20. https://doi.org/10.1067/mob.2000.105962.
191. Pilmis B, Jullien V, Sobel J, Lecuit M, Lortholary O, Charlier C. Antifungal drugs during pregnancy: an updated review. J Antimicrob Chemother. 2015;70(1):14–22. https://doi.org/10.1093/jac/dku355.
192. Namazy J, Cabana MD, Scheuerle AE, Thorp JM Jr, Chen H, Carrigan G, et al. The xolair pregnancy registry (EXPECT): the safety of omalizumab use during pregnancy. J Allergy Clin Immunol. 2015;135(2):407–12. https://doi.org/10.1016/j.jaci.2014.08.025.

Fungal Rhinosinusitis 11

Arunaloke Chakrabarti

Key Points

- Fungal rhinosinusitis (FRS) is common in Asian countries. Large series have been reported from India, Pakistan, Saudi Arabia, and Taiwan.
- Categorization of FRS is difficult due to lot of controversies regarding chronic form, though it is important to categorize as therapy varies among different categories.
- Histopathology can differentiate invasive and noninvasive diseases by tissue invasion of fungi.
- Invasive disease is categorized into acute invasive (immunosuppressed patients), granulomatous invasive (in geographical region from Sudan to India), and chronic invasive (available worldwide).
- Noninvasive disease is categorized into fungal ball (commonly seen in France and Taiwan) and Eosinophil-related FRS including allergic fungal rhinosinusitis (AFRS, common in Asian countries).
- Diagnosis of FRS: imaging, endoscopic biopsy and histopathology, direct microscopy, and culture.
- Management:
  - Acute invasive—surgery, amphotericin B, control of immunosuppression, and immunomodulation.
  - Chronic invasive and granulomatous—surgery and antifungal agents.
  - Eosinophil-related FRS including AFRS—surgery, steroid, and immunotherapy.
  - Fungal ball—surgery.

A. Chakrabarti (✉)
Department of Medical Microbiology, Postgraduate Institute of Medical Education and Research (PGIMER), Chandigarh, India

A. Chakrabarti (ed.), *Clinical Practice of Medical Mycology in Asia*,
https://doi.org/10.1007/978-981-13-9459-1_11

11.1 Introduction

Rhinosinusitis is the inflammation of nose and sinuses. In the disease process, the inflamed and swelled mucous membrane of nose and paranasal sinuses obstructs the sinus opening and prevents mucous from draining normally, leading to pain, nasal blockade, swelling, fetid discharge. The course of the disease may be acute or chronic depending on the etiological agents and host immunity. Fungus as a cause of rhinosinusitis has gained importance in last two decades. It may cause rhinosinusitis either by allergic inflammatory process or by direct invasion. Fungal rhinosinusitis (FRS) is common in Asian countries especially India, Pakistan, and Saudi Arabia [1–8]. The status of the disease in other Asian countries is not known, due to limitation of studies. In a study in the villages of North India, it was observed that 1.4% of young adults suffer from chronic rhinosinusitis (CRS). The prevalence of FRS was 0.11% of population and 8.1% of all CRS cases [9]. A great deal of controversy exists regarding etiology and pathogenesis of CRS. The claims of scientists range from fungi are only bystanders to all CRS cases are due to fungi [2, 3]. Attempts have been made by researchers to resolve the controversy, as therapy varies in different categories of rhinosinusitis. CRS affects nearly 20% of population at some time in their lives [3, 10, 11]. Scientists broadly classify FRS into invasive and noninvasive diseases depending on the invasion of nasal and paranasal sinus tissues by fungi. Depending on the immune status and histopathology, invasive disease is further differentiated into acute invasive, granulomatous invasive, and chronic invasive type. The noninvasive FRS is described in four different clinical forms: localized colonization, fungal ball, allergic fungal rhinosinusitis (AFRS), and eosinophilic fungal rhinosinusitis (EFRS) [2, 3, 12]. The descriptions of all these entities are summarized in Table 11.1. In Asian countries the common clinical form are AFRS, EFRS, and granulomatous invasive types in immunocompetent hosts [1–8].

The distinction between acute and chronic diseases is on the basis of duration of illness: acute within 4 weeks and chronic more than 12 weeks. The host immune status and vascular invasion play important role in the determination of the course of the disease. However, description of any situation with the duration of illness between 4 and 12 weeks is not clear. Occasionally suboptimal treatment may change the course of the illness from acute invasive to chronic or indolent status. The "Fungal Rhinosinusitis Working Group" under International Society for Human and Animal Mycology (ISHAM) proposed the term "subacute" to define such patients, though any change in management strategy is not proposed [3].

11.2 Invasive FRS

The acute invasive type occurs in immunosuppressed hosts especially in patients with hematological malignancy undergoing chemotherapy, transplant recipients, and uncontrolled diabetes. The entity is well described in the chapter on "Mucormycosis" and "Aspergillosis" in this book.

Table 11.1 Different types of fungal rhinosinusitis: epidemiology, pathology, diagnosis, and management

	Acute invasive FRS	Chronic invasive FRS	Granulomatous FRS	Fungal ball	Allergic FRS	Eosinophilic FRS
Susceptible host	Immunocompromised especially • Hematological malignancies undergoing chemotherapy • Transplant recipients • Uncontrolled diabetes	Mild to moderate immunocompromisation • Diabetes • Steroid therapy • Even in apparently healthy host	Immunocompetent	Immunocompetent	Atopic may be systemic or localized	Majority non-atopic
Host demography	No age or sex restriction. Common in patients in critical care	Adult population	Young adult, commonly villagers	Middle-aged and elderly female in France, but no such age restriction in Asian countries	Urban population in the USA, young villagers in Asian countries	Any person
Geographic distribution	Worldwide	Worldwide	India, Sudan, Pakistan, Saudi Arabia	Worldwide, more common in southern France and Taiwan	Southwestern part and Mississippi basin of the USA; India and Pakistan in Asia	Worldwide
Fungi involved	Mucorales commonly, *Aspergillus* species next common, *A. fumigatus* more common in the USA *A. flavus* in India and other Asian countries	*Aspergillus* species	*A. flavus*	*Aspergillus* species more common	Dematiaceous fungi in the USA. *Aspergillus* species more common in India and other Asian countries	Dematiaceous fungi in the USA. *Aspergillus* in India

(continued)

Table 11.1 (continued)

	Acute invasive FRS	Chronic invasive FRS	Granulomatous FRS	Fungal ball	Allergic FRS	Eosinophilic FRS
Role of fungus	Pathogen	Pathogen	Pathogen	Saprobe	Allergen	Not clear
Pathology	Hyphal invasion of blood vessels, thrombosis, infarction, acute neutrophilic infiltrate	Dense accumulation of hyphae, mixed inflammatory reaction	Fibrosis, non-caseating granuloma, hyphae scanty, involvement of one or more sinuses	Dense conglomeration of hyphae, no involvement of sinus mucosa by hyphae, nonspecific chronic inflammation of mucosa	Eosinophilic mucin with few fungal hyphae, no mucosal invasion	Eosinophilic mucin with few fungal hyphae, no mucosal invasion
Course of disease	Acute <4 weeks	Chronic >12 weeks	Indolent, chronic >12 weeks	Chronic >12 weeks	Chronic >12 weeks	Chronic >12 weeks
Clinical presentation	Nonspecific sinonasal symptoms and/or fever. Eschar formation in nose, extension to eye, brain, palate, and facial region	Usually the infection affects ethmoid and sphenoid sinuses. Orbital involvement common	Enlarging mass in cheek and nose, extension to orbit or brain common (orbital apex syndrome)	Nasal obstruction, purulent discharge from nose, facial pain, fetish smell perception and post-nasal discharge	Nasal obstruction, discharge, facial pain and hyposmia may present with orbital globe involvement, cavernous sinus thrombosis, otic complication, occasional asthma	Nasal obstruction, rhinorrhoea, facial pain, or fullness

Diagnosis	Endoscopic biopsy of ischemic and necrotic tissue—direct microscopy and culture. Typically underlying tissue does not bleed while biopsied, CT—maxillary and ethmoid sinuses involved, soft tissue mass, bone erosion, facial soft tissue thickening	Endoscopic biopsy—direct microscopy and culture CT—sphenoid and ethmoid sinus involvement, soft tissue mass Histopathology differentiation from granulomatous FRS	Endoscopic biopsy— direct microscopy and culture CT images similar to granulomatous FRS Histopathology differentiation from chronic invasive FRS	Endoscopic biopsy—direct microscopy and culture Mucopurulent and cheesy or clay like material, radiological evidence of sinus opacification with or without calcification	1. Type I hypersensitivity 2. Nasal polyposis 3. Eosinophilic mucin without mucosal invasion 4. Positive fungal stain 5. Characteristic CT finding of heterogeneous opacities	1. Nonallergic eosinophilic mucin collection 2. Positive fungal stain
Treatment	1. Aggressive surgery 2. Conventional or lipid preparation amphotericin B followed by posaconazole or isavuconazole 3. Control of immunosuppression 4. Immunopotentiation	1. Surgery 2. Systemic antifungals 3. Immune reconstitution	1. Surgery 2. Systemic antifungals	Surgery	1. Surgery 2. Oral and/or local steroid (oral steroid better) 3. Immunotherapy	1. Surgery 2. Occasional steroid therapy 3. Antifungal therapy may be used
Prognosis	High mortality if not managed early also called fungal emergency, as the disease progress in hours	Better prognosis, though recurrence can occur	Better prognosis, though recurrence can occur	Very good cure rate	Recurrence common	Not clear

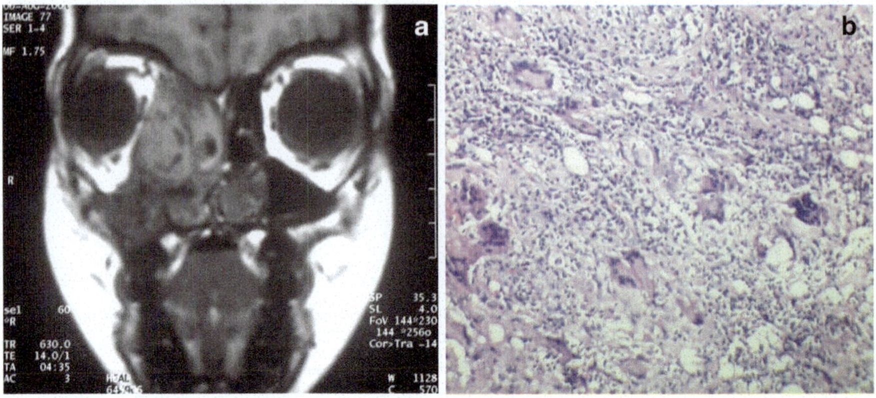

Fig. 11.1 (**a** and **b**) Granulomatous fungal rhinosinusitis; (**a**) CT scan showing blocked paranasal sinuses and extension to the orbital globe, (**b**) histopathology showing granuloma with scanty hyphae

The granulomatous invasive type has been reported in immunocompetent patients of Sudan, India, Pakistan, and Saudi Arabia [2–4, 7, 12, 13]. The patients have a chronic course with enlarging mass in the cheek, orbit, nose, and paranasal sinuses (Fig. 11.1a). Histopathology demonstrates non-caseating granuloma with dense fibrosis, foreign body or Langerhans giant cells, occasional vasculitis, vascular fibrosis, and scanty hyphae (Fig. 11.1b). In contrast to granulomatous invasive type, the chronic invasive type has dense accumulation of hyphae with occasional vascular invasion and mixed inflammatory reaction. *A. flavus* is commonly isolated from granulomatous FRS and *A. fumigatus* from chronic invasive FRS cases. The clinical presentations of both clinical types may be similar, though chronic invasive FRS type is seen in patients with low to moderate immunosuppression due to diabetes or steroid therapy [2, 3, 14, 15]. The clinicopathological distinctions between the two types are not sharp, as both take chronic course with prominent orbital involvement. Therapy and prognosis of both diseases are similar. The difference of prevalent fungi may be due to separate geographical distribution of the disease [2].

11.3 Noninvasive FRS

Asymptomatic colonization of fungi over remaining mucous crust after endoscopic surgery has been observed in few patients. The significance of such colonization is not clear, though certain researchers predict the condition as initiation of fungal ball formation [16].

Fungal ball is defined as the presence of noninvasive accumulation of fungal hyphal conglomeration in maxillary sinus or rarely multiple sinuses [17]. Occasionally flocculent calcium has been observed in hyphal concretion; associated reactive sclerosis of sinus wall is also noticed. The patients usually have radiological evidence of sinus opacification with or without radiographic heterogenicity, presence of mucopurulent cheesy or clay-like materials containing hyphae within the sinus, non-specific inflammation of the mucosa. The disease is common in middle-aged and elderly females of Southern France, though occasionally the disease has been reported in all age group worldwide. Recently a large number of patients with fungal ball in sinus is reported from Taiwan [18]. Rarely fungal ball may become invasive after immunosuppression, and even allergic mucin may be seen along with fungal ball [16, 19, 20]. The disease has been described with various terminologies like mycetoma, aspergilloma, and chronic noninvasive granuloma. Fungal Rhinosinusitis Working Group under International Society for Human and Animal Mycology (ISHAM) unanimously decided to name it as "Fungal ball" [3].

11.4 Eosinophil-Related FRS Including AFRS and EFRS

As this clinical type is common in Asian countries, this disease will be discussed in greater detail.

Historical perspective with the controversies: In 1976, Safirstein first described this clinical entity along with allergic bronchopulmonary aspergillosis (ABPA) in a 24-year-old woman who had recurrent nasal obstruction, mucosal ulceration, edema, and rhinorrhea [21]. Then, in 1981 Miller et al. and in 1983 Katzeinstein et al. described independently few patients who had chronic rhinosinusitis associated with mucosal plug in the sinuses resembling pathology of ABPA. They named the disease as allergic *Aspergillus* sinusitis (AAS) [22, 23]. Later, as fungi other than *Aspergillus*, especially dematiaceous fungi, are found to be associated with this clinical entity, the disease is described as allergic fungal sinusitis (AFS). Bent and Kuhn defined allergic fungal rhinosinusitis (AFRS) with five major and six minor criteria (Table 11.2) [24]. In the pathogenesis of AFRS cases, the hallmark of the

Table 11.2 Bent and Kuhn criteria for diagnosis of AFRS [22]

Major criteria	
1.	A history of type I hypersensitivity described by skin test or in vitro testing
2.	Nasal polyposis
3.	Characteristics of CT findings (Fig. 11.2a, b): unilateral or asymmetric involvement of the sinuses presenting as heterogeneous signal intensity. Central areas of hyperattenuation on CT correspond to hypo-intensity on T1-weighted MR images, and signal void on T2-weighted MR images
4.	Allergic (eosinophilic) mucin without tissue invasion (Fig. 11.2c)
5.	Positive fungal stain
Minor criteria	
1.	Asthma
2.	Unilateral disease
3.	Bone erosion
4.	Fungal culture
5.	Presence of Charcot–Leyden crystals (Fig. 11.2d)
6.	Serum eosinophilia

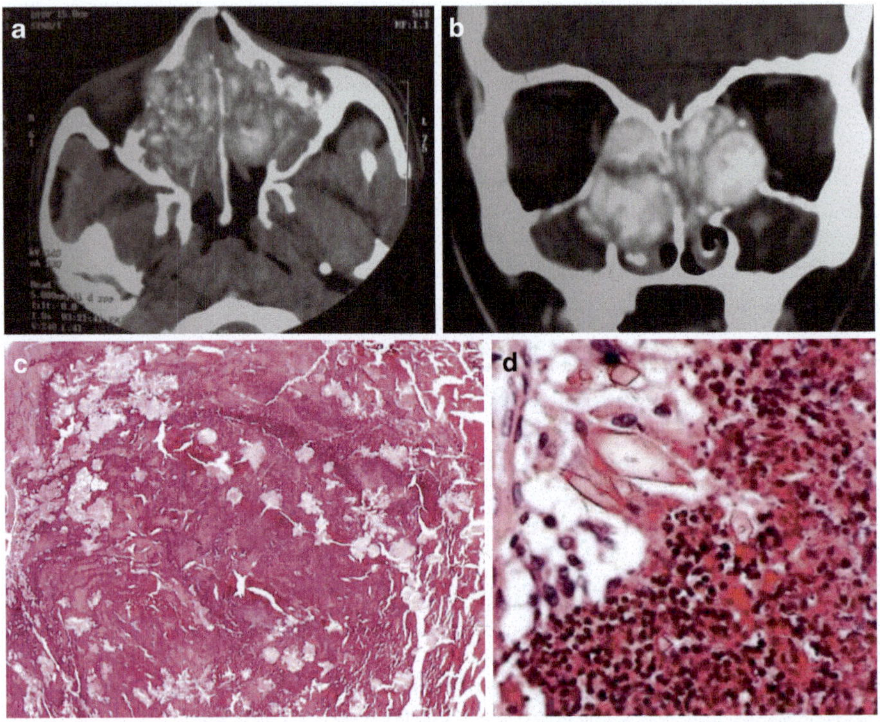

Fig. 11.2 (**a**–**d**) Allergic fungal rhinosinusitis; (**a**) CT scan showing cotton wool pattern opacity, (**b**) CT scan showing concretion pattern, (**c**) eosinophilic (allergic) mucin, (**d**) Charcot–Leyden crystals

disease is Th2 cytokines (IL4, IL5, IL13) production in atopic patients, which leads to ABPA pattern of pathology in nasal sinuses. Although the detection of fungi is important to fulfill the definition of AFRS cases, hyphae may be sparse in sinus content and requires considerable screening time to visualize under microscope.

The definition of AFRS was seriously challenged by Ponikau et al. [25] and subsequently by other workers [26] with the demonstration of fungi in eosinophilic mucin from many cases of CRS independent of type 1 hypersensitivity. They coined the term eosinophilic fungal rhinosinusitis (EFRS) to describe the disease with the striking role of eosinophils in pathogenesis. They claimed that the majority of cases with CRS are due to fungi, as fungi could be detected in nearly all patients using sensitive techniques. However, fungi may be detected in the nose of healthy hosts as well. They proposed that in certain group of individuals, colonizing fungi attract eosinophils in sinuses, which liberate major basic protein (MBP). The large amount of MBP in sinuses damages the nasal epithelium from the luminal side. The damaged epithelium may become portal for bacterial infection [27]. The eosinophilic inflammatory response is claimed to be due to both Th2 and Th1 cytokine production and independent of hypersensitivity reaction [28]. However, this view was confronted by several workers. Ferguson mentioned "eosinophilia or eosinophilic mucin is not synonymous with allergic mucin. Allergies may be associated with eosinophilic mucin, but eosinophilic mucin can be present without evidence of allergies" [16]. Later, Orlandi et al. demonstrated in few patients that IL5 responses to fungus were not predictive of all CRS cases [29]. Therefore, the question arises whether AFRS and EFRS are two distinct entities—AFRS is in patients with atopy and EFRS is independent of atopy.

The confusion was further heightened with the description of a disease called eosinophilic mucin rhinosinusitis (EMRS) by Ferguson [30]. She recorded few cases with eosinophilic mucin in sinuses without any presence of fungal hyphae, and the patients have asthma, increased aspirin sensitivity, and IgG1 deficiency. She considered systemic dysregulation of immunological control plays important role in the pathogenesis of this disease. However presence of fungi in AFRS/EFRS is rare and scattered in eosinophilic mucin. The sensitivity of detection of fungal hyphae depends on the method of sample collection and detection techniques. Enzymatic methods utilizing antibody and PCR technique improve sensitivity [31–33]. In such situation EMRS cases will be diagnosed as EFRS using these sensitive techniques. Further, no difference in expression profile between AFRS and EMRS was found in DNA microarray [34].

Collins et al. proposed a compromised theory of the two extremes by demonstrating specific IgE in the eosinophilic mucin of AFRS as well as non-AFRS patients. They claimed that the pathogenesis is a result of local hypersensitivity in the sinuses rather than systemic hypersensitivity [35]. Pant et al. distinguished eosinophilic mucin CRS (polypoid rhinosinusitis and eosinophilic mucin with or without fungi) and AFRS patients from other form of CRS patients by demonstrating fungal-specific IgG3, rather than IgE. They also raised the question of the role of fungal allergy in AFRS [36]. The confusion with the definition of AFRS is further intensified with the well-documented reports of histologic tissue invasion in few cases of AFRS [12, 37].

A considerable overlap between AFRS, EFRS, and EMRS patients was observed in a study from India [5]. The clear-cut distinction between the entities under eosinophil-related FRS patients remains an enigma, though the difference in therapy in these conditions is predicted. Many consensus definitions were attempted [3, 10, 11], but controversies still exist. The studies on pathogenesis provide contradictory views. Multiple models are proposed for the pathophysiology of the disorder including putative role of allergens, fungal derived antigens, bacteria, and bacteria-derived superantigens [2, 38]. Among different causative agents, it is generally believed that fungi play important role in considerable number of CRS patients. deSazo et al. proposed a workable definition of AFRS [13, 39]. The criteria include (1) presence of CRS (nearly always with nasal polyposis), (2) presence of allergic (eosinophilic) mucin containing noninvasive fungal hyphae in one or more sinus cavities, (3) immune-competence, and (4) fungal allergy (though it is not clear whether local or systemic allergy). A study from India reported a mixed Th1 and Th2 response in eosinophil-related FRS. In contrast to incrementing fungus *Alternaria alternata,* in western world, *Aspergillus flavus* causes immune response in eosinophil-related FRS, and the categorization of the group appears arbitrary [40].

When to suspect AFRS?: The patients are usually young immunocompetent individuals who give a history of long-standing sinus disease (often more than 12 weeks), strongly recalcitrant to traditional medical, and surgical therapy (usually patients are on antibacterial therapy with little success). They have unilateral or asymmetric involvement of paranasal sinuses, a history of atopy, nasal crusts, and polyposis without any significant pain [41]. Nasal crusts are composed of green, brown, or black mucin, displaying the consistency of clay with gray brown-laminated cut surfaces, ranging from a scanty amount to copious volume. On microscopy mucin-containing eosinophils appear as tight clusters and imparting a laminated, scalloped-edge shape. The degenerative products of eosinophils in the form of smudged, elongated nuclei, and basophilic nuclear debris and Charcot–Leyden crystals may also be seen in mucin.

The course of the disease in AFRS patients is usually considered to be subtle, though occasional dramatic presentation of the disease has been reported in the form of acute visual loss, proptosis, gross facial dysmorphia, and telecanthus [42, 43]. The reason for acute presentation is not clear. Perhaps those patients are over-sensitive to fungi or they are heavily exposed to fungal spores.

Responsible fungi: The spectrum of agents causing AFRS is diverse. In the western world, *Alternaria* spp., *Bipolaris* spp., and *Curvularia* spp. are predominantly isolated from these patients [15, 40, 41]. In contrast, *A. flavus* is commonly isolated from Asian patients [2, 5, 7, 12].

Treatment: Like pathogenesis of this entity, controversy exists in the management of AFRS, especially on the mode and dose of corticosteroid therapy, antifungal use, and immunotherapy. None of the management protocol has been found to be ideal, as patients often return with recurrence of the disease. General principles of management include [41]:

1. Avoidance of allergen, if the allergen can be identified.
2. Control of allergy with the use of corticosteroids and antihistamines.
3. Corticosteroids may be used orally or as nasal spray. Multiple studies have shown better benefit with oral corticosteroids. The benefits include increased cure rate, milder disease in patients with recurrence, and increased time for revision surgery [40, 44, 45].
4. Surgery to remove eosinophilic mucin and promote sinus drainage.
5. Immunotherapy directed at both fungal and non-fungal allergens.

11.5 Conclusion

Fungal rhinosinusitis is a common disease in Asian countries especially in India. The disease is complex and understanding of the pathogenesis is still limited. The clear distinction of different types is important as management varies with each category. AFRS is the most common presentation in India with high proportion of the disease in young rural population. A consensus management protocol is still awaited for this disease. Granulomatous invasive FRS is also Asia- and

Africa-specific disease with *A. flavus* as the causative agent. Increased awareness and early diagnosis may help in prompt management of the cases before extension of the disease in orbit or brain.

References

1. Zakirullah, Nawaz G, Sattar SF. Presentation and diagnosis of allergic fungal sinusitis. J Ayub Med Coll Abbottabad. 2010;22:53–7.
2. Chakrabarti A, Das A, Panda NK. Controversies surrounding the categorization of fungal sinusitis. Med Mycol. 2009;47(Suppl I):S299–308.
3. Arunaloke C, Denning David W, Ferguson Berrylin J, Jens P, Walter B, Hirohito K, Bradley M, Naresh P, Stephan V, Catherine K-L, Ashim D, Paramjeet S, Taj-Aldeen Saad J, Serda KA, Handa Kumud K, Ashok G, Thungapathra M, Shivaprakash Mandya R, Amanjit B, Annette F, Radotra Bishan D. Fungal rhinosinusitis: a categorization and definitional schema addressing current controversies. Laryngoscope. 2009;119:1809–18. Telmesani LM. Prevalence of allergic fungal sinusitis among patients with nasal polyps. Ann Saudi Med. 2009; 29: 212-4.
4. Saravanan K, Panda NK, Chakrabarti A, Das A, Bapuraj RJ. Allergic fungal rhinosinusitis: an attempt to resolve the diagnostic dilemma. Arch Otolaryngol Head Neck Surg. 2006;132:173–8.
5. Siddiqui AA, Shah AA, Bashir SH. Craniocerebral aspergillosis of sinonasal origin in immunocompetent patients: clinical spectrum and outcome in 25 cases. Neurosurgery. 2004;55:602–11.
6. Panda NK, Sharma SC, Chakrabarti A, Mann SBS. Paranasal sinus mycoses in north India. Mycoses. 1998;41:281–6.
7. Chakrabarti A, Sharma SC, Chander J. Epidemiology and pathogenesis of paranasal sinus mycoses. Otolaryngol Head Neck Surg. 1992;107:745–50.
8. Chakrabarti A, Rudramurthy SM, Panda N, Das A, Singh A. Epidemiology of chronic fungal rhinosinusitis in rural India. Mycoses. 2015;58:294–302.
9. Meltzer E, Hamilos D, Hadley J, et al. Rhinosinusitis: establishing definitions for clinical research and patient care. J Allergy Clin Immunol. 2004;114(suppl):S155–212.
10. International Rhinosinusitis Advisory Board. Infectious rhinosinusitis in adults: classification, etiology and management. Ear Nose Throat J. 1997;76:5–22.
11. Das A, Bal A, Chakrabarti A, Panda N, Joshi K. Spectrum of fungal rhinosinusitis; histopathologist's perspective. Histopathology. 2009;54:854–9.
12. Veress B, Malik OA, el-Tayeb AA, el-Daoud S, Mahgoub ES, el-Hassan AM. Further observations on primary paranasal Aspergillus granuloma in the Sudan. A morphological study of 46 cases. Am J Trop Med Hyg. 1973;2:765–72.
13. deShazo RD, Chapin K, Swain R. Fungal sinusitis. N Engl J Med. 1997;337:254–9.
14. Milroy CM, Blanshard JD, Lucas S, Michaels L. Aspergillosis of the nose and paranasal sinuses. J Clin Pathol. 1989;42:123–7.
15. Ferguson BJ. Definitions of fungal rhinosinusitis. Otolaryngol Clin North Am. 2000;33:227–35.
16. Grosjean P, Weber R. Fungus balls of the paranasal sinuses: a review. Eur Arch Otorhinolaryngol. 2007;264:461–70.
17. Jiang RS, Huang WC, Liang KL. Characteristics of sinus fungus ball: a unique form of rhinosinusitis. Clin Med Insights Ear Nose Throat. 2018;11:1179550618792254.
18. Gungor A, Adusumilli V. Fungal sinusitis: progression of diseases in immunosuppression—a case report. Ear Nose Throat J. 1998;77:207–15.
19. Graham SM, Ballas ZK. Postoperative steroids confuse the diagnosis of allergic fungal sinusitis. J Allergy Clin Immunol. 1998;101:139–40.
20. Safirstein B. Allergic broncho-pulmonary aspergillosis with obstruction of the upper respiratory tract. Chest. 1976;70:788–90.
21. Millar JN, Johnston A, Lamb D. Allergic aspergillosis of the maxillary sinuses. Thorax. 1981;36:710.

22. Katzenstein AA, Sole SR, Greenberger PA. Allergic Aspergillus sinusitis: a newly recognized form of sinusitis. J Allergy Clin Immunol. 1983;72:82–93.
23. Bent JP, Kuhn FA. Diagnosis of allergic fungal sinusitis. Otolaryngol Head Neck Surg. 1994;111:580–8.
24. Ponikau JU, Sherris DA, Kern EB, Homburger HA, Frigas E, Gaffey TA. The diagnosis and incidence of allergic fungal sinusitis. Mayo Clin Proc. 1999;74:877–84.
25. Braun H, Buzina W, Freudenschuss K, Beham A, Stammberger H. "Eosinophilic fungal rhinosinusitis": a common disorder in Europe? Laryngoscope. 2003;113:264–9.
26. Ponikau JU, Sherris DA, Kephart GM, et al. Striking deposition of toxic eosinophil major basic protein in mucus: implications for chronic rhinosinusitis. J Allergy Clin Immunol. 2005;116:362–9.
27. Shin SH, Ponikau JU, Sherris DA, et al. Chronic rhinosinusitis: an advanced immune response to ubiquitous airborne fungi. J Allergy Clin Immunol. 2004;114:1369–75.
28. Orlandi RR, Marple BF, Georgelas A, Durtschi D, Barr L. Immunologic response to fungus is not universally associated with rhinosinusitis. Otolaryngol Head Neck Surg. 2009;141:750–6.
29. Ferguson BJ. Eosinophilic mucin rhinosinusitis: a distinct clinicopathological entity. Laryngoscope. 2000;110:799–813.
30. Lackner A, Stammberger H, Buzina W, et al. Fungi: a normal content of human nasal mucus. Am J Rhinol. 2005;19:125–9.
31. Murr AH, Goldberg AN, Pletcher SD, Dillehay K, Wymer LJ, Vesper SJ. Some chronic rhinosinusitis patients have elevated populations of fungi in their sinuses. Laryngoscope. 2012;122:1438–45.
32. Guo C, Ghaderoshi S, Kephart GM, et al. Improving the detection of fungi in eosinophilic mucin: seeing what we could not see before. Otolaryngol Head Neck Surg. 2012;147:943–9.
33. Orlandi RR, Thibeault SL, Ferguson BJ. Microarray analysis of allergic fungal sinusitis and eosinophilic muin rhinosinusitis. Otolaryngol Head Neck Surg. 2007;136:707–13.
34. Collins M, Nair S, Smith W, Kette F, Gillis D, Wormald PJ. Role of local immunoglobulin E production in the pathophysiology of noninvasive fungal sinusitis. Laryngoscope. 2004;114:1242–6.
35. Pant H, Kette FE, Smith WB, Wormald PJ, Macardle PJ. Fungal-specific humoral response in eosinophilic mucus chronic rhinosinusitis. Laryngoscope. 2005;115:601–6.
36. Thakar A, Sarkar C, Dhiwakar M, Bahadur S, Dahiya S. Allergic fungal sinusitis: expanding the clinicopathological spectrum. Otolaryngol Head Neck Surg. 2004;130:209–16.
37. Borish L, Rosenwasser L, Steinke JW. Fungi in chronic hyperplastic eosinophilic sinusitis. Clin Rev Allergy Immunol. 2006;30:1–9.
38. deShazo RD, Swain RE. Diagnostic criteria for allergic fungal sinusitis. J Allergy Clin Immunol. 1995;96:24–35.
39. Glass D, Amedee RG. Allergic fungal rhinosinusitis: a review. Ochsner J. 2011;11:271–5.
40. Kale P, Rudramurthy SM, Panda N, Das A, Chakrabarti A. The inflammatory response of eosinophil-related fungal rhinosinusitis varies with inciting fungi. Med Mycol. 2015;53:387–95.
41. Marple BF, Gibbs SR, Newcomer MT, Mabry RL. Allergic fungal sinusitis-induced visual loss. Am J Rhinol. 1999;13:191–5.
42. Manning SC, Schaefer SD, Close LG, Vuitch F. Culture positive allergic fungal sinusitis. Arch Otolaryngol. 1991;117:174–8.
43. Cody DT, Neel HB, Ferreiro JA, Roberts GD. Allergic fungal sinusitis: the Mayo Clinic experience. Laryngoscope. 1994;104:1074–9.
44. Kuhn FA, Javer AR. Allergic fungal rhinosinusitis: our experience. Arch Otolaryngol Head Neck Surg. 1998;124:1179–80.
45. Ryan MW, Marple BF. Allergic fungal rhinosinusitis: diagnosis and management. Curr Opin Otolaryngol Head Neck Surg. 2007;15:18–22.

Part IV

Diagnosis

Diagnostic Algorithm for Invasive Fungal Infections

12

Ziauddin Khan and Suhail Ahmad

Key Points

- The increased spectrum of fungal pathogens and a diversity of clinical and radiological presentations pose a major diagnostic challenge for invasive fungal infections.
- None of the currently available diagnostic tests provide sufficient sensitivity and specificity, thus the optimal approach should rely on a combination of diagnostic strategies, including imaging, fungal biomarkers, and molecular tools.
- A better understanding of the clinicians regarding the availability of new diagnostic tools to achieve rapid and accurate diagnosis is highly warranted.
- Lateral flow devices for aspergillosis and cryptococcosis and T2Candida for candidemia are some noteworthy advances in the rapid diagnosis.
- Serum/bronchoalveolar lavage galactomannan (GM) assay is recommended for the diagnosis of invasive aspergillosis (IA) in high-risk patients (hematologic malignancy, bone marrow transplant recipients).
- GM test is not recommended for routine screening of patients receiving mold-active antifungal therapy/prophylaxis.
- Serum (1-3)-β-D glucan (BDG) assay, a panfungal marker, can be used alone or in combination (with mannan/galactomannan) for diagnosis, particularly for excluding fungal infections.
- Molecular platforms offer promise for specific detection and identification of fungal pathogens in clinical specimens as well as in cultures.
- Results of GM, BDG, and PCR tests should be interpreted in conjunction with clinical, microbiologic, and radiological findings to increase the probability of correct diagnosis.

Z. Khan (✉) · S. Ahmad
Department of Microbiology, Faculty of Medicine, Kuwait University, Safat, Kuwait
e-mail: zkhan@hsc.edu.kw; suhail_ah@hsc.edu.kw

A. Chakrabarti (ed.), *Clinical Practice of Medical Mycology in Asia*,
https://doi.org/10.1007/978-981-13-9459-1_12

12.1 Introduction

Invasive fungal infections (IFI) are a major cause of morbidity and mortality among severely immunocompromised patients, particularly in developing world, where diagnostic and therapeutic resources are limited [1]. Early diagnosis of IFI is central to achieving improved prognosis [2–5]. Currently available approaches can be categorized as conventional (direct microscopy, culture, and histopathology) and biomarker-based [detection of 1, 3-β-D-glucan (BDG), galactomannan (GM), *Candida* mannan (Mn), *Candida*-anti-mannan antibodies (A-Mn) and genus/species-specific DNA] diagnostic methods [2, 5–7]. The biomarker-based approach has the potential to lead to an early diagnosis before a full-blown disease develops and can be used for monitoring response to therapy [8, 9]. High-resolution computed tomography (CT) and magnetic resonance imaging (MRI) scans are other helpful tools for the early diagnosis of IFI, particularly those caused by molds in neutropenic patients [10]. This article provides an updated overview of available modalities for early diagnosis of invasive candidiasis (IC) and invasive mold diseases with particular focus on invasive aspergillosis (IA) and outlines the role of biomarkers in the overall diagnostic strategy.

12.2 How to Suspect Invasive Fungal Infections?

Invasive candidiasis (IC): Candida species are part of normal microbiota and thus may give rise to systemic IC when integrity of skin or mucosa is compromised. A number of risk factors have been identified, which predispose hospitalized patients for developing IC [11]. The likelihood of acquiring candidemia is higher in patients with prolonged stay in intensive care unit (ICU), receiving total parenteral nutrition (TPN), central venous catheter placement, colonization with *Candida* at multiple anatomical sites, receiving multiple antimicrobial agents, or those undergoing abdominal surgery or hemodialysis [11–16]. Clinical prediction criteria for identifying patients who could benefit from either prophylaxis or empirical antifungal therapy against IC have also been developed with varying sensitivity, specificity, positive predictive value (PPV), and negative predictive value (NPV) [12]. These criteria have been as simple as determining *Candida* colonization index to more complex criteria involving multiple risk factors [12–15]. However, colonizing index may fail to identify patient at risk for candidemia in developing countries where nearly all patients in intensive care unit have *Candida* colonization due to overuse of antibiotics [6]. A predictive rule with low PPV and high NPV has also been developed to identify patients who are unlikely to develop IC [16].

IC is also an important cause of late-onset septicemia in premature neonates. The incidence of IC ranges from 2.6 to 12.9% in neonates ≤1500 g birth weight and

6–20% in those with birth weight ≤1000 g [17]. Additional risk factors include gestational age (<32 weeks), use of ≥2 antibiotics, central venous catheter placement, administration of TPN for >5 days, prior *Candida* colonization, and low platelet count [17–19].

Invasive aspergillosis (IA): Among invasive mold diseases, IA is the most dreaded complication of immunocompromised patients causing considerable mortality. Individuals with hematologic malignancies and allogeneic hematopoietic stem cell transplantation (HSCT) have the highest risk [20, 21]. Other high-risk groups include lung or heart transplant recipients, chronic granulomatous disease patients, and HIV-infected individuals with <50 $CD4^{+}$ cells/μL. Initial clinical manifestations of IA are nonspecific, and about 30% patients may remain asymptomatic. Hence, early diagnosis of IA is challenging and needs to be approached from the characteristics of at-risk patients. Clinical features, including resolving pulmonary infiltrates despite usual antibacterial antibiotics and the possible presence of skin, bone, genitourinary, and central nervous system manifestations, should raise the possibility of an invasive mold infection [5]. The duration of neutropenia is the most important risk factor predicting onset, which may be highest if neutrophil count drops below 0.10×10^9 [20, 21]. However, it is important to recognize that IA may also occur in critically ill non-immunocompromised/non-neutropenic hosts, such as those with chronic obstructive pulmonary disease, chronic liver disease, or as a post-influenza complication [22, 23]. Polymorphisms in Toll-like and some other receptor genes also enhance the risk of developing IA [21, 24].

Mucormycosis: Mucormycosis (earlier called zygomycosis) is caused by the members of the order Mucorales. It is a devastating disease of immunocompromised patients with emerging significance [25, 26]. Its incidence is seemingly increasing in patients with hematologic malignancies and solid organ transplant recipients and cases of breakthrough infection during voriconazole and caspofungin therapy have also been reported [25]. Patients with diabetic ketoacidosis exhibit exceptional susceptibility. Metabolic acidosis dissociates iron from iron-binding protein (transferrin), thus enhancing the availability of free iron for the growth of the fungus. Similarly, patients on iron chelation therapy are susceptible to mucormycosis. High iron concentrations interfere with neutrophil chemotaxis as well as reduce their ability to adhere to fungal hyphae [21]. Since invasive mucormycosis runs a rapidly fatal course, a better understanding of the underlying conditions and associated risk factors is prerequisite for achieving early diagnosis and favorable outcome. Since culture positivity is low, and BDG and GM markers are not useful, DNA-based detection methods are essential. In this context, Millon et al. [26] developed three quantitative PCRs for the detection of *Mucor/Rhizopus*, *Lichtheimia* and *Rhizomucor* in serum samples of high-risk hematology patients.

12.2.1 Imaging

Introduction of high-resolution CT and MRI scans has brought about great improvement in imaging-based diagnosis of IFI. Unfortunately, the diagnostic potential of these new imaging techniques still remains underutilized. High-resolution CT scans may show halo sign (nodule or mass surrounded by a ground-glass opacity) and a reversed halo sign (focal rounded area of ground-glass opacity surrounded by a crescent or complete ring of consolidation) among patients with IA and mucormycosis, respectively [27]. Halo signs appear to depict angio-invasive nature of the fungus, but can also be seen in non-fungal diseases [27]. The presence of multiple ($\geq$10) nodules and pleural effusion in CT scans in the absence of other radiographic findings have been reported to be predictive of pulmonary mucormycosis in neutropenic patients [28]. The Halo sign, air-crescent sign, and cavitation in chest CT scan have been included in the clinical criteria for probable invasive fungal disease (IFD) in European Organization for Research and Treatment of Cancer/Mycosis Study Group (EORTC/MSG) guidelines [29]. The use of different imaging modalities has proven to be more beneficial in delineating the number, type, and extent of mycotic lesions [30].

12.2.2 Microscopic and Histopathologic Diagnosis

Direct microscopic examination of clinical specimens provides a distinct advantage over culture as it is a rapid method for presumptive diagnosis of fungal infections. Delayed diagnosis of an invasive fungal infection can be lethal. Microscopy can distinguish whether an infection is caused by a yeast, such as *Candida*, a septate mold, such as *Aspergillus* spp. or a non-septate mold, such as *Mucorales* (Table 12.1) [31, 32]. Direct microscopy is particularly important for infections caused by non-septate fungi because fragile nature of their hyphae can easily be damaged during refrigeration or homogenization of tissues, thus leading to poor recovery in culture. Many other pathogenic fungi can be provisionally identified by direct microscopy (capsule of *Cryptococcus* spp., spherules of *Coccidioides* spp., or small intracellular yeasts of *Histoplasma capsulatum* or *Talaromyces* [*Penicillium*] *marneffei*). It is also important that besides hematoxylin and eosin (H&E) stains, tissue sections are also stained in parallel with at least one specialized fungal stain, such as Grocott methenamine silver (GMS) stain or periodic acid–Schiff (PAS), to avoid delay. These stains should be used routinely in samples from immunocompromised patients (such as those with HIV; on glucocorticoid therapy; with malignant disease, including leukemia; on cancer chemotherapy; receiving solid organ or bone marrow transplantation; with congenital immune-deficiency; and those receiving therapy with immunosuppressive agents, such as antitumor necrosis factor, immunomodulators, or methotrexate). For visualization of fungi in tissue, GMS stain is more sensitive than PAS, and *Mucorales* might need longer staining times, than other fungi. Although demonstration of fungal elements in tissue or other sterile specimens is an

Table 12.1 Characteristic morphological features of specific fungi for presumptive identification in clinical specimens

Fungal pathogen	Size	Morphological characteristics	Comments
Cryptococcus neoformans/C. gatti	5–15 μm	Clear mucoid capsule surrounding yeast cells	India ink detects polysaccharide capsule. Mucicarmine stains capsule pink. Fontana-Masson stain is used for melanin detection
Histoplasma capsulatum	3–5 μm	Intracellular yeasts with halo around	Differentiated by *Leishmania*, *Talaromyces marneffei*, *C. neoformans*, *Candida glabrata*
Emergomyces species	2–7 μm	Intracellular as well as extracellular yeast forms	Histopathologic findings alone are not sufficient to distinguish *Emergomyces* sp. from other dimorphic fungi
Coccidioides immitis/ Coccidioides posadasii	15–100 μm	Large yeast-like structures containing endospores	
Pneumocystis jirovecii	3–5 μm	Cysts with trophozoites, fine honeycomb	Fibrin exudates, alveolar proteinosis
Sporothrix schenckii	3–15 μm	Elongated "cigar-shaped" yeast-like forms	Can be very scarce; pseudoepitheliomatous hyperplasia
Candida spp.	3–15 μm	Usually hyphae-like structures and yeasts	
Aspergillus spp.	5–15 μm	Septate; dichotomous branching at 45° angle	Less common hyphae; e.g., *Fusarium* spp., *Scedosporium* spp. (hyaline), *Cladosporium* spp. (pigmented)
Molds of the order *Mucorales*	15–100 μm; irregular diameter hyphae	Usually broad ribbon-like hyphae, rarely septate	

Modified from Schelenz et al. [31]

evidence of "proven" mycosis (EORTC criteria), it is often not attempted due to fear of complications or bleeding, particularly in patients with severe thrombocytopenia [33]. However, sample collection by CT-guided fine-needle aspiration from deep tissue improves the diagnostic yield [30].

12.2.3 Isolation and Identification of Fungal Pathogens

Although most yeasts can be isolated from BACTEC blood culture bottles and blood culture is "gold standard" for the diagnosis of IC/candidemia, ~50% of patients with IC may yield negative results [11, 34]. Growth of *Candida glabrata* in BACTEC™ medium is slow requiring longer incubation period of >5 days. Use of lysis-centrifugation method may yield higher blood culture positivity, but the technique is prone to contamination [35]. Recently, T2Candida platform (T2 Biosystem) that uses T2 magnetic resonance to detect *Candida* directly in the whole blood samples has been used for the diagnosis of *Candida* bloodstream infections. It has high sensitivity (~90%) and specificity (~98%) for diagnosing candidemia and also has potential to be used as a prognostic tool [36, 37]. It is superior to cultures or serum BDG in identifying patients with candidemia. T2Candida may improve patient care by shortening time required for *Candida* isolation and species identification as compared to conventional blood culture methods. The mean time to *Candida* detection and species identification in T2Candida platform is about 4.4 ± 1.0 h [36, 37]. However, the technique can identify only five *Candida* species and cannot replace conventional culture method due to need of in vitro susceptibility testing (a more detailed role of T2Candida in the diagnosis of invasive candidiasis is described later).

Some molds (*Fusarium* spp.) are more frequently isolated while *Aspergillus* and some other molds do not grow well in BACTEC blood culture bottles. Isolation of *Aspergillus* species from respiratory specimens mixed with *Candida* can be enhanced with peptone glucose fluconazole agar [38]. As stated above, agents of mucormycosis often fail to grow from specimens positive by direct microscopy due to fragile nature of fungal hyphae; hence, the diagnosis is largely dependent on histopathological evidence [39]. Prolonged refrigeration and aggressive grinding of tissues may make these fungi nonviable due to coenocytic nature of their hyphae [40]. Since there are no validated biomarkers available for the diagnosis of mucormycosis, molecular methods can be attempted when culture is negative [26, 41]. Recent molecular techniques including direct DNA sequencing and high-throughput multiplex assays using Luminex® xMAP technology offer rapid and accurate identification of important fungal pathogens [2, 3, 42]. However, these methods still require multicenter evaluation and standardization.

Matrix-assisted laser desorption ionization-time of flight mass spectrometry (MALDI-TOF MS) is now being increasingly used for rapid identification of yeasts including *Candida auris*, a recently described multidrug-resistant species [43–45]. The MALDI-TOF MS analysis identifies organisms based on their protein fingerprints. However, some rare but clinically significant yeast species are not accurately identified by MALDI-TOF MS systems due to limitations of their databases. Expansion of database of their library by addition of less common species is required to improve their performance, as shown recently for *C. auris* [45]. With progress in extraction protocols and the composition of comparative protein fingerprinting libraries, MALDI-TOF MS has also been used for the identification of filamentous fungi including *Mucorales* in recent years [46, 47]. In addition to pure cultures, MALDI-TOF MS can also be applied for the identification of fungi in blood specimens. However, detection of mixed isolates is still a challenge. MALDI-TOF MS has also been used for the detection of antifungal resistance [48].

12.2.4 Biomarkers

Lack of specific signs and symptoms and limitations associated with conventional diagnostic procedures have led to the development of non-culture-based methods (e.g., detection of biomarkers) for early diagnosis of invasive mycoses. Biomarkers can be panfungal or group-specific and include (1→3)-β-D-glucan (BDG), galactomannan (GM), *Candida* mannan (Mn), anti-Mn antibodies (A-Mn), and species-specific DNA. Biomarkers can be easily detected in small amount of body fluids (serum; plasma; blood; bronchoalveolar lavage [BAL] or cerebrospinal fluid [CSF]), quantified, and are usually not affected by patient's immune status. However, detection of GM in serum and BAL and detection of BDG in serum are only approved by the United States (US) Food and Drug Administration (FDA) for diagnostic laboratories (Table 12.2) [49]. Serial biomarker detection can also be used for monitoring

Table 12.2 Biomarker-based tests used for the diagnosis of invasive aspergillosis

Test	BDG	GM	LFD
Method	Biological cascade-based assay	Anti-GM monoclonal antibody (mAb EB A2)	Anti-GM monoclonal antibody (mAb JF-5)
Commercial assay	Fungitell[a]	Platelia Aspergillus EIA	Aspergillus LFD
Result interpretation	Negative result: <60 pg/mL Intermediate result: 60–79 pg/mL Positive result: ≥80 pg/mL	Negative result: <0.5 ODI Positive result: ≥0.5 ODI[d]	Qualitative method (positive/negative results)
Clinical applications	Used for the early detection of IFI	Used for the early diagnosis of invasive aspergillosis in adult patients	Point-of-care testing for early detection of invasive aspergillosis
FDA approval	Serum	Serum, BAL	Not approved
Test performance for the diagnosis of invasive aspergillosis	Sensitivity: 77% (67–84%) Specificity: 85% (80–90%)	Serum-GM[b] Sensitivity: 41–78% Specificity: 60–95% BAL-GM[b] Sensitivity: 87% (79–92%) Sensitivity: 89% (85–92%)	Serum-LFD[c] Sensitivity: 20–68% Specificity: 72–98% BAL-LFD Sensitivity: 80–100% Specificity: 81–95%

FDA food and drug administration, *BDG* 1,3-β-D-glucan, *IFI* invasive fungal infections, *GM* galactomannan, *EIA* enzyme immunoassay, *ODI* optical density index, *BAL* bronchoalveolar lavage, *LFD* lateral flow device

Modified from Miceli and Maertens [49]

[a]Other kits used for the detection of BDG include Fungitec-G test MK (G-MK), beta-glucan test Wako (Curdlan), and the BGSTAR beta-glucan test Maruha which are available in Japan

[b]Galactomannan test performance may vary depending on the patient population and cutoff point used. Table shows test performance using cutoff point 0.5 ODI

[c]Lateral flow test performance may vary depending on the patient population

[d]BAL samples with index value 0.5–1.0 have a lower predictive value than BAL samples with >1.0 index value

prognosis. Although fungal biomarkers represent promising adjuncts to the diagnostic armamentarium for invasive fungal disease, yet substantial gaps exist in the correct use and interpretation of these diagnostic tools in different patient populations.

(1→3)-β-D-Glucan (BDG): The serum BDG assay has been extensively evaluated for the diagnosis of IFI including IA and IC [8, 50–52]. Clinically significant levels of BDG may appear several days before the mycological diagnosis is achieved. In critically ill ICU patients with sepsis, a single positive BDG test was superior to *Candida* score and *Candida* colonization index for IC. A meta-analysis of studies involving patients with hematological malignancies showed that use of two consecutive positive results had very high specificity and PPV [51]. The BDG assay has been included in mycological criteria as probable evidence for IFD in EORTC/MSG consensus definitions document [29]. The test is also recommended for use as moderate evidence for hepatosplenic candidiasis by European Conference on Infections in Leukemia (ECIL) Laboratory Working Group [52]. Recently, a simple clinical prediction rule for the diagnosis of *Pneumocystis jirovecii* pneumonia in the World Health Organization's algorithm for seriously ill HIV-infected patients has been proposed needing external validation [53]. Apart from the diagnostic role of BDG test as a panfungal marker [54], it also has greater utility for excluding IFI due to its high NPV [2, 34]. BDG test may be falsely positive in patients receiving hemodialysis or receiving blood products with cellulose-containing materials (Table 12.3).

Candida mannan (Mn) and anti-mannan antibody (A-Mn) assays: Detection of Mn and A-Mn has also been used for diagnosing IC in surgical and hematological cancer patients with an overall sensitivity of 58% and 59%, respectively, and a combined sensitivity of 83% when both Mn and A-Mn are detected [55–57]. Species-related differences are noted in detection of Mn and A-Mn with sensitivity being highest for *C. albicans* (80–100%) and lowest for *C. parapsilosis* and *C. krusei* (40–50%) [56]. The ECIL Laboratory Working Group has recommended combined detection of Mn and A-Mn as moderate evidence for diagnosing hepatosplenic candidiasis in leukemic patients and HSCT recipients [52]. Bio-Rad Laboratories

Table 12.3 False positivity of biomarker tests

Source(s)	Beta-D glucan	Galactomannan[a]
Medications	Ampicillin-clavulanate, ampicillin-sulbactam	Piperacillin-tazobactam, Beta lactams
Infusions	Immunoglobulin, cellulose filter, albumin	Plasma-Lyte, sodium gluconate
Medical interventions	Hemodialysis with cellulose filter, gauze	Soybean proteins, cardboard
Bacterial infection	Gram-positive bacterial septicemia, *Alcaligenes faecalis*	*Bifidobacterium* spp. from gut
Environmental		Presence of non-Aspergillus fungi such as *Penicillium, Alternaria, Paecilomyces, Geotrichum, Histoplasma, Fusarium*
Food intake		Pasta, yoghurt, ice-pop

[a]Also see PLATELIA™ *ASPERGILLUS* Ag insert (BIO-RAD)

(France) has recently introduced improved versions of these two tests (Platelia *Candida* Ag Plus™ and Platelia *Candida* Ab Plus™) and prospective randomized studies are needed to evaluate their performance in different high-risk patients. Recently, Clancy and Nguyen have presented comparative positive and negative predictive values for mannan/anti-mannan and BDG, PCR, and T2Candida tests in the diagnosis of candidemia in different patient populations (Table 12.4) [58, 59]. Data on the effect of immunosuppression and heavy *Candida* colonization on the performance of these assays in terms of false-negative and false-positive results are very limited [50, 55, 56].

Detection of galactomannan (GM): Sequential GM (Platelia Aspergillus Ag, Bio-Rad, France) detection with an index cutoff value >0.5 in thrice-weekly samples or >0.8 for a single sample enables early (10 ± 4 days) diagnosis of IA before a clinical disease develops [60, 61]. Variable sensitivity (60–100%) and specificity (81–99%) of GM detection is reported in patients depending upon the samples tested and cut-off index values used [33, 62, 63]. A meta-analysis of GM assay (0.5 cutoff value) in BAL for the diagnosis of IA demonstrated pooled sensitivity, specificity, and positive and negative likelihood ratio of 87%, 89%, 80%, and 15%, respectively [64]. A monoclonal antibody-based point-of-care test has also been developed and showed comparable positivity with GM assay for diagnosis of IA [65]. GM assay may cross-react with sera of patients with penicilliosis/histoplasmosis/blastomycosis.

Table 12.4 Prevalence of candidemia in different populations and anticipated PPVs and NPVs of non-culture tests

Prevalence (%)[a]	Representative patient	T2Candida[b]		Mannan/anti-mannan and BDG[c]		PCR[d]	
		PPV	NPV	PPV (%)	NPV (%)	PPV	NPV
0.4	Any hospitalized patient from whom a blood culture is collected	15	>99.9	1	99.9	3	>99.9
1	Patient admitted to ICU	31	99.9	4	99.7	8	99.9
2	Patient with febrile neutropenia and baseline rate of candidemia prior to empirical antifungal treatment	47	99.8	7	99.5	16	99.8
3	Patient with sepsis, shock, or >3 7 day stay in ICU	67	99.7	11	99.2	22	99.6
10	Patient at increased risk for candidemia-based clinical prediction models	82	99	31	97	50	98.8

Adopted from Clancy and Nguyen [58]

[a]References for the prevalence of candidemia in various patient populations are summarized in Clancy et al. [36, 59]. The sensitivity and specificity of each assay for candidemia are estimated from meta-analyses of combined mannan/anti-mannan, BDG, and PCR assays and the T2Candida DIRECT and DIRECT2 studies

[b]Sensitivity/specificity, 90%/98%

[c]Sensitivity/specificity, 80%/80%

[d]Sensitivity/specificity, 90%/90%

BAL from patients colonized with *Aspergillus/Bifidobacterium* or those receiving piperacillin/tazobactam, plasma-Lyte solutions or cyclophosphamide may also show false-positive result (Table 12.3) [2, 33, 66].

12.3 Molecular Identification of Blood Culture Isolates of *Candida* Species

In diagnostic mycology laboratory, the identification of fungal pathogens is mainly relied upon microscopic examination, tissue morphology, and culture. Such identification approaches are time-consuming and require high level of expertise in phenotypic characteristics of fungal pathogens. With increasing range of fungi associated with invasive infections, particularly in immunocompromised patients, the application of molecular identification methods has become a necessity. Besides being rapid, the molecular methods can be used in the absence of live cells, even in formalin-fixed tissues. Among different fungal pathogens, the detection and identification of *Candida* species in clinical specimens have witnessed considerable progress [2, 59, 66]. Identification of specific *Candida* species is also required even if blood cultures are positive for proper patient management. Molecular methods offer rapid species-specific identification of blood culture isolates while phenotypic tests may take one to several days [2, 66]. Conventional PCR with panfungal primers followed by species-specific detection of amplicons (using probe primers) by enzyme immunoassay or uniplex/multiplex PCR with species-specific primers followed by gel electrophoresis is simple and cost-effective for identifying most frequently isolated *Candida* species [67–71]. Panfungal real-time PCR assays using species-specific probe primers yield faster results in a single step; however, practical application of using distinct probe primers in a single reaction is limited [2, 66]. Panfungal PCR followed by sequencing (or pyrosequencing) of species-specific regions or hybridization with specific probe primers on a microarray is suitable for rapid detection of common and rare pathogenic *Candida* species [72–74]. Broad-range PCR amplification of loci containing species-specific sequences (such as 18S, 5.8S, or 28S rRNA genes for fungal pathogens), by electrospray ionization/mass spectrometry (PCR/ESI-MS), has also been developed for the identification of several medically important *Candida* spp. [2, 66].

12.3.1 Molecular Diagnosis

Nucleic acid-based amplification techniques detect fungal DNA/RNA in suitable samples for the diagnosis of IFI [4, 61, 62, 66, 67, 75]. Most PCR-based assays have focused on the detection of IC and IA [56, 66, 75]. Semi-nested/nested PCR, multiplex PCR, or multiplex PCR followed by DNA microarray have been used for diagnosing IC [2, 57, 66–68]. Quantitative real-time PCR assays exhibit higher sensitivity and specificity (>90%) and minimize false-positive results [34, 67, 75]. Combined detection of fungal nucleic acid with another panfungal or group-specific biomarker has offered greater sensitivity and specificity [50]. Detection of fungal DNA and BDG was more sensitive than blood cultures among patients with deep-seated candidiasis and also enhanced the ability to diagnose IC in blood culture-negative patients [34, 75]. European *Aspergillus* PCR Initiative (EAPCRI) working group has developed standard methodology for improving performance of *Aspergillus* PCR assays [76]. A bivariate meta-analysis has reported a pooled sensitivity and specificity of 91% and 92%, respectively, in BAL samples for diagnosis of IA [77]. Again, combined detection of fungal nucleic acid with GM has offered greater sensitivity and specificity. Diagnostic performance of PCR in GM-positive BAL samples was comparable, and performance of both tests resulted in optimal sensitivity and specificity, resulting in early diagnosis and proper management of IA [9, 78].

The first commercially available PCR-based test (LightCycler SeptiFast from Roche Diagnostics) rapidly (within few hours) detects five *Candida* species, directly from blood drawn at the same time as for blood culture [79]. The test exhibited 83% concordance with blood culture results with most discrepant results originating from samples obtained from clinically suspected patients who were PCR-positive but tested negative by culture. More recent studies have shown that detection of *C. albicans* and other *Candida* species from blood samples of patients with suspected systemic bacterial or fungal infection by SeptiFast was much superior compared to culture and other in-house PCR assays [80, 81].

Another commercial test (T2Candida panel) recently approved by the US FDA rapidly detects and identifies five *Candida* species, viz. *C. albicans, C. tropicalis, C. parapsilosis, C. krusei*, and *C. glabrata* in a culture-independent manner [82, 83]. The test performed on the fully automated T2Dx instrument (T2 Biosystems) combines magnetic resonance with molecular diagnostics by amplifying target DNA followed by the detection of the amplified products by amplicon-induced agglomeration of supermagnetic particles and T2 magnetic resonance (T2MR) measurement for the diagnosis of candidemia with a mean time to species identification of less than 5 h [82, 83]. The T2Candida can be used to efficiently diagnose or rule out candidemia using low-volume blood specimens from pediatric and adult patients with sensitivity and specificity of ~90% and ~98%, respectively, for the detection of candidemia [37, 82, 83]. The T2Candida panel was superior to cultures or serum BDG detection in identifying patients with complicated candidemia, in predicting the outcome of empirical antifungal therapy for suspected candidiasis patients and avoiding empirical antifungal therapy in ~60% of T2Candida-negative patients [37, 84–86]. A multicenter, prospective study of the T2Candida panel reported that T2Candida and companion blood cultures were positive in 69 of 152 (45%) and 36 of 152 (24%) patients, respectively [36]. Combined test results were positive for both T2Candida and blood cultures in 32 of 152 (21%) patients, T2Candida alone was positive in 37 of 152 (24%) patients, blood cultures alone were positive in 4 of

152 (3%) patients while 79 of 152 (52%) patients were negative for both T2Candida and blood cultures [36]. Interestingly, candidemia by *C. albicans* was significantly associated with T2Candida positivity, however, some highly suspected candidemia patients yielded T2Candida positive results but companion blood culture-negative results. The data showed that T2Candida improves care by shortening the time to detection of candidemia together with species identification compared to blood cultures and also rendered active candidemia unlikely when the results were negative [36]. The higher sensitivity of these molecular assays is not surprising since blood culture considered as the "gold standard" of sepsis remains negative in ~50% of all clinical cases of sepsis including those caused by *Candida* species [34].

12.3.2 Point-of-Care Diagnostic Tests

A new generation of point-of-care (POC) tests for the diagnosis of IFI have shown promising results in various studies with significant reduction in turnaround time and cost [87]. These include *Aspergillus*-specific lateral-flow device (LFD) test for IA, cryptococcal lateral flow assay for cryptococcosis, and loop-mediated isothermal amplification assay for histoplasmosis [88, 89]. As compared to culture, LFD test for cryptococcosis showed sensitivity of 99.5% and specificity of 98%. In comparison to other commercially available tests for cryptococcal antigen, the LFD test was equal or superior in sensitivity and specificity in CSF, plasma, and serum samples. The LFD test is particularly useful for early screening of cryptococcal infection before clinical disease develops. The search for POC tests for other fungal infections including mucormycosis is in progress.

12.3.3 A Summary of Algorithm Best Practiced

Biomarker-driven strategies have now become routine for supporting early and specific diagnosis of IFI and are included in revised EORTC/MSG consensus definitions of IFD. A practical approach for the diagnosis of IC and IA is proposed in Fig. 12.1. The diagnostic performance of twice-weekly BDG detection for IC and IA yielding negative results has a high NPV for IFI. Sequential BDG detection in serum may also be used for outcome evaluation in IC [90]. Similarly, GM monitoring is used for patients at high risk (probability >5–10%) of developing IA, and an index value of ≥0.8 in single serum sample or ≥0.5 in two consecutive samples should prompt a twice-weekly diagnostic work-up with clinical, microbiological, and radiological evaluation [40]. Clinical outcome of IA may be predicted by following the trends in GM index during the first 2 weeks of antifungal therapy [91]. Combined detection of Mn and A-Mn can be used as a moderate evidence for deep-seated candidiasis in leukemic patients [52]. However, PCR-based assays are not yet included in ECIL recommendations or revised EORTC/MSG criteria of IFD due to variations in inter-laboratory evaluations but may be used as an adjunct with other biomarkers.

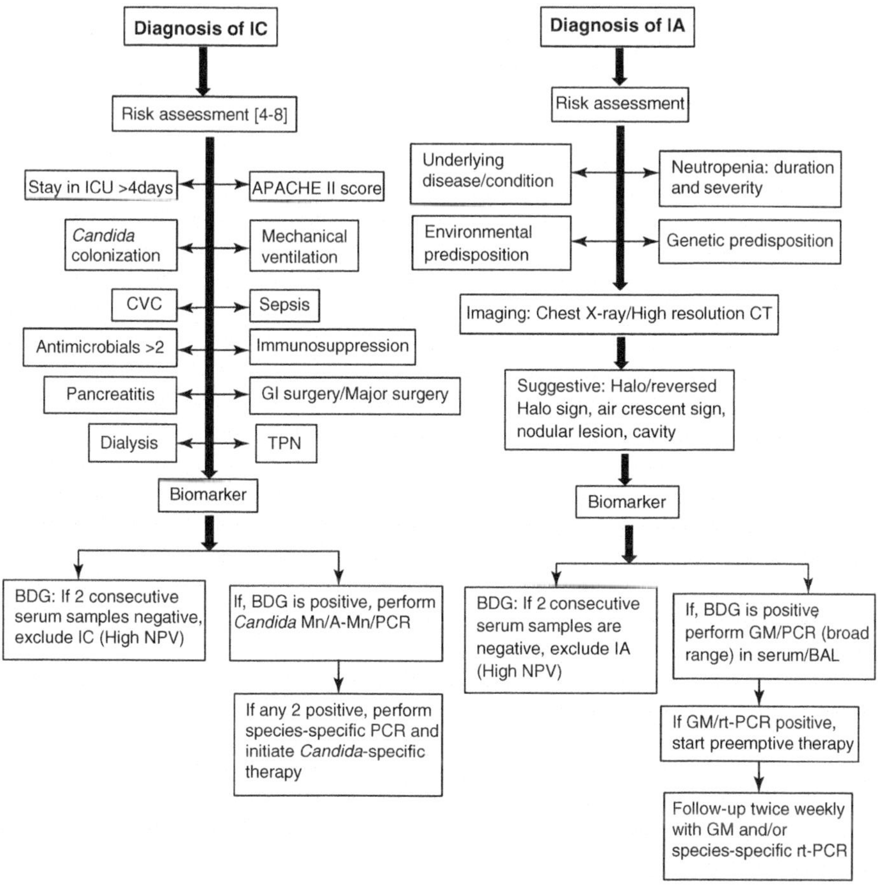

Fig. 12.1 A practical approach for the diagnosis of invasive candidiasis (IC) and invasive aspergillosis (IA). *CVC* central venous catheter, *TPN* total parenteral nutrition, *BDG* β-D-glucan, *GM* galactomannan, *rt-PCR* real-time PCR, *Mn* mannan, *A-Mn* anti-mannan antibody, *NPV* negative predictive value

12.3.4 How to Improve Diagnostic Potential

A high index of suspicion and careful assessment of well defined risk factors are important first steps toward early diagnosis. Combined detection of BDG and Mn + A-Mn provide useful tools for screening patients at high risk of developing IC/candidemia. Likewise, GM detection in serum or BAL specimens alone or in combination with either BDG or broad-range real-time PCR (to be followed with species-specific real-time PCR) in high-risk patients are preferable options to direct treatment strategies for IA [6, 9, 77, 78]. Since sensitivity of GM detection in serum is generally low, BAL is the preferred specimen, particularly in non-neutropenic patients. However, results of biomarker assays should always be interpreted cautiously with clinical, radiological, and microbiological findings in an integrated manner [10]. A better understanding of the genetic markers that are related to susceptibility to IFI is required, and further research on finding new diagnostic targets for IFI is underway [21, 24]. In this context, a recent report of detection of antibody to thioredoxin reductase (TR) of *Aspergillus fumigatus* in serum of non-neutropenic IA patients is noteworthy [92]. The sensitivity of the test was 81% as against 52% for GM. Combined detection of anti-TR antibody and GM appear promising but need further prospective evaluation.

12.4 Conclusions

IFI in immunocompromised patients are usually fatal unless diagnosed and treated promptly. Conventional diagnostic methods are time-consuming and lack sensitivity, yet they are useful as isolation of etiologic agent, still considered as the "gold standard" for diagnosis, is often negative. However, isolation of fungal pathogen facilitates antifungal susceptibility as different species/strains may differ in their susceptibility profiles, necessitating therapeutic adjustments. Although demonstration of fungal elements in tissue provides a rapid diagnosis, it fails to provide species-specific identification of the pathogen and requires invasive procedures. With progress in imaging techniques and established role of biomarkers as surrogates for diagnosis, an integrated approach is the key for early and specific diagnosis of IFI. Biomarker detection is less invasive and may be positive before actual disease manifests and sequential detection may indicate prognosis. It is time that clinicians avail these new tools in overall diagnostic and therapeutic strategies for improved prognosis. It is also important that clinicians are aware of the local epidemiology and the nature of the immunosuppression while considering the most likely fungal organisms that may infect a given patient to achieve maximum benefit from these laboratory-based diagnostic approaches.

References

1. Slavin MA, Chakrabarti A. Opportunistic fungal infections in the Asia-Pacific region. Med Mycol. 2012;50:18–25.
2. Khan ZU, Ahmad S. Non-culture-based diagnostic methods for the diagnosis of invasive candidiasis: are they helpful to clinicians? J Kuwait Med Assoc. 2013;45:4–14.
3. Ramanan P, Wengenack NL, Theel ES. Laboratory diagnostics for fungal infections: a review of current and future diagnostic assays. Clin Chest Med. 2017;38:535–54.
4. Halliday CL, Kidd SE, Sorrell TC, Chen SC. Molecular diagnostic methods for invasive fungal disease: the horizon draws nearer? Pathology. 2015;47:257–69.
5. Batzlaff CM, Limper AH. When to consider the possibility of a fungal infection: an overview of clinical diagnosis and laboratory approaches. Clin Chest Med. 2017;38:385–91.
6. Ostrosky-Zeichner L, Sable C, Sobel J, Alexander BD, Donowitz G, Kan V, Kauffman CA, Kett D, Larsen RA, Morrison V, Nucci M, Pappas PG, Bradley ME, Major S, Zimmer L, Wallace D, Dismukes WE, Rex JH. Multicenter retrospective development and validation of a clinical prediction rule for nosocomial invasive candidiasis in the intensive care setting. Eur J Clin Microbiol Infect Dis. 2007;26:271–6.

7. Cornely OA, Bassetti M, Calandra T, Garbino J, Kullberg BJ, Lortholary O, Meersseman W, Akova M, Arendrup MC, Arikan-Akdagli S, Bille J, Castagnola E, Cuenca-Estrella M, Donnelly JP, Groll AH, Herbrecht R, Hope WW, Jensen HE, Lass-Flörl C, Petrikkos G, Richardson MD, Roilides E, Verweij PE, Viscoli C, Ullmann AJ, ESCMID Fungal Infection Study Group. ESCMID∗ guideline for the diagnosis and management of *Candida* diseases 2012: non-neutropenic adult patients. Clin Microbiol Infect. 2012;18(Suppl 7):19–37.
8. Neofytos D, Railkar R, Mullane KM, Fredricks DN, Granwehr B, Marr KA, Almyroudis NG, Kontoyiannis DP, Maertens J, Fox R, Douglas C, Iannone R, Kauh E, Shire N. Correlation between circulating fungal biomarkers and clinical outcome in invasive aspergillosis. PLoS One. 2015;10(6):e0129022.
9. Morrissey CO, Chen SC, Sorrell TC, Milliken S, Bardy PG, Bradstock KF, Szer J, Halliday CL, Gilroy NM, Moore J, Schwarer AP, Guy S, Bajel A, Tramontana AR, Spelman T, Slavin MA, for the Australasian Leukaemia Lymphoma Group and the Australia and New Zealand Mycology Interest Group. Galactomannan and PCR versus culture and histology for directing use of antifungal treatment for invasive aspergillosis in high-risk haematology patients: a randomised controlled trial. Lancet Infect Dis. 2013;13:519–28.
10. Ruhnke M, Behre G, Buchheidt D, Christopeit M, Hamprecht A, Heinz W, et al. Diagnosis of invasive fungal diseases in haematology and oncology. 2018 update of the recommendations of the infectious diseases working party of the German Society for Hematology and Medical Oncology (AGIHO). Mycoses. 2018;61(11):796–813. https://doi.org/10.1111/myc.12838.
11. McCarty TP, Pappas PG. Invasive candidiasis. Infect Dis Clin North Am. 2016;30:103–24.
12. Eggimann P, Bille J, Marchetti O. Diagnosis of invasive candidiasis in the ICU. Ann Intensive Care. 2011;1:1–37.
13. Ahmed A, Baronia AK, Azim A, Marak RSK, Yadav R, Sharma P, Gurjar M, Poddar B, Singh RK. External validation of risk prediction scores for invasive candidiasis in a medical/surgical intensive care unit: an observational study. Indian J Crit Care Med. 2017;21:514–20.
14. León C, Ruiz-Santana S, Saavedra P, Galván B, Blanco A, Castro C, Balasini C, Utande-Vázquez A, González de Molina FJ, Blasco-Navalproto MA, López MJ, Charles PE, Martín E, Hernández-Viera MA, Cava Study Group. Usefulness of the "*Candida* score" for discriminating between *Candida* colonization and invasive candidiasis in non-neutropenic critically ill patients: a prospective multicenter study. Crit Care Med. 2009;37:1624–33.
15. Ostrosky-Zeichner L, Pappas PG, Shoham S, Reboli A, Barron MA, Sims C, Wood C, Sobel JD. Improvement of a clinical prediction rule for clinical trials on prophylaxis for invasive candidiasis in the intensive care unit. Mycoses. 2011;54:46–51.
16. Hermsen ED, Zapapas MK, Maiefski M, Rupp ME, Freifeld AG, Kalil AC. Validation and comparison of clinical prediction rules for invasive candidiasis in intensive care unit patients: a matched case-control study. Crit Care. 2011;15:R198.
17. Chapman RL. *Candida* infections in the neonate. Curr Opin Pediatr. 2003;15:97–102.
18. Al-Sweih N, Khan Z, Khan S, Devarajan LV. Neonatal candidaemia in Kuwait: a 12-year study of risk factors, species spectrum and antifungal susceptibility. Mycoses. 2009;52:518–23.
19. Hammoud MS, Al-Taiar A, Fouad M, Raina A, Khan Z. Persistent candidemia in neonatal care units: risk factors and clinical significance. Int J Infect Dis. 2013;17:e624–8
20. Herbrecht R, Bories P, Moulin JC, Ledoux MP, Letscher Bru V. Risk stratification for invasive aspergillosis in immunocompromised patients. Ann N Y Acad Sci. 2012;1272:23–30.
21. Pagano L, Akova M, Dimopoulos G, Herbrecht R, Drgona L, Blijlevens N. Risk assessment and prognostic factors for mould related diseases in immunocompromised patients. J Antimicrob Chemother. 2011;66(Suppl 1):i5–14.
22. Samarakoon P, Soubani A. Invasive pulmonary aspergillosis in patients with COPD: a report of five cases and systematic review of the literature. Chron Respir Dis. 2008;5:19–27.
23. Stevens DA, Melikian GL. Aspergillosis in the 'nonimmunocompromised' host. Immunol Invest. 2011;40:751–66.
24. Mezger M, Einsele H, Loeffler J. Genetic susceptibility to infections with *Aspergillus fumigatus*. Crit Rev Microbiol. 2010;36:168–77.

25. Meis JF, Chakrabarti A. Changing epidemiology of an emerging infection: zygomycosis. Clin Microbiol Infect. 2009;15(Suppl 5):10–4.
26. Millon L, Herbrecht R, Grenouillet F, Morio F, Alanio A, Letscher-Bru V, Cassaing S, Chouaki T, Kauffmann-Lacroix C, Poirier P, Toubas D, Augereau O, Rocchi S, Garcia-Hermoso D, Bretagne S, French Mycosis Study Group. Early diagnosis and monitoring of mucormycosis by detection of circulating DNA in serum: retrospective analysis of 44 cases collected through the French Surveillance Network of Invasive Fungal Infections (RESSIF). Clin Microbiol Infect. 2016;22:810.e1–8.
27. Georgiadou SP, Sipsas NV, Marom EM, Kontoyiannis DP. The diagnostic value of halo and reversed halo signs for invasive mold infections in compromised hosts. Clin Infect Dis. 2011;52:1144–55.
28. Chamilos G, Marom EM, Lewis RE, Lionakis MS, Kontoyiannis DP. Predictors of pulmonary zygomycosis versus invasive pulmonary aspergillosis in patients with cancer. Clin Infect Dis. 2005;41:60–6.
29. De Pauw B, Walsh TJ, Donnelly JP, Stevens DA, Edwards JE, Calandra T, et al.; European Organization for Research and Treatment of Cancer/Invasive Fungal Infections Cooperative Group; National Institute of Allergy and Infectious Diseases Mycoses Study Group (EORTC/MSG) Consensus Group. Revised definitions of invasive fungal disease from the European Organization for Research and Treatment of Cancer/Invasive Fungal Infections Cooperative Group and the National Institute of Allergy and Infectious Diseases Mycoses Study Group (EORTC/MSG) Consensus Group. Clin Infect Dis. 2008;46:1813–1821.
30. Katragkou A, Fisher BT, Groll AH, Roilides E, Walsh TJ. Diagnostic imaging and invasive fungal diseases in children. J Pediatric Infect Dis Soc. 2017;6(suppl. 1):S22–31.
31. Schelenz S, Barnes RA, Barton RC, Cleverley JR, Lucas SB, Kibbler CC, Denning DW. British Society for Medical Mycology Best Practice recommendations for the diagnosis of serious fungal diseases. Lancet Infect Dis. 2015;15:461–74.
32. Guarner J, Brandt ME. Histopathologic diagnosis of fungal infections in the 21st century. Clin Microbiol Rev 2011;24:247–280.mxf
33. Beirão F, Araujo R. State of the art diagnostic of mold diseases: a practical guide for clinicians. Eur J Clin Microbiol Infect Dis. 2013;32:3–9.
34. Clancy CJ, Nguyen MH. Finding the "missing 50%" of invasive candidiasis: how nonculture diagnostics will improve understanding of disease spectrum and transform patient care. Clin Infect Dis. 2013;56:1284–92.
35. Sinha K, Tendolkar U, Mathur M. Comparison of conventional broth blood culture technique and manual lysis centrifugation technique for detection of fungemia. Indian J Med Microbiol. 2009;27:79–80.
36. Clancy CJ, Pappas PG, Vazquez J, Judson MA, Kontoyiannis DP, Thompson GR 3rd, Garey KW, Reboli A, Greenberg RN, Apewokin S, Lyon GM 3rd, Ostrosky-Zeichner L, Wu AHB, Tobin E, Nguyen MH, Caliendo AM. Detecting infections rapidly and easily for candidemia trial, part 2 (DIRECT2): a prospective, multicenter study of the T2Candida panel. Clin Infect Dis. 2018;66:1678–86.
37. Clancy CJ, Nguyen MH. T2 magnetic resonance for the diagnosis of bloodstream infections: charting a path forward. J Antimicrob Chemother. 2018;73(suppl_4):iv2–5.
38. Randhawa HS, Chowdhary A, Preeti Sinha K, Kowshik T, Vijayan VK. Evaluation of peptone glucose fluconazole agar as a selective medium for rapid and enhanced isolation of *Aspergillus fumigatus* from the respiratory tract of bronchopulmonary aspergillosis patients colonized by *Candida albicans*. Med Mycol. 2006;44:343–8.
39. Chakrabarti A, Das A, Sharma A, Panda N, Das S, Gupta KL, Sakhuja V. Ten years' experience in zygomycosis at a tertiary care centre in India. J Infect. 2001;42:261–6.
40. Lass-Flörl C. Zygomycosis: conventional laboratory diagnosis. Clin Microbiol Infect. 2009;15(Suppl 5):60–5.
41. Skiada A, Lanternier F, Groll AH, Pagano L, Zimmerli S, Herbrecht R, Lortholary O, Petrikkos GL, European Conference on Infections in Leukemia. Diagnosis and treatment of mucormycosis in patients with hematological malignancies: guidelines from the 3rd European Conference on Infections in Leukemia (ECIL 3). Haematologica. 2013;98:492–50.

42. Preuner S, Lion T. Species-specific identification of a wide range of clinically relevant fungal pathogens by the Luminex® xMAP technology. Methods Mol Biol. 2013;968:119–39.
43. Jamal WY, Ahmad S, Khan ZU, Rotimi VO. Comparative evaluation of two matrix-assisted laser desorption/ionization time-of-flight mass spectrometry (MALDI-TOF MS) systems for the identification of clinically significant yeasts. Int J Infect Dis. 2014;26:167–70.
44. Lee HS, Shin JH, Choi MJ, Won EJ, Kee SJ, Kim SH, Shin MG, Suh SP. Comparison of the Bruker biotyper and VITEK MS matrix-assisted laser desorption/ionization time-of-flight mass spectrometry systems using a formic acid extraction method to identify common and uncommon yeast isolates. Ann Lab Med. 2017;37:223–30.
45. Bao JR, Master RN, Azad KN, Schwab DA, Clark RB, Jones RS, Moore EC, Shier KL. Rapid, accurate identification of *Candida auris* by using a novel matrix-assisted laser desorption ionization-time of flight mass spectrometry (MALDI-TOF MS) database (library). J Clin Microbiol. 2018;56. pii: e01700-17.
46. Shao J, Wan Z, Li R, Yu J. Species identification and delineation of pathogenic mucorales by matrix-assisted laser desorption ionization-time of flight mass spectrometry. J Clin Microbiol. 2018;56. pii: e01886-17.
47. Stein M, Tran V, Nichol KA, Lagacé-Wiens P, Pieroni P, Adam HJ, Turenne C, Walkty AJ, Normand AC, Hendrickx M, Piarroux R, Karlowsky JA. Evaluation of three MALDI-TOF mass spectrometry libraries for the identification of filamentous fungi in three clinical microbiology laboratories in Manitoba, Canada. Mycoses. 2018;61:743–53.
48. Vella A, De Carolis E, Mello E, Perlin DS, Sanglard D, Sanguinetti M, Posteraro B. Potential use of MALDI-TOF mass spectrometry for rapid detection of antifungal resistance in the human pathogen *Candida glabrata*. Sci Rep. 2017;7:9099.
49. Miceli MH, Maertens J. Role of non-culture-based tests, with an emphasis on galactomannan testing for the diagnosis of invasive aspergillosis. Semin Respir Crit Care Med. 2015;36:650–61.
50. Mokaddas E, Burhamah MH, Khan ZU, Ahmad S. Levels of (1→3)-β-D-glucan, *Candida* mannan and *Candida* DNA in serum samples of pediatric cancer patients colonized with *Candida* species. BMC Infect Dis. 2010;10:292.
51. Lamoth F, Cruciani M, Mengoli C, Castagnola E, Lortholary O, Richardson M, Marchetti O, Third European Conference on Infections in Leukemia (ECIL-3). β-glucan antigenemia assay for the diagnosis of invasive fungal infections in patients with hematological malignancies: a systematic review and meta-analysis of cohort studies from the Third European Conference on Infections in Leukemia (ECIL-3). Clin Infect Dis. 2012;54:633–43.
52. Marchetti O, Lamoth F, Mikulska M, Viscoli C, Verweij P, Bretagne S, European Conference on Infections in Leukemia (ECIL) Laboratory Working Groups. ECIL recommendations for the use of biological markers for the diagnosis of invasive fungal diseases in leukemic patients and hematopoietic SCT recipients. Bone Marrow Transplant. 2012;47:846–54.
53. Maartens G, Stewart A, Griesel R, Kengne AP, Dube F, Nicol M, Rangaka MX, Mendelson M. Development of a clinical prediction rule to diagnose *Pneumocystis jirovecii* pneumonia in the World Health Organization's algorithm for seriously ill HIV-infected patients. South Afr J HIV Med. 2018;19:851.
54. White PL, Posso RB, Gorton RL, Price JS, Wey E, Barnes RA. An evaluation of the performance of the Dynamiker® fungus (1-3)-β-D-glucan assay to assist in the diagnosis of pneumocystis pneumonia. Med Mycol. 2018;56:778–81.
55. Alam FF, Mustafa AS, Khan ZU. Comparative evaluation of (1, 3)-β-D-glucan, mannan and anti-mannan antibodies, and *Candida* species-specific snPCR in patients with candidemia. BMC Infect Dis. 2007;7:103.
56. Mikulska M, Calandra T, Sanguinetti M, Poulain D, Viscoli C, Third European Conference on Infections in Leukemia Group. The use of mannan antigen and anti-mannan antibodies in the diagnosis of invasive candidiasis: recommendations from the Third European Conference on Infections in Leukemia. Crit Care. 2010;14:R222.
57. Mokaddas E, Khan ZU, Ahmad S, Nampoory MR, Burhamah M. Value of (1-3)-β-d-glucan, *Candida* mannan and *Candida* DNA detection in the diagnosis of candidaemia. Clin Microbiol Infect. 2011;17:1549–53.

58. Clancy CJ, Nguyen MH. Diagnosing invasive candidiasis. J Clin Microbiol. 2018;56: pii: e01909-17.
59. Clancy CJ, Nguyen MH. Non-culture diagnostics for invasive candidiasis: promise and unintended consequences. J Fungi (Basel). 2018;4. pii: E27.
60. Maertens J, Theunissen K, Verbeken E, Lagrou K, Verhaegen J, Boogaerts M, Eldere JV. Prospective clinical evaluation of lower cut-offs for galactomannan detection in adult neutropenic cancer patients and haematological stem cell transplant recipients. Br J Haematol. 2004;126:852–60.
61. Cuenca-Estrella M, Bassetti M, Lass-Flörl C, Rácil Z, Richardson M, Rogers TR. Detection and investigation of invasive mould disease. J Antimicrob Chemother. 2011;66(Suppl 1):15–24.
62. Khan ZU, Ahmad S, Mokaddas E, Said T, Nair MP, Halim MA, Nampoory MR, McGinnis MR. Cerebral aspergillosis diagnosed by detection of *Aspergillus flavus*-specific DNA, galactomannan and (1-3)-β-D-glucan in clinical specimens. J Med Microbiol. 2007;56:129–32.
63. Mokaddas E, Burhamah MH, Ahmad S, Khan ZU. Invasive pulmonary aspergillosis due to *Aspergillus terreus*: value of DNA, galactomannan and (1-3)-β-D-glucan detection in serum samples as an adjunct to diagnosis. J Med Microbiol. 2010;59:1519–23.
64. Zou M, Tang L, Zhao S, Zhao Z, Chen L, Chen P, Huang Z, Li J, Chen L, Fan X. Systematic review and meta-analysis of detecting galactomannan in bronchoalveolar lavage fluid for diagnosing invasive aspergillosis. PLoS One. 2012;7:e43347.
65. White PL, Parr C, Thornton C, Barnes RA. Evaluation of real-time PCR, galactomannan enzyme-linked immunosorbent assay (ELISA), and a novel lateral-flow device for diagnosis of invasive aspergillosis. J Clin Microbiol. 2013;51:1510–6.
66. Ahmad S, Khan Z. Invasive candidiasis: a review of non-culture-based laboratory diagnostic methods. Indian J Med Microbiol. 2012;30:264–9.
67. Ahmad S, Khan Z, Mustafa AS, Khan ZU. Semi-nested PCR for diagnosis of candidemia: comparison with culture, antigen detection, and biochemical methods for species identification. J Clin Microbiol. 2002;40:2483–9.
68. Ahmad S, Mustafa AS, Khan Z, Al-Rifaiy AI, Khan ZU. PCR-enzyme immunoassay of rDNA in the diagnosis of candidemia and comparison with amplicon detection by agarose gel electrophoresis. Int J Med Microbiol. 2004;294:45–51.
69. Asadzadeh M, Ahmad S, Hagen F, Meis JF, Al-Sweih N, Khan Z. Simple, low-cost detection of *Candida parapsilosis* complex isolates and molecular fingerprinting of *Candida orthopsilosis* strains in Kuwait by ITS region sequencing and amplified fragment length polymorphism analysis. PLoS One. 2015;10:e0142880.
70. Al-Obaid K, Asadzadeh M, Ahmad S, Khan Z. Population structure and molecular genetic characterization of clinical *Candida tropicalis* isolates from a tertiary-care hospital in Kuwait reveal infections with unique strains. PLoS One. 2017;12:e0182292.
71. Khan Z, Ahmad S, Al-Sweih N, Joseph L, Alfouzan W, Asadzadeh M. Increasing prevalence, molecular characterization and antifungal drug susceptibility of serial *Candida auris* isolates in Kuwait. PLoS One. 2018;13:e0195743.
72. Ahmad S, Al-Mahmeed M, Khan ZU. Characterization of *Trichosporon* species isolated from clinical specimens in Kuwait. J Med Microbiol. 2005;54:639–46.
73. Khan ZU, Al-Sweih NA, Ahmad S, Al-Kazemi N, Khan S, Joseph L, Chandy R. Outbreak of fungemia among neonates caused by *Candida haemulonii* resistant to amphotericin B, itraconazole and fluconazole. J Clin Microbiol. 2007;45:2025–7.
74. Al-Sweih N, Ahmad S, Khan S, Joseph L, Asadzadeh M, Khan Z. *Cyberlindnera fabianii* fungemia outbreak in preterm neonates in Kuwait and literature review. Mycoses. 2019;62(1):51–61. https://doi.org/10.1111/myc.12846.
75. Nguyen MH, Wissel MC, Shields RK, Salomoni MA, Hao B, Press EG, Shields RM, Cheng S, Mitsani D, Vadnerkar A, Silveira FP, Kleiboeker SB, Clancy CJ. Performance of *Candida* real-time polymerase chain reaction, β-D-glucan assay, and blood cultures in the diagnosis of invasive candidiasis. Clin Infect Dis. 2012;54:1240–8.

76. White PL, Mengoli C, Bretagne S, Cuenca-Estrella M, Finnstrom N, Klingspor L, Melchers WJ, McCulloch E, Barnes RA, Donnelly JP, Loeffler J, European Aspergillus PCR Initiative (EAPCRI). Evaluation of *Aspergillus* PCR protocols for testing serum specimens. J Clin Microbiol. 2011;49:3842–8.
77. Sun W, Wang K, Gao W, Su X, Qian Q, Lu X, Song Y, Guo Y, Shi Y. Evaluation of PCR on bronchoalveolar lavage fluid for diagnosis of invasive aspergillosis: a bivariate meta-analysis and systematic review. PLoS One. 2011;6:e28467.
78. Avni T, Levy I, Sprecher H, Yahav D, Leibovici L, Paul M. Diagnostic accuracy of PCR alone compared to galactomannan in bronchoalveolar lavage fluid for diagnosis of invasive pulmonary aspergillosis: a systematic review. J Clin Microbiol. 2012;50:3652–8.
79. Lucignano B, Ranno S, Liesenfeld O, Pizzorno B, Putignani L, Bernaschi P. Multiplex PCR allows rapid and accurate diagnosis of bloodstream infections in newborns and children with suspected sepsis. J Clin Microbiol. 2011;49:2252–8.
80. Fernández-Cruz A, Marín M, Kestler M, Alcalá L, Rodriguez-Créixems M, Bouza E. The value of combining blood culture and SeptiFast data for predicting complicated bloodstream infections caused by gram-positive bacteria or *Candida* species. J Clin Microbiol. 2013;51:1130–6.
81. Elges S, Arnold R, Liesenfeld O, Kofla G, Mikolajewska A, Schwartz S. Prospective evaluation of the SeptiFAST multiplex real-time PCR assay for surveillance and diagnosis of infections in haematological patients after allogeneic stem cell transplantation compared to routine microbiological assays and an in-house real-time PCR method. Mycoses. 2017;60:781–8.
82. Pfaller MA, Wolk DM, Lowery TJ. T2MR and T2Candida: novel technology for the rapid diagnosis of candidemia and invasive candidiasis. Future Microbiol. 2016;11:103–17.
83. Zervou FN, Zacharioudakis IM, Kurpewski J, Mylonakis E. T2 magnetic resonance for fungal diagnosis. Methods Mol Biol. 2017;1508:305–19.
84. Muñoz P, Vena A, Machado M, Martínez-Jiménez MC, Gioia F, Gómez E. T2MR contributes to the very early diagnosis of complicated candidaemia. A prospective study. J Antimicrob Chemother. 2018;73(suppl 4):iv13–9.
85. Muñoz P, Vena A, Machado M, Gioia F, Martínez-Jiménez MC, Gómez E. T2Candida MR as a predictor of outcome in patients with suspected invasive candidiasis starting empirical antifungal treatment: a prospective pilot study. J Antimicrob Chemother. 2018;73(suppl 4):iv6–iv12.
86. Patch ME, Weisz E, Cubillos A, Estrada SJ, Pfaller MA. Impact of rapid, culture-independent diagnosis of candidaemia and invasive candidiasis in a community health system. J Antimicrob Chemother. 2018;73(suppl 4):iv27–30.
87. Prattes J, Heldt S, Eigl S, Hoenigl M. Point of care testing for the diagnosis of fungal infections: are we there yet? Curr Fungal Infect Rep. 2016;10:43–50.
88. Heldt S, Hoenigl M. Lateral flow assays for the diagnosis of invasive Aspergillosis: current status. Curr Fungal Infect Rep. 2017;11:45–51.
89. Tang MW, Clemons KV, Katzenstein DA, Stevens DA. The cryptococcal antigen lateral flow assay: a point-of-care diagnostic at an opportune time. Crit Rev Microbiol. 2016;42:634–42.
90. Sims CR, Jaijakul S, Mohr J, Rodriguez J, Finkelman M, Ostrosky-Zeichner L. Correlation of clinical outcomes with β-glucan levels in patients with invasive candidiasis. J Clin Microbiol. 2012;50:2104–6.
91. Chai LY, Kullberg BJ, Johnson EM, Teerenstra S, Khin LW, Vonk AG, Maertens J, Lortholary O, Donnelly PJ, Schlamm HT, Troke PF, Netea MG, Herbrecht R. Early serum galactomannan trend as a predictor of outcome of invasive aspergillosis. J Clin Microbiol. 2012;50:2330–6.
92. Shi LN, Li FQ, Lu JF, Kong XX, Wang SQ, Huang M, Shao HF, Shao SH. Antibody specific to thioredoxin reductase as a new biomarker for serodiagnosis of invasive aspergillosis in non-neutropenic patients. Clin Chim Acta. 2012;413:938–43.

Difficulties Faced in Asian Countries for the Diagnosis of Fungal Infections and Possible Solutions

13

Arunaloke Chakrabarti

Key Points

- Fungal infection rate is very high in Asian countries, but there is lack of awareness among medical personnel and deficiency of laboratory facility.
- Many rare fungi caused outbreaks in those countries, which require expertise to identify the causative agents early.
- In a survey of seven Asian countries, it was observed that advanced diagnostic tests (Galactomannan, beta-D-glucan, PCR, therapeutic drug monitoring, antifungal susceptibility testing) were limited to few laboratories only. Those tests were almost non-existent in laboratories of Indonesia, the Philippines and Thailand.
- As majority of country administrators still do not recognize the importance of fungal diseases and separate country control program may be expensive, the fungal disease diagnosis may be integrated with HIV (diagnosis of opportunistic infection), tuberculosis (diagnosis of chronic pulmonary aspergillosis), blindness (diagnosis of fungal keratitis) control programmes and antimicrobial (antifungal susceptibility testing) stewardship programmes.
- WHO has included cryptococcal antigen tests, blood culture, microscopy, fungal culture and antimicrobial susceptibility testing in the first Model List of Essential in vitro Diagnostics (EDL). This would help in advocacy with government for the development of mycology laboratories.
- Ideal four categories of laboratories (local, clinical, regional and reference) are also proposed for each country. Bigger countries like China and India may require reference laboratories at each of its provinces.

A. Chakrabarti (✉)
Department of Medical Microbiology, Postgraduate Institute of Medical Education and Research (PGIMER), Chandigarh, India

A. Chakrabarti (ed.), *Clinical Practice of Medical Mycology in Asia*,
https://doi.org/10.1007/978-981-13-9459-1_13

13.1 Introduction

It is estimated that Asia has the largest burden of fungal diseases per capita in the world, and more than 50% population of the world live in this continent. The largest groups affected by serious infection include patients in intensive care unit, cancer, HIV/AIDS, diabetes, post-tuberculosis patients, asthma and chronic obstructive pulmonary disease [1, 2]. Though the mortality due to fungal diseases is comparable to tuberculosis and malaria, very little attention is focused in the control and management of fungal infections [3]. To overcome the neglect and to make visible changes in morbidity and mortality due to fungal infections, awareness building and development of competent diagnostic mycology laboratories are the initial steps [4].

Estimated burden of the disease in South-East Regional countries (some of the data are collected from the website of Global Action Fund for Fungal Infection [GAFFI] at https://www.gaffi.org/)

- HIV-infected patients (500,000) are at risk, and 30,000 develop cryptococcal meningitis and another 80,000 *Pneumocystis* pneumonia with an estimated 27,000 and 67,000 deaths, respectively.
- Endemic disease—at least 1000 patients suffer from disseminated histoplasmosis or talaromycosis in those HIV-infected patients [1].
- Invasive aspergillosis—in leukaemia, lymphoma, lung cancer, post-transplantation, AIDS, COPD patients admitted to hospital and numerous others including severe influenza, estimated at 196,000 patients, of whom probably 176,000 die. Indian recent data showed a prevalence of 9.5 cases/1000 ICU admissions [5, 6].
- Mucormycosis—is a very common disease in diabetics with over 200,000 cases annually, mortality >50%. China and India have reported very high incidence of mucormycosis [7].
- Invasive candidiasis and intra-abdominal candidiasis—in hospitalized patients, post-surgical or in intensive care probably exceed 745,000 patients annually [8, 9].
- Chronic pulmonary aspergillosis—post-tuberculosis around 670,000, with an estimated 100,000 deaths [10, 11].
- Fungal sinusitis—north India village data showed 1 in 1000 of villagers suffer from fungal sinusitis [11, 12].
- Fungal asthma—2,785,000 in the 55 million asthmatic adults, of whom 60–80% might respond to antifungal therapy [10].
- Fungal keratitis—probably affects 1.1 million people annually, of whom 768,000 are from South Asia; perhaps 60–75% lose their sight in one eye or the eye has to be removed.

13.1.1 Present Status of Mycology Laboratories in Asian Countries

- An online survey of mycology laboratories in seven Asian countries was conducted, and 241 laboratories from China, India, Indonesia, the Philippines, Singapore, Taiwan and Thailand participated in the study [13].
- Overall, 53.5% mycology laboratories operate as separate designated mycology laboratories.
- 31.1% laboratories have regular formal staff training, 42.7% are accredited, and 56.1% participate in external quality assurance scheme (EQAS) programmes.
- Microscopy and culture methods are available in nearly all laboratories.
- Only 16.9% laboratories perform DNA sequencing and 12.3% laboratories use matrix-assisted laser desorption/ionization time-of-flight mass spectroscopy (MALDI-TOF MS) for isolate identification.
- Antifungal susceptibility testing is performed by 58.9% laboratories, mainly for yeasts.
- Serology—Cryptococcal antigen testing is performed in 66 laboratories, galactomannan testing in 55 laboratories, and beta D glucan testing in 24 laboratories (almost no access to galactomannan and beta-D-glucan test in Indonesia, the Philippines and Thailand).
- Polymerase chain reaction (PCR) used in diagnosis of fungal infections in 37 laboratories.
- Therapeutic drug monitoring is conducted in 21 laboratories.
- Among South-east Asian region Bhutan, Maldives, Myanmar, North Korea and Timor-Leste have very poor mycology laboratory service.

With the present status of mycology laboratories, management of fungal disease is difficult in Asian countries, as

- Clinicians do not know which patient to be treated due to lack of diagnosis and epidemiological data
- Prophylaxis—do not know the magnitude in a risk group
- Do not know when to stop empiric therapy

The situation is further complicated with the outbreak due to rare fungi in Asian countries [14–17].

- Epidemiology of those rare fungal diseases is not known—do not know environmental reservoirs, modes of transmission, and ways to detect them.
- Laboratory diagnosis is a challenge.

- Specific identification requires expertise.
- Antifungal susceptibility testing—no breakpoint known. So, do not know which antifungal to use.
- Diagnosis requires reference laboratories.
- Reference laboratory facilities are not available in all regions and countries.

13.1.2 Possible Solution

- Recognition of fungal disease as public health threat. Public health responses should be upgraded for fungal outbreaks and, for cryptococcal meningitis in patients with AIDS, mycetoma and chromoblastomycosis (last two diseases have been recognized as neglected tropical diseases by the World Health Organization).
- Integration of fungal diseases into existing HIV, tuberculosis, diabetes, respiratory diseases and blindness control programmes would help in improvement of the laboratories (HIV-associated opportunistic fungal infections within care and treatment programmes for HIV infection, chronic pulmonary aspergillosis within tuberculosis control or chronic respiratory disease programmes, Aspergillus and Candida acquired resistance within antimicrobial resistance and antimicrobial stewardship programs, fungal keratitis within blindness control programmes) [4].
- The integration would also help in staff training in the field of fungal diagnosis.
- Advocacy is the major important step to draw the attention of government of each country, academia and other stakeholders about the serious concern on fungal infections.
- Surveillance and epidemiology study in Asian countries would help recognition of the burden of the problem. Under-recognition of the burden of fungal diseases leads to decreased resource allocation for diagnosis.
- In 2018, the first Model List of Essential in vitro Diagnostics (EDL) issued by the World Health Organization has included cryptococcal antigen tests, blood culture, microscopy, fungal culture and antimicrobial susceptibility testing. This year Histoplasma antigen detection is also included. The inclusion of tests in the list will help in advocacy with the government of each country to include those tests at least in fungal diagnosis.
- With government support, the development of new quality mycology laboratories and the improvement of existing laboratories with regular staff training may be fulfilled.
- Quality assurance is an important step and accreditation of laboratories would help in the improvement of quality of laboratories.
- Inclusion of essential advanced rapid biomarker and point-of-care tests.

13.2 An Outline on the Establishment of Mycology Reference and Other Laboratories

13.2.1 Diagnostic Portfolio of Mycology Reference Laboratories

A modern mycology laboratory offers the following portfolio of tests, and these will form the core diagnostic capabilities of each newly constituted laboratory.

Test	Infection	Diagnostic sensitivity (%)	Turnaround time[a]
Direct microscopy	Invasive infections, skin, hair and nails, vulvo-vaginal candidiasis	30–90	2 h
Antigen	Cryptococcal meningitis	99	2 h
PCR on respiratory samples	*Pneumocystis* pneumonia	98	1 day
Antigen (ELISA) on serum and respiratory samples	Invasive aspergillosis and hisotoplasmosis (antigen test in urine better)	80	1–2 days
Beta-glucan detection	Most fungal infections, high NPV allowing therapy to be stopped	65–77	1–2 days
Aspergillus IgG antibody	Chronic pulmonary aspergillosis	80–95	1 day
Aspergillus IgE	Screen for ABPA in asthma	>95	1–2 days
Fungal culture and identification	All except *Pneumocystis*	10–50	3–14 days
Molecular identification from histopathology positive, culture negative	All, especially mould infections	50–60	7 days
Itraconazole, voriconazole and posaconazole blood levels	Aspergillosis, and other invasive fungal infections	100	1–3 days

[a]Turnaround time includes transport to laboratory, test time (including batching), reporting and assumes a normal working day

The newly constituted laboratories may be properly equipped with standard methods. Each laboratory should be led by an experienced medical microbiologist with a special interest in mycology and a PhD scientist with good fungal research credentials.

In addition, five technical staff need to be recruited to perform the diagnostic tests. At least one of these staff must have extensive experience in direct microscopy to rapidly diagnose fungal disease and in fungal pathogen identification. Some variations in how the service is configured may depend on the existing expertise in biochemistry/pharmacology for drug levels, identification using MALDI-TOF, etc. All staff of the Mycology Laboratory may be groomed to generate the critical mass required to offer expert advice and education of clinical staff and students and to properly assemble and interpret surveillance data.

Each mycology laboratory may have a dedicated IT person to utilize sample tracking and reporting systems, manage the laboratory's website and play a key part in capturing and assembling surveillance data.

13.2.2 Quality Control

Internationally many laboratories subscribe to microbiology quality assurance schemes, which include fungal isolates, such as NEQAS [www.ukneqas.org.uk/], Scandinavia [www.folkhalsomyndigheten.se/documents/projektwebbar/ram/neqamm-2009-report.pdf], Australia [www.rcpaqap.com.au/microbiology/] and in India (Mycology Reference Laboratory at Postgraduate Institute of Medical Education and Research, Chandigarh).

In addition, an international proficiency testing programme for azole antifungals was established in Nijmegen, the Netherlands [www.ncbi.nlm.nih.gov/pmc/articles/PMC2612190/].

Integration of country EQAS programme with international agencies will help improve the performance of mycology laboratories.

13.2.3 Four-Tier Laboratory Development

The following table explains the distinction between different mycology laboratory capabilities.

Tests	Local clinical microbiology laboratory	Clinical microbiology laboratory at each medical college and centres handling specialized patients	Regional mycology laboratory (city having population more than two million)	Reference mycology laboratory (state capital of each province)
Tests	• Microscopy • Primary fungal culture • Differentiate *C. albicans* vs. non-albicans • Dermatophyte	AND • Fluorescent microscopy with optical brightener • India ink and other specialized fungal stains • Identification of common *Candida*, *Aspergillus*, *Mucorales* by conventional techniques • Antifungal susceptibility testing • Common serological tests for crypto, GM test, *Aspergillus* antibody and antigen	AND • Identification of unusual fungi by MALDI and sequencing • Beta-glucan test • Therapeutic drug monitoring	AND • Molecular typing technique for outbreak investigation • Molecular diagnostic tests • All specialized serological tests • Molecular resistance detection • Culture collection • National standards • Training programme

References

1. Chakrabarti A, Slavin MA. Endemic fungal infections in Asia-Pacific region. Med Mycol. 2011;49:337–44.
2. Slavin MA, Chakrabarti A. Opportunistic fungal infections in the Asia-Pacific region. Med Mycol. 2012;50:18–25.
3. Editorial. Stop neglecting fungi. Nat Microbiol. 2017;2:17120.
4. Cole DC, Govender NP, Chakrabarti A, Sacarlal J, Denning DW. Improvement of fungal disease identification and management: combined health systems and public health approaches. Lancet Infect Dis. 2017;17:e412–9.
5. Chakrabarti A, Kaur H, Savio J, et al. Epidemiology and clinical outcomes of invasive mould infections in Indian intensive care units (FISF study). J Crit Care. 2019;51:64–70.
6. Rotjanapan P, Chen YC, Chakrabarti A, et al. Epidemiology and clinical characteristics of invasive mould infections: a multicenter, retrospective analysis in five Asian countries. Med Mycol. 2018;56:186–96.
7. Hariprasath P, Arunaloke C. Global epidemiology of mucormycosis. J Fungi. 2019;5:26. https://doi.org/10.3390/jof5010026.
8. Tan BH, Chakrabarti A, Li RY, et al. Incidence and species distribution of candidaemia in Asia: a laboratory-based surveillance study. Clin Microbiol Infect. 2015;21:946–53.
9. Chakrabarti A, Sood P, Rudramurthy SM, et al. Incidence, characteristics and outcome of ICU-acquired candidemia in India. Intensive Care Med. 2015;41:285–95.
10. Agarwal R, Denning DW, Chakrabarti A. Estimation of the burden of chronic and allergic pulmonary aspergillosis in India. PLoS One. 2014;9:e114745.
11. Denning DW, Chakrabarti A. Pulmonary and sinus fungal diseases in non-immunocompromised patients. Lancet Infect Dis. 2017;17:e357–66.
12. Chakrabarti A, Rudramurthy SM, Panda N, Das A, Singh A. Epidemiology of chronic fungal rhinosinusitis in rural India. Mycoses. 2015;58:294–302.
13. Chindamporn A, Chakrabarti A, Li R, et al. Survey of laboratory practices for diagnosis of fungal infection in seven Asian countries: an Asia Fungal Working Group (AFWG) initiative. Med Mycol. 2018;56:416–25.
14. Chakrabarti A, Singh K, Narang A, et al. Outbreak of Pichia anomala in the pediatric service of a tertiary care center in northern India. J Clin Microbiol. 2001;39:1702–6.
15. Chakrabarti A, Shivaprakash MR, Curfs-Breuker I, Baghela A, Klaassen CH, Meis JF. Apophysomyces elegans: epidemiology, AFLP typing, and in vitro antifungal susceptibility pattern. J Clin Microbiol. 2010;48:4580–5.
16. Chakrabarti A, Singh R. The emerging epidemiology of mould infections in developing countries. Curr Opin Infect Dis. 2011;24:521–6.
17. Chakrabarti A, Rudramurthy SM, Kale P, et al. Epidemiological study of a large cluster of fungaemia cases due to Kodamaea ohmeri in an Indian tertiary care centre. Clin Microbiol Infect. 2014;20:O83–9.

Fungal Outbreak Investigations

14

Anup Ghosh and Sanjay Bhattacharya

Key Points

- **Nosocomial (or healthcare associated) fungal outbreaks** are evolving at a fast pace.
- Besides **common fungi**, **rare fungi** can cause outbreaks.
- **Man to man** transmission of fungi is limited to **yeast and *Pneumocystis***.
- **Hospital air quality maintenance** is important for the prevention of ***Aspergillus*** infections.
- Special care should be taken and practices followed as per evidence-based guidelines during **demolition, construction, and renovation** activities in healthcare environments.
- Though there is a paucity of guidelines, ***Aspergillus* spore count in air of <1 cfu/m^3** is recommended especially in high-risk patients (transplant units, critical care units, and wards for immunocompromised patients).
- It is important we have a **continuous monitoring and surveillance system** for fungal outbreaks using appropriate statistical tools such as the **cumulative sum test (CUSUM).**
- **Standard precautions** such as hand hygiene, environmental cleaning and disinfection, appropriate segregation, and disposal of biomedical and general waste need to be in place for the prevention and control of fungal outbreaks.

A. Ghosh
Department of Medical Microbiology, Postgraduate Institute of Medical Education and Research (PGIMER), Chandigarh, India

S. Bhattacharya (✉)
Department of Microbiology, Tata Medical Center, Kolkata, India
e-mail: sanjay.bhattacharya@tmckolkata.com

A. Chakrabarti (ed.), *Clinical Practice of Medical Mycology in Asia*,
https://doi.org/10.1007/978-981-13-9459-1_14

14.1 Fungal Outbreak Investigations

14.1.1 Introduction

Outbreak of fungal infection either in the community or in the healthcare setting can be an important cause of morbidity, mortality, hospital admission, and increased healthcare expenditure. There are also indirect social costs associated with outbreaks such as loss of economic productivity, job loss, and psychological stress. Outbreaks may begin as a smoldering, hidden, insidious entity which may not be obvious or noticeable in its early phases. The efficiency of the public health surveillance system can be assessed by its ability to detect outbreaks at an early stage. It is, therefore, critical that mechanisms and processes are established and made operational to detect, evaluate, analyze, contain, and prevent fungal infection outbreaks.

14.1.2 Outbreak Definition and Case Definitions

An outbreak is defined as a sudden increase of incidence of a disease. For the purpose of evaluating an outbreak, a case definition needs to be defined. A case definition is critical for effective investigation of an outbreak. A case definition allows for the standardization of cases that may occur at different time periods and in different geographical locations. The criteria used for case definition should be specific to the outbreak under investigation. The common components of case definition include demographic details of patients (age, gender, occupation, ethnicity, geographic location) date of onset of illness, clinical criteria, and laboratory criteria associated with illness (https://www.cdc.gov/urdo/downloads/CaseDefinitions.pdf; [1]).

14.1.3 Controversy: Dermatophytosis in India—Outbreak or Hyperendemicity or Extensive Disease

It is possible that infections which are endemic or hyperendemic may not be always recognized as outbreaks. An example is the Indian epidemic of superficial dermatophytosis which is common in many parts of the country across India. It affects patients of all age groups. There are many indiscriminate use of topical fixed dose combination (FDC) ointment including steroid with antifungal and antibacterial compounds in India. This has been attributed to the hyperendemicity resulting from inappropriate or inadequate treatment of dermatophytosis. However, extensive and disseminated clinical form has also been observed. Dermatologist in India had come up with a number of beneficial suggestions to prevent occurrence and dissemination of dermatophytosis. These suggestions have included the following recommendations [2]:

(a) Strict avoidance of antifungal preparation where steroids are present (avoidance of fixed-dose combination or FDC having steroids and antifungal agents)

(b) Following the "*rule of two*" with regard to the application of antifungal agents topically (antifungal agents to be applied for at least 2 weeks twice a day and from 2 cm beyond the margin of lesion to the center of lesion)
(c) Advice against wearing of tight garments
(d) Discouraging sharing of bed linen
(e) Wearing clothes only after thoroughly drying the body following regular shower
(f) Washing clothes and bed linen in hot water and drying them in sunlight by putting them inside out
(g) Washing contaminated clothes separately from the non-contaminated clothes
(h) Preferring non-occlusive footwear
(i) Environmental cleaning and disinfection

14.1.4 Epidemiology of Fungal Infection Outbreaks in Asia

Outbreaks caused by fungi are likely to have occurred in human societies from time immemorial; however, the documentation and analysis of the outbreaks are a much more recent phenomenon and has happened after establishment of medical mycology as a distinct specialty within medicine. Many global outbreaks have been detected including those in Asia (Table 14.1) and developed countries such as the United States as late as 2012 when contaminated methyl prednisolone injection led to multistate outbreaks of fungal meningitis from *Exserohilum rostratum*. By August 2013, more than 700 cases of fungal meningitis cases were reported from 20 states in the USA causing about 63 deaths [3].

Table 14.1 Examples of fungal infection outbreaks reported from some Asian countries

Year of outbreak or reporting	Fungus involved	Number of cases reported	Reported from	Type of infection	Sources of infection or risk factors
1996–1998	*Pichia anomala*	379	India	Blood stream infection	Hands of healthcare workers
2000	*Aspergillus*: 9 *Candida*: 2 *Mucor*: 1	12	India	Endophthalmitis	5% dextrose
2005	*Aspergillus fumigatus*	3	Sri Lanka	Meningitis	Contaminated plastic syringes
2009–2011	*Mold*	76	Afghanistan	Wound contamination	South location, lower elevation, warm temperature, isothermality
2017	*Candida auris*	74	India	Blood stream infection	Anti-fungal exposure, low APACHE II score, respiratory illness, public sector hospitals, vascular surgery

Box 14.1: Common Sources of Fungal Infection Outbreaks

Human to Human Transmission
- *Candida*
- *Pichia*
- *Pneumocystis jirovecii*

Transmission from the Environment
- Air: *Aspergillus*
- Water: *Fusarium*

Iatrogenic Transmission
- Contaminated medicines: *Aspergillus*, *Mucorales*, etc.
- Fungal endophthalmitis after contaminated infusion

Risk Factors of Fungal Infection Outbreaks
1. Failure to contain dust and spores during demolition, construction, renovation in healthcare facilities
2. Failure to implement standard precautions
3. Failure to maintain cleanliness through good housekeeping activities
4. Contamination of medicines, food
5. Vulnerable cohort: Immunocompromised patients, neonates, diabetics

14.1.4.1 Human to Human Transmission
- *Candida*
- *Pichia*
- *Pneumocystis jirovecii*

14.1.4.2 Outbreaks Due to *Pneumocystis jirovecii*
Pneumocystis jirovecii infections are thought to occur due to human to human transmission from an infectious patient source [4]. Outbreaks of this infection have occurred in India. In one report from the army hospital in New Delhi, India, nine cases of *P. jirovecii* infection was reported within a 4 month period among patients who were renal transplant recipients. Mortality occurred in one patient (11%). The cause of the outbreak was lack of co-trimoxazole prophylaxis, which was discontinued in these patients 6 months after the renal transplant. The outbreak was halted after co-trimoxazole prophylaxis was re-instituted universally to all patients with renal transplantation [5].

14.1.4.3 *Pichia anomala* Outbreak in *India*
Chakrabarti et al. reported from Chandigarh in northern India an outbreak of *Pichia anomala* infection in pediatric wards over a period of 23 months during 1996–1998. Altogether 379 neonates and children (4.2% of total admission) were infected by this fungus. Carriage on the hands of healthcare personnel was identified as probable

source of fungus. The mortality rate from *Pichia anomala* infection in this outbreak was 42.4%. The outbreak was investigated using a case–control study model. *Pichia* isolates were typed using multi-locus enzyme electrophoresis (MLEE). Environmental investigations were done using mycology cultures from environment and hands of healthcare workers. The outbreak could only be controlled after a health education campaign to improve hand-washing practices was instituted and after nystatin-fluconazole prophylaxis to all premature neonates and high-risk infants was introduced. Further investigations traced the source of agent in the hand of a resident doctor. With the change of posting, the staff carried the unusual yeast from one ward to other. The lessons learnt from this outbreak included importance of standard precautions (in this case hand hygiene); recognition of *P. anomala* as an agent competent to cause outbreak; outbreak increases morbidity and mortality of patients and cost of medical management; and importance of laboratory diagnosis and molecular typing methods in identifying possible source of the outbreak [6]. In a follow-up study, the same team of investigators showed that PCR-based identification and strain typing of *Pichia anomala* was possible using the ribosomal intergenic spacer region IGS1 [7].

14.1.4.4 *Candida auris* Outbreak: From Local to Global

Global outbreak of fungal infection was unheard. But, with the global outbreak of *Candida auris,* it is now reality. The infection was reported for the first time from Japan in 2009 in a patient with otitis media. Within a decade it spread to many countries in six continents. In Asia large number of cases have been reported from Japan, Kuwait, India, Pakistan, Qatar, Singapore, and South Korea [8].

A recent meta-analysis stated that most cases were reported from four countries India, South Africa, the USA, and the UK. There was a male predominance (~65%) among the infections reported and fungemia related isolates comprised about 67% of the cases. Crude mortality or all-cause mortality reported in this meta-analysis was about 30%. Infections were most commonly noted among patients with comorbidities such as diabetes and lung and kidney diseases. In patients with sepsis, the possibility of *Candida auris* infection in these countries should be taken into consideration. Fluconazole resistance was not universal but highest (~44%), but resistance to other broader spectrum antifungal agents such as amphotericin B (~15%), voriconazole (~13%), and caspofungin (~3.5%) were detected. For the identification and confirmation of this multi-drug-resistant fungi, a variety of different techniques have been used which included PCR (~30%), Bruker MALDI-TOF MS (14%), Vitek 2 YST ID (~12%), AFLP or amplified fragment length polymorphism analysis (~12%), and WGS or whole genome sequencing analysis (~10%). The two novel antifungal agents in the pipeline to treat this fungus included SCY-078 and VT-1598. Recommended infection control precautions are contact precautions, periodic surveillance, and cleaning and disinfection of the environmental surfaces with chlorine-based agents [9].

In India in a multicenter study of 27 ICUs, the incidence of *C. auris* candidemia was reported to be 5.3% of all candidemia cases [10, 11]. In a case–control analysis the following risk factors were noted with regard to *Candida auris* candidemia: duration of ICU stay (25 days median versus 15 days non-auris isolates), admission to North Indian ICUs and public sector hospitals (these may be related to overcrowding and deviations in infection control practices), underlying respiratory diseases, vascular surgical interventions, previous antifungal drug exposure, and low APACHE II score. Antifungal resistance in this study was reported not just against fluconazole (58.1%) but also against amphotericin B (13.5%) and caspofungin (9.5%) [11].

It is important to note that *Candida auris* may be confused with *Candida haemulonii* and *Candida famata* by the Vitek systems. Biochemical misidentification has also been reported with API 20C-AUX (*C. auris* misidentified as *Candida sake* or *Rhodotorula glutinis*). There are reports of misidentification by Microscan Walkaway system. Correct identification requires the use of either MALDI-TOF or DNA sequencing. While using DNA sequencing, ITS region or D1-D2 region has most commonly been targeted. It is clear from the experience of *Candida auris* in India and elsewhere that appropriate system for fungal identification along with correct MIC testing strategy is an essential part of outbreak investigation

14.1.4.5 Interventions to Control *Candida auris* Outbreak

The lessons of fungal infection outbreaks as learnt during the *Candida auris* experience are noteworthy [12, 13]. Certain interventions proposed to contain the outbreak have been identified to have undoubted usefulness. These have included:

1. Notification of public health agency and the hospital administration
2. Isolation precaution for an infected or colonized patient
3. Contact precaution for an infected or colonized patient
4. Reinforcement of environmental cleaning thrice daily with chlorine-based disinfectants (1000 ppm or parts per million of free chlorine) and/or vaporized hydrogen peroxide
5. Reduction of invasive procedures in colonized patients
6. Other preventative measures which have helped contain outbreaks have included:
   - Improved hand hygiene
   - Certain other interventions like screening of contacts or skin decolonization with 4% w/v Chlorhexidine are of doubtful efficacy [13].

14.1.4.6 Transmission from the Environment

- Air: *Aspergillus*
- Water: *Fusarium*

14.1.4.7 Fungal Infection Outbreak After Construction and Renovation Activities

Outbreaks of fungal infection can occur after the construction and renovation activities in healthcare setting although documented reports from Asia are difficult to find in medical literature. These generally occur among patients with hematological malignancies and in patients who are immunocompromised. The causative pathogens of these outbreaks are usually *Aspergillus*, but *Mucorales* and other uncommon fungi are also occasionally reported. The commonest sites involved are usually the lungs and mortality can be as high as 50% [14]. The minimum number of fungal spores that may result in the acquisition of fungal infection after construction or renovation remains undetermined. Control measures which should include physical separation of the area undergoing construction or renovation, use of air filters, and good housekeeping may help in containing the outbreaks. Defective ventilation systems, colonization of ventilation airway ducts, damaged or ill-fitting HEPA, and other air filters (coarse and fine air filters) along the HVAC (heating ventilation air conditioning) system, inadequate air flow or air exchange (ACH—air changes per hour), poor housekeeping, and inappropriate ambient temperature and relative humidity regulation can enhance mold growth in hospital environment and result in outbreaks especially in high-risk settings such as hemato-oncology and intensive care unit. In a study from Chandigarh in India, it was reported that there existed nearly 100 cfu/m^3 of fungal spore count in air irrespective of whether the area was air conditioned (AC) or non-AC. The predominant species isolated were *Aspergillus flavus* and *Aspergillus fumigatus* [15]. In another study from Kolkata in India, the common fungal species detected in air were *Cladosporium,* unidentified *Ascospores,* unidentified *Basidiospores, Aspergilli/Penicilli, Nigrospora, Chaetomium, Drechslera,* and *Alternaria.* Higher spore count was recorded in winter. The highest fungal species variability was observed in early monsoon (June). The total airborne concentration of fungi recorded in the study was 16×10^3 spores per m^3 of air [16]. The above studies demonstrate that there is no substitute for good hospital engineering, HVAC (heating ventilation air conditioning) system, good housekeeping, along with source containment through planning and barrier for the prevention of fungal infection in vulnerable patients. Fungi, especially molds, are omnipresent in the environment. When we interpret mycology results and take corrective measures, the facts about normal environmental mycology need to be taken into consideration.

14.1.4.8 Fungal Infection Outbreaks After Natural Disaster

Outbreaks of invasive fungal infection can occur after natural disaster [17]. The disaster-associated fungal infection has included outbreaks of *Coccidioides immitis* (pulmonary and disseminated forms) after earthquake and dust storm in the USA; *Aspergillus fumigatus* meningitis after Indian Ocean tsunami in Sri Lanka; incidence of *Cladophialophora bantiana* soft tissue infection in Thailand after tsunami; *Scedosporium apiospermum* infection of lung and brain after earthquake and tsunami in Japan; *Apophysomyces elegans* infection reported from Sri Lanka and Thailand after tsunami; and *Fusarium* and *Mucor* infection of soft tissue reported from South East Asia after tsunami. During the war in Afghanistan between 2001 and 2014, several cases of fungal wound contamination after combat trauma were reported. The environmental risk factors identified with regard to mold contamination of battle wounds were warmer temperature and lower elevation of the region. Invasive fungal infections which are trauma related may result in substantial morbidity (limb amputation) and mortality (rate as high as 38% has been reported) [18].

14.1.4.9 Iatrogenic Transmission

- Contaminated medicines: *Aspergillus*, *Mucor*, etc.
- Fungal endophthalmitis

14.1.4.10 Fungal Infection Outbreaks from Contaminated Medicines

Contaminated medicines may occasionally be the cause of fungal infection outbreaks; examples include outbreaks caused by methyl prednisolone injection in the USA and infections caused by contaminated ondansetron [3, 19]. Sterility testing of the suspected brands and medicine lots by culture and molecular methods may help identify the sources.

14.1.4.11 *Aspergillus* Meningitis Outbreak in Sri Lanka

An outbreak of *Aspergillus* meningitis was reported from Sri Lanka in 2006. Meningitis was reported in five women after spinal anesthesia for cesarean section. The incubation period was about 11 days. Papilledema, lateral rectus palsy, cerebral infarction, and hemorrhage were noted. In this series three out of five patients died (mortality rate: 60%). CSF showed pleocytosis with decreased glucose, and *Aspergillus fumigatus* was isolated [20]. The reason of outbreak was the receipt of an overwhelming amount of medications through donation after the Indian Ocean tsunami of 2004. The warehouse for medicines was saturated, and some medicines could not be properly stored. This lead to the contamination of some medications (including a spinal anesthetic) with *Aspergillus spp.* The outbreak demonstrated that storage of medication was as important as its proper manufacture, transport, and administration.

14.1.4.12 Fungal Endophthalmitis Outbreak in India

An analysis of 14 years of experience reported from PGIMER Chandigarh in northern India revealed 113 patients with fungal endophthalmitis. Out of these, majority were post-cataract (53 out of 113) and post-trauma (48 out of 113) related. *Aspergillus* was the commonest species (54%) followed by yeasts (24%) and black fungi (11%). Visual acuity after treatment remained less than 20/400 in 77%, 64%, and 50% of patients infected with *Aspergillus*, yeasts, and black fungi, respectively [21]. In 2000, 12 cases of culture-positive (9 *Aspergillus*, 2 *Candida*, 1 *Mucor*) fungal endophthalmitis were reported from the same institute (PGIMER Chandigarh, India). The patients had to undergo pars plana vitrectomy, intravitreal antimicrobial agents, and oral antifungal therapy for 4–6 weeks. Environmental investigations revealed that 11 of the 72 samples of 5% dextrose infusion bottles were culture-positive for fungi: six for *Aspergillus fumigatus*, three for *Aspergillus niger*, and two for *Candida albicans* [22]. Fungal endopthalmitis after cataract or other ophthalmic surgery is a preventable calamity. This requires rigorous quality control and sterility checks in pharmaceutical manufacturing processes besides upgradation of the cleaning, disinfection, and sterilization systems in the Central Sterile Supply Department. Hospital administrators, pharmaceutical industry stakeholders, ophthalmic surgeons, pharmacists, operation theater technologists, operating room nurses, and housekeeping staff need to be adequately trained about the importance of aseptic precautions, quality control of medicines, environmental cleanliness, good ventilation, air quality, and sterile surgical instruments.

14.1.4.13 Management of Fungal Infection Outbreak in Community and Healthcare Settings

For the investigation and management of any fungal outbreak, there is a need to convene an outbreak control team. In the community setting, this should include a public health professional, a local administrator (bureaucrat or responsible government official), representative from public health laboratory, an epidemiologist, a physician experienced in management of fungal infection and representatives of other relevant departments. In the hospital or healthcare setting, the outbreak control team should consist of the hospital infection control officer, hospital administrator, nursing superintendent, infection control nurse, maintenance engineer, housekeeping manager, physician experienced in management of fungal infection, microbiologist, and representative of other relevant departments (e.g., pharmacist for medicine-related outbreaks). The outbreak needs to be monitored on daily basis during the initial phases and subsequently weekly thereafter during the phase of resolution. An epidemic curve needs to be constructed on daily basis with records kept about new cases, ongoing cases, number of deaths/disabilities, discharges, ICU admission, and complications. It is very important that the necessary investigations are conducted to identify the fungus involved, the source of spread identified and contained, and antifungal susceptibility of the isolates done as quickly as possible. Help from external experts, reference laboratories, and public health professionals may be required from an early stage, and relevant notification to public health should be done as mandated. The detection of the source may require inspection of premises (HVAC system, water treatment plant), environmental surveillance (air quality monitoring, water quality checks), sterility testing of medicines and review of practices (hand hygiene, insertion and maintenance of central lines, etc.). Availability of essential medicines needed for the management of fungal infection in outbreak situation needs to be ensured. This is especially important if expensive and unusual antifungal agents are to be used. The pharmacy stocks may need enhancement during the crisis period [23, 24].

14.1.4.14 Technical (Mycological) Investigation of Fungal Outbreaks

The technical investigation of fungal outbreak relies on the isolation of fungus from patients as well as non-patient samples (air, water, surfaces, medicines, IV fluid, etc.) [25]. The type of samples used for the isolation of fungus depend upon the nature of fungus causing the outbreak, clinical features of index patients, and nature of the suspected sources presumed to be involved. Following isolation of the fungus, specific identification and genotyping may be required. For specific identification, advanced techniques such as MALDI-TOF or DNA sequence-based identification are preferable. This is because conventional identification method based on morphology and biochemical reaction (even using automated system like VITEK, Micro scan, or API 20C-AUX) may give erroneous identification [26, 27].

Box 14.2: Outbreak Investigation Process

- Confirm presence of outbreak: consider using CUSUM
- Establish case definition: needs to be sensitive and adequately specific
- Describe epidemiologic features of cases: create an epidemic curve
- Scrutinize patient care activities: audit practices
- Determine environmental involvement: air, water, and surface microbiology
- Mapping the location of potential sources: seek help of epidemiologist; use molecular typing (MLST: multi-locus sequence typing; WGST—whole genome sequence typing)
- Implement control and prevention measures: use multidisciplinary approach
- Alert key partners: administrators, clinician, nursing, housekeeping, microbiologists, infection control team, engineers, pharmacy, food and beverages, public health, etc.

Adapted from: Davoudi S, Graviss LS, Kontoyiannis DP. **Healthcare-associated outbreaks due to Mucorales and other uncommon fungi. Eur J Clin Invest. 2015** Jul; 45 (7):767–73.

14.1.4.15 Air Sampling for Fungi

A single air sample will often underestimate the fungal contamination in the air, and multiple air sampling has to be performed. There are no universally acceptable numerical guidelines with regard to acceptable fungal spore count. For deciding appropriateness in a particular location, the following threshold levels have been recommended with respect to area of air sampling:

1. Outdoor air (Note: seasonal variation has been recognized):
   - Total fungal colony count: 10^3–10^5 CFU/m^3,
   - *Aspergillus*: spore count: 0.2–3.5 conidia/m^3
2. HEPA filtered air (99.97% efficiency and >10 air changes per hour): <0.1 CFU/m^3

   If total fungal count exceeds 1 CFU/m^3 on several occasions, the air systems or procedural practice in patient areas requires intensive evaluation. Further investigation of sources of contamination is warranted in the following circumstances:
   - Total indoor spore counts are greater than outdoor counts.
   - Comparison of indoor and outdoor levels of fungal organisms show one of the following:
     - Organisms are present in the indoor sample and not in the outdoor sample.
     - The predominant organisms found in the indoor sample are different from the predominant organisms in the outdoor sample.
     - A monoculture of an organism is found in the indoor sample. It may be absent from samples taken in other areas of the building.
     - Persistently high counts.

If persistently high counts are recorded, or nosocomial invasive aspergillosis suspected or confirmed, it is important to identify the source of contamination by sampling:

- Dust
- Fabrics
- Ventilation ducts/ventilation screens (air curtains)/fans
- Ceiling voids
- Kitchen areas
- Excreta of roosting birds in close proximity of windows

It is important to monitor airflow patterns and monitor these on a daily basis by using flutter strips or smoke tubes in existing protective environment units [15].

14.1.5 CUSUM (Cumulative Sum Test)

Initially developed for quality control in industrial settings, the cumulative sum test (or CUSUM) has been used in epidemiological surveillance including monitoring of fungal and other healthcare-associated infection outbreaks. In a study from France, using the CUSUM methodology, significant links were found between nosocomial invasive aspergillosis incidence and fungal contamination of in hematology wards. The principle of the CUSUM methodology is as follows. The CUSUM computes at each month n, a score T_n defined by $T_n = \max\ (0, T_{n-1+} W_n)$ where $T_0 = 0$ and W_n is the log-likelihood ratio sample weight. This weight is a measure of the deviation of the observed count from the target or expected count. At the end of each month n, the CUSUM tests the null hypothesis against the alternative hypothesis. If the process is in control, it implies that the incidence of an epidemiological event (in this case fungal infection incidence) is at an acceptable level. If the process is out of control (which in this example means the incidence of nosocomial fungal infection has reached an unacceptable level), the null hypothesis is rejected. In the outbreak situation, the CUSUM score crosses a predefined limit [28].

14.2 Conclusion

The field of nosocomial (or healthcare associated) fungal outbreaks is evolving at a fast pace. Besides common fungi, rare fungi cause many outbreaks. Man to man transmission of fungi is limited to yeast and *Pneumocystis*. Hospital air quality maintenance is important for the prevention of *Aspergillus* and *Mucor* infections. Special care should be taken and practices followed as per evidence-based guidelines during demolition, construction, and renovation in healthcare environments. Though there is a paucity of guidelines *Aspergillus* spore count in air, a spore count of <1 cfu/m^3 is recommended especially in high-risk patient areas (transplant recipients, immunocompromised patients, and critical care units). It is important we have a continuous monitoring and surveillance system for fungal outbreak detection and monitoring using the cumulative sum test. Standard infection control practices such as hand hygiene, environmental cleaning and disinfection, appropriate segregation, and disposal of biomedical and general waste need to be in place for the prevention and control of fungal outbreaks. With the increase in the number of vulnerable patients (diabetics, immunocompromised, steroid users, and antibiotics users), global climate change, increased international and transcontinental movement of people goods and animals, as well as a change in environmental conditions from construction and renovation activities, and also due to global warming, it is likely that an increasing number of fungal outbreaks would be reported in future. Our capability to detect and contain fungal outbreaks at an early stage would depend upon many factors, most importantly the robustness of fungal infection detection and surveillance system in hospitals and communities. It is in our long-term economic and healthcare interest that we develop outbreak management systems in all healthcare facilities and administrative units. Development of diagnostic mycology services, networking between surveillance centers, and allocation of adequate resources along with coordination of current and future plans will determine the outbreak management preparedness of various healthcare facilities.

References

1. CDC. Outbreak case definitions. https://www.cdc.gov/urdo/downloads/CaseDefinitions.pdf. Accessed 14 Sept 2018.
2. Verma S, Madhu R. The great Indian epidemic of superficial dermatophytosis: an appraisal. Indian J Dermatol. 2017;62(3):227–36.
3. Litvintseva AP, Hurst S, Gade L, Frace MA, Hilsabeck R, Schupp JM, Gillece JD, Roe C, Smith D, Keim P, Lockhart SR, Changayil S, Weil MR, MacCannell DR, Brandt ME, Engelthaler DM. Whole-genome analysis of Exserohilum rostratum from an outbreak of fungal meningitis and other infections. J Clin Microbiol. 2014;52(9):3216–22.
4. Alanio A, Gits-Muselli M, Mercier-Delarue S, Dromer F, Bretagne S. Diversity of Pneumocystis jirovecii during infection revealed by ultra-deep pyrosequencing. Front Microbiol. 2016;7:733.
5. Jairam A, Dassi M, Chandola P, Lall M, Mukherjee D, Hooda AK. Pneumocystis jiroveci outbreak in a renal transplant center: lessons learnt. Indian J Nephrol. 2014;24(5):276–9.
6. Chakrabarti A, Singh K, Narang A, Singhi S, Batra R, Rao KL, Ray P, Gopalan S, Das S, Gupta V, Gupta AK, Bose SM, McNeil MM. Outbreak of Pichia anomala infection in the pediatric service of a tertiary-care center in Northern India. J Clin Microbiol. 2001;39(5):1702–6.
7. Bhardwaj S, Sutar R, Bachhawat AK, Singhi S, Chakrabarti A. PCR-based identification and strain typing of Pichia anomala using the ribosomal intergenic spacer region IGS1. J Med Microbiol. 2007;56(Pt 2):185–9.
8. Chowdhary A, Sharma C, Meis JF. Candida auris: a rapidly emerging cause of hospital-acquired multidrug-resistant fungal infections globally. PLoS Pathog. 2017;13(5):e1006290.
9. Osei Sekyere J. Candida auris: a systematic review and meta-analysis of current updates on an emerging multidrug-resistant pathogen. Microbiology. 2018;7(4):e00578. https://doi.org/10.1002/mbo3.578. Epub 2018 Jan 18.
10. Chakrabarti A, Sood P, Rudramurthy SM, Chen S, Kaur H, Capoor M, Chhina D, Rao R, Eshwara VK, Xess I, Kindo AJ, Umabala P, Savio J, Patel A, Ray U, Mohan S, Iyer R, Chander J, Arora A, Sardana R, Roy I, Appalaraju B, Sharma A, Shetty A, Khanna N, Marak R, Biswas S, Das S, Harish BN, Joshi S, Mendiratta D. Incidence, characteristics and outcome of ICU-acquired candidemia in India. Intensive Care Med. 2015;41(2):285–95.
11. Rudramurthy SM, Chakrabarti A, Paul RA, Sood P, Kaur H, Capoor MR, Kindo AJ, Marak RSK, Arora A, Sardana R, Das S, Chhina D, Patel A, Xess I, Tarai B, Singh P, Ghosh

A. Candida auris candidaemia in Indian ICUs: analysis of risk factors. J Antimicrob Chemother. 2017;72(6):1794–801.
12. Biswal M, Rudramurthy SM, Jain N, Shamanth AS, Sharma D, Jain K, Yaddanapudi LN, Chakrabarti A. Controlling a possible outbreak of Candida auris infection: lessons learnt from multiple interventions. J Hosp Infect. 2017;97(4):363–70.
13. Lockhart SR, Etienne KA, Vallabhaneni S, Farooqi J, Chowdhary A, Govender NP, Colombo AL, Calvo B, Cuomo CA, Desjardins CA, Berkow EL, Castanheira M, Magobo RE, Jabeen K, Asghar RJ, Meis JF, Jackson B, Chiller T, Litvintseva AP. Simultaneous emergence of multidrug-resistant Candida auris on 3 continents confirmed by whole-genome sequencing and epidemiological analyses. Clin Infect Dis. 2017;64(2):134–40.
14. Kanamori H, Rutala WA, Sickbert-Bennett EE, Weber DJ. Review of fungal outbreaks and infection prevention in healthcare settings during construction and renovation. Clin Infect Dis. 2015;61(3):433–44.
15. Rudramurthy SM, Singh G, Hallur V, Verma S, Chakrabarti A. High fungal spore burden with predominance of Aspergillus in hospital air of a tertiary care hospital in Chandigarh. Indian J Med Microbiol. 2016;34(4):529–32.
16. Das S, Gupta-Bhattacharya S. Monitoring and assessment of airborne fungi in Kolkata, India, by viable and non-viable air sampling methods. Environ Monit Assess. 2012;184(8):4671–84.
17. Benedict K, Park BJ. Invasive fungal infections after natural disasters. Emerg Infect Dis. 2014;20(3):349–55.
18. Tribble DR, Rodriguez CJ, Weintrob AC, Shaikh F, Aggarwal D, Carson ML, Murray CK, Masuoka P, Infectious Disease Clinical Research Program Trauma Infectious Disease Outcomes Study Group. Environmental factors related to fungal wound contamination after combat trauma in Afghanistan, 2009–2011. Emerg Infect Dis. 2015;21(10):1759–69.
19. Etienne KA, Roe CC, Smith RM, Vallabhaneni S, Duarte C, Escadon P, Castaneda E, Gomez BL, de Bedout C, López LF, Salas V, Hederra LM, Fernandez J, Pidal P, Hormazabel JC, Otaiza F, Vannberg FO, Gillece J, Lemmer D, Driebe EM, Englethaler DM, Litvintseva AP. Whole-genome sequencing to determine origin of multinational outbreak of *Sarocladium kiliense* bloodstream infections. Emerg Infect Dis. 2016;22(3):476–81.
20. Gunaratne PS, Wijeyaratne CN, Chandrasiri P, Sivakumaran S, Sellahewa K, Perera P, Fernando R, Wanigasinghe J, Jayasinghe S, Ranawala R, Riffsy MT, Seneviratne HR. An outbreak of Aspergillus meningitis following spinal anaesthesia for caesarean section in Sri Lanka: a post-tsunami effect? Ceylon Med J. 2006;51(4):137–42.
21. Chakrabarti A, Shivaprakash MR, Singh R, Tarai B, George VK, Fomda BA, Gupta A. Fungal endophthalmitis: fourteen years' experience from a center in India. Retina. 2008;28(10):1400–7.
22. Gupta A, Gupta V, Dogra MR, Chakrabarti A, Ray P, Ram J, Patnaik B. Fungal endophthalmitis after a single intravenous administration of presumably contaminated dextrose infusion fluid. Retina. 2000;20(3):262–8.
23. WHO. How to detect and investigate outbreaks in the healthcare setting. http://www.who.int/gpsc/information_centre/moro-maria-luisa_outbreaks.pdf. Accessed 15 Sept 2018.
24. WHO. Infection prevention and control in health care for preparedness and response to outbreak. http://www.who.int/csr/bioriskreduction/infection_control/background/en/. Accessed 15 Sept 2018.
25. Davoudi S, Graviss LS, Kontoyiannis DP. Healthcare-associated outbreaks due to Mucorales and other uncommon fungi. Eur J Clin Investig. 2015;45(7):767–73.
26. Bougnoux ME, Brun S, Zahar JR. Healthcare-associated fungal outbreaks: new and uncommon species, new molecular tools for investigation and prevention. Antimicrob Resist Infect Control. 2018;7:45.
27. Litvintseva AP, Brandt ME, Mody RK, Lockhart SR. Investigating fungal outbreaks in the 21st century. PLoS Pathog. 2015;11(5):e1004804.
28. Menotti J, Porcher R, Ribaud P, Lacroix C, Jolivet V, Hamane S, Derouin F. Monitoring of nosocomial invasive aspergillosis and early evidence of an outbreak using cumulative sum tests (CUSUM). Clin Microbiol Infect. 2010;16(9):1368–74.

Part V

Clinical Practice and Management in Asia

Superficial Fungal Infections: Clinical Practices and Management in Asia

15

Shivaprakash M. Rudramurthy and Harsimran Kaur

Key Points

- Dermatophytosis (tinea), *Malassezia* related skin disorders (pityriasis versicolor, seborrheic dermatitis or folliculitis) and fungal keratitis (FK) are common superficial fungal infections.
- Topical therapy, primarily using azoles or allylamines, is recommended for localized lesions of naïve tinea cruris and tinea corporis.
- Combination of both topical and systemic therapy is recommended in cases of dermatophytosis with extensive skin involvement, presence of papules/pustules or recalcitrant, and onychomycosis and tinea pedis.
- Rule of two is applied in topical therapy of dermatophytosis where the drug is applied 2 cm beyond the margin of lesion for at least 2 weeks after the clinical recovery.
- Systemic antifungals commonly include terbinafine, itraconazole and occasionally fluconazole with promising results of pulse therapy.
- Duration of systemic therapy ranges from 2 to 4 weeks and >4 weeks in naïve and recalcitrant cases of dermatophytosis, respectively.
- There is no role of steroids in the management of dermatophytosis.
- *Malassezia*-related skin disorders are treated with topical antifungals except in case of folliculitis where systemic therapy with itraconazole is required.
- For fungal keratitis, topical application of voriconazole, natamycin and chlorhexidine have all shown promising response.

S. M. Rudramurthy (✉) · H. Kaur
Department of Medical Microbiology, Postgraduate Institute of Medical Education and Research (PGIMER), Chandigarh, India

A. Chakrabarti (ed.), *Clinical Practice of Medical Mycology in Asia*,
https://doi.org/10.1007/978-981-13-9459-1_15

15.1 Introduction

The fungal infections limited to epidermis, mucosa, hair and nail fall into the category of superficial infections. The common types of superficial fungal infections include dermatophytosis (tinea) and diseases caused by *Malassezia* (pityriasis versicolor, seborrheic dermatitis or folliculitis). Recently, there has been emergence of fungal keratitis which is an implantation infection due to either injury or contact lens [1]. The exact burden of the superficial fungal infection is not known especially in developing nations due to under-diagnosis [2]. The global burden of skin and appendage fungal infections and fungal keratitis is estimated to be one billion and one million annual cases, respectively [2]. Superficial fungal infections may affect both immunocompetent and immunocompromised patients. These infections rarely cause serious complications but exhibit chronicity and high frequency of recurrence [3]. Due to similar clinical presentation of dermatitis and related inflammatory disorders, the diagnosis of dermatophytosis is delayed and results in overuse and misuse of antifungals [3]. The diagnosis and management of superficial fungal infections face challenges especially in resource limited settings. There exist a set of guidelines of these infections in Western countries which assist the clinicians in making decisions. But due to the variation in epidemiology of these infections between developing and developed nations, these guidelines may not be applicable for managing patients in Asian region. Even in this region, differences in clinical presentation, etiological agents and antifungal susceptibility profile have been noted, which necessitates the formulation of region-specific guidelines for the management of superficial fungal infections. Although data is scarce across the region, we discuss here the current clinical practices and management of superficial fungal infections in Asia.

15.2 Current Guidelines for Superficial Fungal Infections

A Medline search of management guidelines of superficial fungal infections in PubMed revealed few guidelines including dermatophytosis (n = 8), *Malassezia*-related skin disorders (n = 4) and infectious keratitis (n = 2) (Table 15.1). Two additional guidelines from WHO (HIV patients) and European expert panel are available for the management of superficial mycoses. Most of these guidelines are from the United States, Europe and the United Kingdom. Among Asian countries, only India and Japan have certain recommendations for the management of dermatophytosis and/or infectious keratitis. The Japanese guidelines of dermatophytosis and infectious keratitis are described in their local language only. The physicians in India have become sensitized to the challenges of management of superficial fungal infections in the recent past. This has resulted in upsurge of literature with increased recognition of challenges in the management of these infections.

Table 15.1 Different guidelines available on the management of superficial fungal infections

S. No.	Disease	Guidelines	Region	Author Year
1	Superficial mycoses	Guidelines on the treatment of skin and oral HIV-associated conditions in children and adults. WHO [4]	Worldwide	2014
		Topical antifungal-corticosteroid combination therapy for the treatment of superficial mycoses: Conclusions of an expert panel meeting [5]	Europe	Schaller et al. 2016
2	Dermatophytosis	Guidelines of care for superficial mycotic infections of the skin: tinea corporis, tinea cruris, tinea faciei, tinea manuum and tinea pedis. Guidelines/Outcomes Committee American Academy of Dermatology [6]	USA	Drake et al. 1996
		Guidelines of care for superficial mycotic infections of the skin: tinea capitis, tinea barbae. Guidelines/ Outcomes Committee American Academy of Dermatology [7]	USA	Drake et al. 1996
		Guidelines of care for superficial mycotic infections of the skin: onychomycosis. Guidelines/Outcomes Committee. American Academy of Dermatology [8]	USA	1996
		Treatment of onychomycosis caused by dermatophytes—an opinion proposed by the Committee for Standardization of the Japanese Society for Medical Mycology 2007 [9]	Japan	Mohri et al. 2007
		European society for Paediatric Dermatology Guidelines for the management of tinea capitis in children [10]	Europe	Kakourou et al. 2010
		British Association of Dermatologists' guidelines for the management of onychomycosis [11]	Britain	Ameen et al. 2014
		British Association of Dermatologists' guidelines for the management of tinea capitis [12]	Britain	Fuller et al. 2014
		Expert Consensus on The Management of Dermatophytosis in India (ECTODERM India) [13]	India	Rajagopalan et al. 2018

(continued)

Table 15.1 (continued)

S. No.	Disease	Guidelines	Region	Author Year
3	Malassezia-related Skin Diseases	Guidelines of care for superficial mycotic infections of the skin: Pityriasis (tinea) versicolor. Guidelines/Outcomes Committee. American Academy of Dermatology [14]	USA	Drake et al. 1996
		ESCMID and ECMM joint clinical guidelines for the diagnosis and management of rare invasive yeast infections [15]	Europe	Arendrup et al. 2013
		Evidence-based Danish guidelines for the treatment of *Malassezia*-related skin diseases [16]	Denmark	Hald et al. 2015
		Treatment of Seborrhoeic Dermatitis in Asia: A Consensus Guide [17]	Asia	Cheong et al. 2015
4	Keratitis	Guidelines for the clinical management of infectious keratitis [18]	Japan	2007
		Guidelines for the clinical management of infectious keratitis (2nd edition) [19]	Japan	2013

15.3 Clinical Practices and Management of Superficial Fungal Infections in Asia

The data on clinical practices and management of superficial fungal infections is insufficient across the Asian countries. Most of the studies available discuss the changing trends of epidemiological features of these infections. There are stark differences within and between countries in the Asian region ranging from skin texture to socioeconomic status, climate, access to treatment, emphasizing the requirement of region-specific guidelines [20]. Certain challenges faced by Asian population include scarcity of qualified dermatologists especially in rural and peripheral areas, prolific use of multiple less efficacious irrational FDCs, unauthorized cosmetics, poor quality generic products and self-treatment/non-compliance of patients and medication from non-healthcare personnel.

15.3.1 Dermatophytosis

Available literature of practices and management are limited to dermatophytosis and that too from India.

15.3.1.1 Challenges Faced by Dermatologists in Asian Countries

Dermatologists in developing countries are fraught with challenges of

- Unusual presentation of dermatophytosis causing difficulty in diagnosis and management of the disease. The lesions are large, multiple and present as ring within ring and are probably modified in appearance due to steroid use.
- The chronicity and increasing resistance among dermatophytes are additional therapeutic challenges. The standard guidelines from western countries are difficult to imply in such situation.
- There is an increasing trend of experience-based treatment rather than standard guidelines available in literature.
- The over-the-counter availability of irrational fixed drug combination (FDC) creams containing steroid along with antifungal and antibacterial agents leads to the development of chronic recurrent and refractory dermatophytosis. Newer formulations like fluconazole/itraconazole powder and amphotericin B gel/cream have been introduced in the market irrespective of their efficacy and safety [21]. The use of these drugs suppresses the normal inflammatory response to the fungi. This misuse of steroids and irrational drug combinations leads to the so-called "double edged tinea" with double concentric rings which is prevalent widely in some of the Asian countries. Additional adverse effects in such cases include striae formation, atrophy and hyperpigmentation after 3–4 weeks of FDC use [21].
- Another trait noticeable in Indian population is a familial tendency of dermatophytosis similar to scabies. Any member in house suffering from the disease transmits to other members especially children due to close association and sharing linens. They also share irrational prescriptions leading to clinical resistance or picture of treatment failure.
- There has also been a noticeable increase in genital dermatophytosis where perineal lesions are often ignored while applying topical agents and the site remains as reservoirs for the recurrence of disease.
- Patients usually self-experiment with over-the-counter drugs.
- There is a dearth of literature regarding antifungal breakpoints of dermatophytes, clinical correlation, pharmacokinetic/pharmacodynamic studies, and epidemiological cut-off MIC values.

15.3.1.2 Expert Consensus on the Management of Dermatophytosis in India (ECTODERM India) [13]

Dermatologists in India have shown a major change in their prescription patterns that varies from Western guidelines. Recently, Indian Expert Forum Consensus Group was formed to formulate evidence-based and experience-driven local guidelines for the management of dermatosis in India (ECTODERM) [13].

Sample Collection and Diagnosis

Samples should be collected from the edge of the lesions where hyphae are expected to be plenty and transportation to be done in dry black strong paper. The examination using 10% KOH mount after 1–30 min of preparation is considered as point-of-care test for the confirmation of diagnosis. Sensitivity and specificity depend on adequate sample collection and expertise of microscopic examination. Fungal culture is recommended only in recalcitrant and multisite cases. Dermoscopic examination for evaluating the involvement of vellus hair is an important adjunct diagnostic modality as positive features implicate systemic therapy. Due to increase in antifungal resistance among dermatophytes, the importance of antifungal susceptibility of the etiologic agents was well recognized by the experts. But due to the lack of data on correlation between in vitro susceptibility and clinical outcome along with unavailability of MIC breakpoint of dermatophytes, the routine performance of the in vitro antifungal susceptibility was not considered feasible at present. Behzadi et al. from Iran also stressed upon the identification of dermatophyte species for accurate management due to increase in antifungal resistance [22].

Management of Tinea Cruris, Tinea Corporis, Tinea Pedis, Tinea Unguium and Tinea Capitis

Experts suggested assessment of a combination of factors like site involved, dry or moist area, prior antifungal use and age of patient to decide antifungal management. Topical therapy is recommended for localized lesions of naïve tinea cruris and tinea corporis. Combination therapy (both topical and systemic) is recommended in extensive skin involvement or lesions with papules/pustules or recalcitrant cases and even naïve cases of tinea pedis. Topical antifungals in the form of solutions, gels or sprays are preferred in case of macerated tinea pedis while cream or ointment is recommended for dry scaly type of disease. Systemic therapy is necessary in cases with the involvement of vellus hair. The combination therapy should include drugs from different classes so as to have a broader coverage, thereby preventing resistance development. Topical agents should be preferred in paediatric patients as rapid turnover favours better clinical response. Only topical agents are given in pregnant females. Terbinafine is pregnancy category B, but data on its safety in pregnancy is scarce. Regarding itraconazole too, it is suggested to maintain contraception for 2 months after its intake. The treatment is individualized in elderly patients where preference is given to topical agents. Systemic therapy is advised only in non-response to topical therapy, extensive lesions and recalcitrant cases.

The duration of therapy ranges from 2 to 4 weeks and >4 weeks in naïve and recalcitrant cases, respectively. The management (topical or systemic) should continue 2 weeks post-clinical cure. Nail lacquers available for tinea unguium require a longer duration of application (amorolfine once weekly for 6–12 months; ciclopirox olamine once daily 9–12 months in onychomycosis).

General measures: The necessity of compliance to the management should be clearly explained to the patient. The use of tight clothing/occlusive footwear, sharing of towels/clothes/combs/hats/scarves/pillows and walking barefoot should be discouraged. The skin folds and toe clefts should be completely dried before wearing socks or shoes. The clothes should be washed in hot water, dried in sun and ironed regularly. The patients with high sweat rate should be advised to change clothing more frequently and use absorbent powders and deodorants to decrease perspiration. The surrounding environment should be kept clean by dusting, mopping and vacuuming. Infection from pets should be considered in patients with dermatophytosis [21].

Topical therapy: Among topical agents, azoles are recommended as first-line of treatment. These include clotrimazole (1% cream/lotion/solution/powder/spray), ketoconazole (2% cream/gel/shampoo), econazole (1% cream), miconazole (2% cream/lotion/powder/gel), oxiconazole (1% cream/lotion), bifonazole (1% cream), sertaconazole (2% cream), eberconazole (1% cream) and luliconazole (1% cream/lotion) [23]. Other topical antifungals include terbinafine (1% cream/powder), naftifine (1% cream/gel), butenafine (1% cream), amorolfine (0.25% cream/5% nail lacquer), ciclopirox olamine (1% cream/shampoo/8%nail lacquer) and selenium sulphide (1%, 2.5% lotion/shampoo) [23].

Additional therapies like antihistaminic, 6% salicylic acid and moisturizers play a supplemental role. Rule of two is applied in topical therapy where the drug is applied 2 cm beyond the margin of lesion for at least 2 weeks after the clinical recovery. In vitro data from India suggests most effective antifungals in the order: luliconazole > butenafine > ciclopirox = naftifine, other azoles > terbinafine [23].

Systemic therapy: Naïve tinea pedis cases should be treated with terbinafine 250 mg daily and recalcitrant or severe disease cases with itraconazole 200–400 mg/day in divided doses. Similarly, naïve tinea cruris or corporis with extensive lesions should be treated with either terbinafine (250 mg once daily) or itraconazole (100–200 mg/day) while recalcitrant cases, deep inflammatory, multisite lesions, non-responders and *T. rubrum* syndrome should be treated with higher dose of itraconazole (200–400 mg/day, in divided doses) along with appropriate topical therapy. In tinea incognito, the use of topical steroids is dissuaded and withdrawal is recommended in case of tinea incognito in addition to itraconazole 200–400 mg daily for 4–6 months. Fluconazole (allowed in infants) and terbinafine (only in ≥2 years) are agents of choice if systemic agents are to be given in children. Terbinafine is a preferred oral drug in elderly due to multiple drug interactions of azoles. In case of treatment failure with these drugs, griseofulvin (250–500 mg twice daily) or fluconazole (150 mg–300 mg/week) can be used.

Management of Onychomycosis

Onychomycosis can be caused by both *Candida* and dermatophytes or non-dermatophytic moulds. Standard guidelines for the management of onychomycosis are lacking in Asian countries. Dermatologists usually prescribe both topical and systemic therapies in onychomycosis either alone or in combination [24]. The drug cannot penetrate the hard keratinized nail plate well, leaving a 1000 times lower amount reaching the inner area of nail [11]. Treatment with topical agents alone is limited to classical superficial white onychomycosis (except in transverse or striate infections), early distal and lateral subungual onychomycosis (DLSO) (except in the presence of longitudinal streaks, central yellow onycholytic area) when <80% of the nail plate is affected without involving lunula or when systemic antifungals are contraindicated [11, 22]

The duration of therapy should range from minimum 6 weeks to 3 months or more [24].

Sample collection and diagnosis: The dermatologists recommend direct microscopy and fungal culture in all cases of onychomycosis and subjecting to antifungal susceptibility testing in view of emerging antifungal resistance [24]. The sample collection varies according to the type of onychomycosis [24]. Nail bed scraping are collected in distal subungal onychomycosis, currated (1–2mm serrated) nail material from proximal subungal onychomycosis, scraping of white areas in white superficial onychomycosis and nail clippings in endonyx/total dystropic onychomycosis [24].

Topical therapy: Various topical agents include 8% ciclopirox solution (daily or twice daily for 48 weeks), 5% amorolfine [once or twice a week for 6 (finger nail) to 12 (toe nail) months], 5% tavaborole (once daily for 48 weeks) and 10% efinaconazole solution (once daily for 48 weeks) [23]. The solvent evaporates and increases the concentration of the active ingredient.

Systemic therapy: The two antifungals, terbinafine and itraconazole, are the most common and effective drugs for the management of onychomycosis. Pulsed manner of treatment has shown promising results [25]. The "Indian Association of Dermatologists, Venereologists and Leprologists" (IADVL) manual for the treatment of dermatophytosis suggests treatment with terbinafine for moulds (continuous dosage: 250 mg daily for 6 weeks for fingernail infection and 12 weeks for toenail infection: pulsed dosage: 250 mg twice daily for 1 week for a month—for 2 and 3 months for fingernail and toenail, respectively; dosage in paediatric population 125 mg in 20–40 kg and 62.5 mg in <20 kg), itraconazole for both moulds and yeasts (continuous dosage: 200 mg daily for 2 and 3 months for finger and toe nail respectively; pulsed dosage: 200 mg twice daily for 1 week a month—for 2 and 3 months for fingernail and toenail respectively) and fluconazole for *Candida* infections [23]. Griseofulvin and ketoconazole are not preferred by most dermatologists due to long duration of treatment and serious side effects respectively. Fluconazole, although less efficacious than terbinafine and itraconazole, is a reserve drug for those who cannot take other oral antifungals [24].

Surgical debridement: Subungual hyperkeratosis needs to be surgically debrided by either chemical removal (40% urea in lacquer base, 50% potassium iodide) or mechanical removal [23].

Newer therapies: Laser, photodynamic therapy and iontophoresis [23].

15.3.1.3 Current Practices

Currently, the dermatologists of India prescribe

(a) Higher dosage of oral antifungals
(b) Longer duration (at least 3 weeks) of both topical and oral antifungals
(c) Periodic monitoring of liver function tests [21].

It has been noticed that withdrawal of treatment before 3 weeks leads to recurrence of lesions. Inadequate results have been noticed with 100 mg itraconazole for 2–4 weeks, and therefore, clinicians go for 200 mg for 3–4 weeks. The practice of prescribing weight-based doses of terbinafine and itraconazole rather than standard recommendation (250 mg terbinafine for 15 days; 100 mg itraconazole for 15 days or 200 mg for 7 days) is found to be more beneficial. The use of older antifungal agents like griseofulvin (500 mg BD for 6 weeks), fluconazole (150 mg thrice weekly for 8 weeks) or topical ciclopirox olamine has shown promising results in recalcitrant dermatophytosis [21]. Newer topical agents like eberconazole and sertaconazole are more efficacious than clotrimazole. For better results, dermatologists follow rule of two.

Behzadi et al. from Iran mentioned the practice of preferring topical agents for the management of tinea and combination of both topical and systemic agents in case of refractory cases. The commonly used antifungals in their region include azoles, griseofulvin and terbinafine [22].

15.3.2 Malassezia-Related Skin Disorders

Malassezia species, an integral member of normal human skin, is associated with various dermatological disorders like pityriasis versicolor, seborrheic dermatitis and folliculitis [26]. Even systemic infections have been reported in patients on lipid supplementation or catheterization [26]. Large population-based studies are lacking in determining the epidemiology of disease in Asia.

15.3.2.1 Seborrheic dermatitis (SD)

Seborrheic dermatitis (SD) is quite common inflammatory skin disorder characterized by scaly brownish itchy lesions in sebaceous gland-rich areas of scalp, face and trunk [17]. Few studies from Asia have shown prevalence rate ranging from 2.1 to 26.5% and higher rate (17–47%) in HIV-positive population [17]. The management in Asian population differs due to significant differences in the texture of skin of these individuals from Caucasians [17]. Asian skin has higher melanin, more prone to post-inflammatory pigmentation, higher stratum corneum water content and lipid levels, higher dermatological response to irritants in topical formulations leading to complications. Irritant products/cosmetics and soaps/creams containing alcohol cause hyperreactivity in Asian population. Evidence-based Danish guidelines recommend use of azoles (2% ketoconazole cream/shampoo, 2% miconazole cream and/or 1.5% ciclopirox olamine up to 4 weeks) as drug of choice in SD with or without supplementary topical steroids, calcineurin inhibitors or oral antifungal agents (itraconazole 200 mg for 7 days followed by maintenance doses 200 mg OD for 2 days every month) in patients with widespread or refractory lesions [16].

An expert consensus panel of 12 dermatologists from Asian countries (India, South Korea, Taiwan, Malaysia, Vietnam, Singapore, Thailand, Philippines, Indonesia, Italy) met in Singapore in 2014 for the formulation of Asia specific management guidelines for SD [17] (Table 15.2).

Table 15.2 Asia-specific management guidelines for seborrheic dermatitis

	Scalp and hairy areas		Non-scalp SD	
Mild SD	Topical antifungals (1–1.5% ciclopirox shampoo; 1–2% ketoconazole shampoo, gel)	2–3 times per week	Topical antifungals (1% ciclopirox cream; 2% ketoconazole cream)	Twice daily × 4 weeks
	AIAFp shampoo	2–3 times per week	AIAFp shampoo	Twice daily × 4 weeks
	Keratolytics (Salicylic acid 3% shampoo; Tar 1–2% shampoo)	2–3 times per week	Additional if no improvement	
			Topical corticosteroids (Class I)	Twice daily × 4 weeks
	Others: Selenium sulphide 2.5% shampoo; Zinc pyrithione 1–2% shampoo	2–3 times per week	Topical calcineurin inhibitors	Twice daily × 4 weeks
Additional if no improvement	Topical corticosteroids (I-II)	Once daily × 4 weeks		
Moderate to severe SD	Steroid added according to severity			
	Topical corticosteroids (I–II)	Once daily × 4 weeks	Topical corticosteroids (class II)	Twice daily × 4 weeks
	Topical corticosteroids (III–IV)	Twice weekly × 2 weeks		
If no improvement with above therapy				
Systemic antifungals	Itraconazole 100 mg caps	First month: 200 mg/day for 1 week, then 200 mg/day for 2 days/month up to 11 months		
	Terbinafine 250 mg caps	Continuous regimen: 250 mg/day for 4–6 weeks Intermittent regimen:250 mg/day for 12 days per month for 3 months		
	Fluconazole 50 mg caps	50 mg/day for 2 weeks or 200–300 mg weekly for 2–4 weeks		
Infants	Topical antifungals (2% ketoconazole shampoo)	Twice per week for 4 weeks	Topical antifungals (2% ketoconazole cream)	Once daily × 7 days
	Emollients	Daily	Topical steroids (Class I)	Once daily × 7 days
	AIAFp shampoo	12 h		

AIAFp anti-inflammatory with antifungal properties

15.3.2.2 Pityriasis versicolor (PV)

PV is a superficial fungal infection of the skin seen in tropical and subtropical regions in which commensal *Malassezia* yeasts turn to mycelia phase which are capable of invading the stratum corneum [14, 16]. The prevalence of PV differs in various geographical regions. There are no guidelines available specific for Asian countries, but a handful of studies available from Asia show the efficacy of various drug dose regimens (Table 15.3). Clinicians in Asia use European and Danish guidelines.

Table 15.3 Studies from Asia showing the efficacy of various drug dose regimens in pityriasis versicolor

S. No.	Year	Author, place	Treatment groups	Number of patients	Complete cure rate	Follow-up cure/relapse rate (*p* value)
1	1989	Kagawa et al., Japan [28]	1% terbinafine cream, 2×/day for 14 days	87	90%	
2	1995	Kose et al., Tekirdag, Turkey [29]	600 mg for 14 days, fluconazole vs. 400 mg for 14 days itraconazole	27 vs. 25	80% vs. 74%	Relapse 14% vs. 20%
3	1996	Balwada et al., Haryana, India [30]	2% ketoconazole cream, 1×/day for 14 days vs. 1% clotrimazole cream	20 vs. 20	90% vs. 80%	100% cure rate in both
4	1997	Sankara et al., Davangre, India [31]	400 mg single dose fluconazole	25	92%	–
5	1999	Balachandran et al., Manipal, India [32]	400 mg single dose fluconazole vs. placebo	18 vs. 12	44% vs. 8%	–
6	1999	Ravikumar et al., Manipal, India [33]	400 mg single dose itraconazole vs. placebo	12 vs. 13	17% vs. 0%	–
7	2000	Chopra et al., Haryana, India [34]	2% ketoconazole cream, 1×/day for 14 days vs. 1% terbinafine cream	25 vs. 25	88% vs. 96%	Relapse: 3 patients vs. 2 patients
8	2001	Bhogal et al., Delhi, India [35]	400 mg single dose fluconazole vs. 150 mg/week, 4 weeks, fluconazole vs. 400 mg single dose ketoconazole vs. 200 mg for 10 days ketoconazole	45 each group	82% vs. 64% vs. 53% vs. 73%	Relapse 0% vs. 7% vs. 25% vs. 4%
9	2002	Kokturk et al., Mersin, Turkey [36]	200 mg for 5 days, itraconazole vs. 400 mg single dose itraconazole vs. 400 mg for 3 days, itraconazole	20 each	70% vs. 20% vs. 75%	$P < 0.001$
10	2002	Kose et al., Ankara, Turkey [37]	400 mg single dose itraconazole vs. 200 mg for 7 days, itraconazole	24 vs. 26	85% vs. 90%	–
11	2003	Aggarwal et al., Haryana, India [38]	2% ketoconazole shampoo, 1×/week for 3 weeks vs. 2.5% selenium sulphide shampoo	20 each	85% vs. 90%	Relapse: 1 patients vs. 2 patients

(continued)

Table 15.3 (continued)

S. No.	Year	Author, place	Treatment groups	Number of patients	Complete cure rate	Follow-up cure/relapse rate (*p* value)
12	2003	Rathi et al., Siliguri, West Bengal [39]	2% ketoconazole shampoo, 1×/day, for 3 days	30	90%	–
13	2004	Partap et al., Chandigarh, India [40]	400 mg single dose fluconazole vs. 400 mg single dose itraconazole	20 each	65% vs. 20%	Relapse 35% vs. 60% $P < 0.01$
14	2005	Karakas et al., Adana, Turkey [41]	300 mg/week, 2 weeks, fluconazole	44	78%	Relapse 0%
15	2007	Yazdanpanah et al., Mashhad, Iran [42]	Single dose 400 mg ketoconazole vs. two doses of 300 mg of fluconazole with 2 weeks interval	47 vs. 43	87.9% vs. 81.5%	Failure 12.1% vs. 18.5%
16	2010	Dehgan et al., Gorgan, Iran [43]	400 mg single dose fluconazole, placebo cream 2×/day, 14 days vs. Placebo pill, 1% clotrimazole cream 2×/day, 14 days	50 vs. 55	82% vs. 95%	92% vs. 82%
17	2015	Shi et al., Zhenghou, China [44]	2% ketoconazole cream +0.1% adapalene gel, 1×/day for 14 days vs. 2% ketoconazole cream, 2×/day for 14 days	50 each	92% vs. 72%	$P < 0.01$

Topical antifungals are considered as drug of choice for the treatment of PV in the form of creams, lotions and shampoos daily or twice daily. Ketoconazole foam is a latest form which can be easily acceptable to patients [27]. The recommendation of topical treatment suggests either (a) once or twice daily for 14 days topical 2% ketoconazole cream or foam and once weekly use of 2% ketoconazole shampoo or (b) twice daily terbinafine cream/gel for 7 days [16, 27]. The combination treatment has shown better efficacy. Other local antifungal options include ciclopirox olamine (1.5% shampoo, two times weekly for 2 weeks), miconazole (cream twice daily) and clotrimazole (cream twice daily for 2 weeks) [16]. The longer duration of treatment has shown better outcome in patients. Multiple non-specific topical treatments like selenium sulphide (2.5% shampoo, once daily for 3 days and repeat after a week), zinc pyrithione (1% shampoo, two to three times weekly), propylene glycol (50% in water, twice daily for 2 weeks) and Whitfield's ointment supplementing the antifungals are effective in treating PV by removing the dead debris rather than acting on *Malassezia* [16, 27]. The systemic antifungals are reserved for severe or recalcitrant cases. These include 200 mg itraconazole daily for 5 or 7 days/100 mg daily for 2 weeks/single dose itraconazole 400 mg, 300 mg fluconazole weekly for 2–3 weeks/single dose fluconazole of 400 mg or 200 mg pramiconazole daily for 2 days [16, 27]. Fluconazole is preferred over itraconazole due to higher toxicity and drug interactions in the latter. Patients should be explained of the hyper or hypopigmentation problems which take months to recover. Multiple applications of topical drugs may decrease patient compliance, specifically PV affecting large body surface. These patients may benefit from short course of oral treatments. As relapse rate is quite high in PV, prophylactic treatment with 200 mg twice daily itraconazole on a single day in a month for 6 consecutive months, selenium sulphide once every third month or 2% ketoconazole shampoo once daily up to 3 days in the beginning of summer months may reduce the chances in severe cases [16, 27].

15.3.2.3 Malassezia Folliculitis

It is an inflammatory condition of sebaceous glands caused by *Malassezia* leading to breach of follicular epithelium. Danish guidelines address the management of folliculitis [16]. The diagnosis is possible clinically along with the demonstration of multiple conidia with unipolar budding and occasional hyphae in the pustular discharge by puncturing with a needle or stripping pustule with tape. The literature on the management of *Malassezia folliculitis* is very scanty. Systemic antifungal treatment appears to be the major mode of treatment due to the better penetration of drug into hair follicle. The drugs include itraconazole 200 mg daily for 3 weeks (93% response) and fluconazole (100–200 mg daily for 1–4 weeks or 300 mg once weekly for 1–2 months). Isotretinoin has been used systemically in a single case due to its sebo-suppressive effect [16]. Danish guidelines recommend use of 2% ketoconazole shampoo twice weekly for 2–4 weeks along with topical acne treatment as first-line of topical therapy. Other antifungal agents include 2% ketoconazole shampoo alone twice weekly for 2–4 weeks and miconazole cream twice daily for 4 weeks. Among topical agents, selenium sulphide (2.5% shampoo, daily for 3 days) and propylene glycol (50% in water, twice daily for 3 weeks) have shown efficacy of 88% and 100%, respectively [16]. Econazole, miconazole and ketoconazole have a variable response rate of 10–80%. Combination therapy may provide added benefit. Maintenance therapy is required for the prevention of relapses (selenium sulphide once a week or propylene glycol twice weekly).

15.3.3 Fungal Keratitis

The majority of fungal keratitis cases are reported from Asian countries with high burden in India (20–44%), Bangladesh (36%) and Nepal (17%) of all keratitis cases [45]. The diagnosis relies upon the demonstration of fungal elements in direct 10% KOH mount, Gram's stain and fungal culture for the identification of the etiologic agent. Due to lack of availability of standard guidelines, there is variability in management. Treatment failures have been reported with topical natamycin which is commonest used antifungal [46]. Topical 1% voriconazole with or without oral drug has shown beneficial results in refractory cases due to its better diffusion into aqueous humour (0.61–3.30 mg/L after 1 h of topical therapy) [47–53]. A good number of clinical trials have been conducted regarding management of fungal keratitis in Asian region (Table 15.4). The summary of conclusions of these trials is given below:

(a) 0.2% chlorhexidine is an acceptable substitute in case of unavailability of natamycin.
(b) Chlorhexidine can even be considered as an initial therapy in peripheral areas of developing countries due to its low cost and easy availability.
(c) Topical natamycin is superior to topical voriconazole (both reconstituted parenteral formulation and commercial drops).
(d) Intrastromal injections of voriconazole are not superior to adding topical voriconazole in severe cases.
(e) There is no benefit of adding oral voriconazole to topical natamycin therapy.
(f) Significant better clinical and microbiological cure noted in *Fusarium* keratitis as compared to *Aspergillus* keratitis in natamycin group (vs. voriconazole group).

A survey to evaluate practice patterns in the management of fungal corneal ulcer was published in 2009 where 92 respondents participated from North America (59%), South America (12%), Asia (21%), Europe (3%) and Australia (3%) [54]. Although overall natamycin (96%) was the most common topical antifungal agent used followed by amphotericin B (75%) and voriconazole (63%), physicians mentioned preference of using voriconazole (if available commercially) over natamycin for both yeast and filamentous fungi. For the management of yeast keratitis, amphotericin B (92%) was preferred choice followed by natamycin (68%) and voriconazole (49%). Half of the respondents preferred combination therapy (natamycin and voriconazole; 41%) followed by natamycin/amphotericin B/voriconazole (13%) and amphotericin B/voriconazole (13%) in filamentous fungal keratitis while amphotericin B and voriconazole in yeast keratitis. Preferred treatment and actual treatment differed due to higher cost of the latter or lack of evidence. The use of systemic treatment was mentioned "sometimes" by 55%, "most of the times" by 27%, "always" by 10% and "never" by 8%.

A subsequent survey of 110 respondents was conducted in 2017 where participation was maximum from North America (66.6%), Asia (14.6%), South America (8.3%), Europe (6.3%), Africa (2.1%), and Australia (2.1%) [55]. This survey was done after the completion of the MUTT trial where natamycin was found to be superior to voriconazole [56]. A significant increase in the use of voriconazole was noticed in 2017 survey as compared to 2007 survey probably due to increased availability of drug formulation. However, in case of preferred treatment, choice of natamycin increased by 19.9% while voriconazole decreased by 30.5% [45].
Therefore, topical therapy forms the primary treatment modality with centre-wise protocol of duration till complete resolution [63]. Systemic therapy should be considered in severe cases with keratoplasty in refractory cases [63].

Table 15.4 Clinical trials on the management of fungal keratitis in Asian region

	Author (enrolled number)	Year	Country	Type of study	Objective	Result summary
1	Rahman et al. [57] ($n = 71$)	1998	Bangladesh	RCT	0.2% chlorhexidine gluconate vs. 2.5% natamycin	0.2% chlorhexidine gluconate good alternative
2	Prajna et al. [58] ($n = 120$)	MUTT 2010	India	Therapeutic exploratory trial	Topical natamycin vs. topical voriconazole (reconstituted parenteral formulation)	Topical natamycin superior
3	Arora et al. [59] ($n = 30$)	2011	India	Prospective randomized pilot study	Topical 5% natamycin vs. 1% topical voriconazole	No difference
4	Prajna et al. [60] ($n = 120$)	2012	India	RCT (subgroup analysis)	*Fusarium* keratitis vs. *Aspergillus* keratitis	No difference in 3 month visual activity Increased perforation in *Fusarium* keratitis voriconazole group
5	Prajna et al. [56] ($n = 368$)	MUTT I 2013	India	RCT (Therapeutic confirmatory trial)	Topical 5% natamycin vs. topical 1% voriconazole (reconstituted parenteral formulation)	Topical natamycin superior
6	Sharma et al. [53] ($n = 40$)	2013	India	RCT	Topical vs. intrastromal 1% voriconazole in addition to 5% natamycin in recalcitrant fungal keratitis	Topical route superior
7	Sharma et al. [45] ($n = 118$)	2015	India	RCT	Topical 1%natamycin vs. topical 1% voriconazole (commercial drops)	Topical natamycin superior
8	Uddaraju et al. [61] ($n = 13$)	2015	India	RCT	Corneal crosslinking as adjuvant therapy in non-resolving deep stromal fungal keratitis	No improvement with this adjuvant therapy
9	Prajna et al. [62] ($n = 240$)	MUTT II 2016	India	RCT (therapeutic confirmatory trial)	Benefit of addition of oral voriconazole	No benefit

15.4 Conclusion

It is indisputable that the epidemiological picture of superficial fungal infections in Asian countries is changing and severe, recalcitrant, chronic infections are being described. The rise in such cases coupled with lack of guidelines for diagnosis and treatment of such infections has resulted in a situation of epidemic proportions. Additionally, the unregulated use of irrational FDCs, self-medication, and poor compliance to treatment are also matter of concern. Topical and systemic antifungals are commonly used for the management in India. The use of higher doses of antifungals with longer treatment duration (at least 3 weeks) has been found beneficial. Surgical debridement of infected area and use of newer therapies such as laser, photodynamic therapy and iontophoresis may be beneficial. Recently, various studies have been conducted to evaluate the efficacy of various treatment regimens for the management of superficial fungal infection, and this information may be useful to guide therapy in the future.

15.5 Summary of Management of Superficial Fungal Infections

1. Dermatophytosis
   (a) Naïve case (duration of therapy 2–4 weeks)
      - Tinea other than tinea pedis
         - Localized lesions: Topical azoles/allylamines/amorolfine/ciclopirox olamine
         - Extensive lesions/papules/pustules/vellus hair involvement/tinea rubrum syndrome: Combination therapy (topical plus oral terbinafine 250 mg once daily or itraconazole 100–200 mg/day)
      - Tinea pedis: Combination therapy (topical plus oral terbinafine 250 mg daily)

   (b) Recalcitrant case (duration of therapy 2–4 weeks)
      Combination therapy (topical plus higher oral dose of itraconazole 200–400 mg/day in divided doses)

   (c) Additional therapies like anti-histaminic, 6% salicylic acid and moisturisers
2. Onychomycosis: Combination therapy[1]
   (a) Topical therapy: 8% ciclopirox solution (daily or twice daily for 48 weeks), 5% amorolfine [once or twice a week for 6 (finger nail) to 12 (toe nail) months]

[1] Only topical therapy is limited to classical superficial white onychomycosis (except in transverse or striate infections), early distal and lateral subungual onychomycosis (DLSO) (except in the presence of longitudinal streaks, central yellow onycholytic area) when <80% of the nail plate is affected without involving lunula or when systemic antifungals are contraindicated.

   (b) Systemic therapy: Terbinafine for moulds (continuous dosage: 250 mg daily for 6 weeks for fingernail infection and 12 weeks for toenail infection: pulsed dosage: 250 mg twice daily for 1 week a month—for 2 and 3 months for fingernail and toenail, respectively; dosage in paediatric population 125 mg in 20–40 kg and 62.5 mg in <20 kg), itraconazole for both moulds and yeasts (continuous dosage: 200 mg daily for 2 and 3 months for fingernail and toenail, respectively; pulsed dosage: 200 mg twice daily for 1 week a month—for 2 and 3 months for fingernail and toenail, respectively) and fluconazole for *Candida* infections

3. Seborrheic dermatitis (SD)
   (a) Topical antifungals (1–2% ciclopirox/1–2% ketoconazole) with AIAFp shampoo/keratolytics/selenium sulphide/zinc (duration 2–3 times a week in scalp/hairy areas; BD for 4 weeks in non-scalp SD)
   (b) If no improvement, topical steroids and calcineurin inhibitors are added which if fail, systemic antifungals are added (itraconazole 100 mg: first month: 200 mg/day for 1 week, then 200 mg/day for 2 days/month up to 11 months; terbinafine 250 mg, continuous regimen: 250 mg/day for 4–6 weeks, intermittent regimen: 250 mg/day for 12 days per month for 3 months; fluconazole 50 mg/day for 2 weeks or 200–300 mg weekly for 2–4 weeks)
4. Pityriasis versicolor
   (a) Non-severe cases: Topical 2% ketoconazole × 14 days/terbinafine BD × 7 days/1.5% ciclopirox olamine 2 times weekly for 2 weeks/miconazole (twice daily), clotrimazole (twice daily) for 2 weeks
   (b) Severe cases: Combination therapy with topical plus 200 mg itraconazole daily for 5 or 7 days/100 mg daily for 2 weeks/single dose itraconazole 400 mg, 300 mg fluconazole weekly for 2–3 weeks/single dose fluconazole of 400 mg, or 200 mg pramiconazole daily for 2 days
5. *Malassezia* folliculitis
   (a) Systemic therapy: Itraconazole 200 mg daily for 3 weeks (93% response) and fluconazole (100–200 mg daily for 1–4 weeks or 300 mg once weekly for 1–2 months)
   (b) Topical may be added for acne: 2% ketoconazole shampoo twice weekly for 2–4 weeks
6. Fungal keratitis
   (a) Topical therapy 1% natamycin, 1% voriconazole till complete resolution

References

1. Hay R. Superficial fungal infections. Medicine (Baltimore). 2017;45(11):707–10.
2. Bongomin F, Gago S, Oladele R, Denning D. Global and multi-national prevalence of fungal diseases—estimate precision. J Fungi. 2017;3(4):57.
3. Steven P, Scott P, Andrea B. Superficial fungal infections. In: Soutor C, Hordinsky MK, editors. Clinical dermatology. 1st ed. New York: McGraw-Hill Companies; 2013.

4. World Health Organization. Guidelines on the treatment of Skin and Oral HIV-associated conditions in children and adults. Guidel treat Ski Oral HIV-associated cond child adults. 2014.
5. Schaller M, Friedrich M, Papini M, Pujol RM, Veraldi S. Topical antifungal-corticosteroid combination therapy for the treatment of superficial mycoses: conclusions of an expert panel meeting. Mycoses. 2016;59(6):365–73.
6. Drake LA, Dinehart SM, Farmer ER, Goltz RW, Graham GF, Hordinsky MK, et al. Guidelines of care for superficial mycotic infections of the skin: tinea corporis, tinea cruris, tinea faciei, tinea manuum, and tinea pedis. J Am Acad Dermatol. 1996;34(2):282–6.
7. Drake LA, Dinehart SM, Farmer ER, Goltz RW, Graham GF, Hordinsky MK, et al. Guidelines of care for superficial mycotic infectionsof the skin: tinea capitis and tinea barbae. J Am Acad Dermatol. 1996;34(2):290–4.
8. Drake LA, Dinehart SM, Farmer ER, Goltz RW, Graham GF, Hordinsky MK, et al. Guidelines of care for superficial mycotic infections of the skin: onychomycosis. J Am Acad Dermatol. 1996;34(1):116–21.
9. Mohri S, Watanabe S, Toshio K, Shibuya K, Nishiyama Y, Abe M, et al. Treatment of onychomycosis caused by dermatophytes—an opinion proposed by committee for standardization of the Japanese Society for Medical Mycology 2007. Nippon Ishinkin Gakkai Zasshi. 2008;49(1):1–3.
10. Kakourou T, Uksal U. Guidelines for the management of tinea capitis in children. Pediatr Dermatol. 2010;27(3):226–8.
11. Ameen M, Lear JT, Madan V, Mohd Mustapa MF, Richardson M. British Association of Dermatologists' guidelines for the management of onychomycosis 2014. Br J Dermatol. 2014;171(5):937–58.
12. Fuller LC, Barton RC, Mohd Mustapa MF, Proudfoot LE, Punjabi SP, Higgins EM. British Association of Dermatologists' guidelines for the management of tinea capitis 2014. Br J Dermatol. 2014;171(3):454–63.
13. Rajagopalan M, Inamadar A, Mittal A, Miskeen AK, Srinivas CR, Sardana K, et al. Expert consensus on the management of dermatophytosis in India (ECTODERM India). BMC Dermatol. 2018;18(1):6.
14. Drake LA, Dinehart SM, Farmer ER, Goltz RW, Graham GF, Hordinsky MK, et al. Guidelines of care for superficial mycotic infections of the skin: pityriasis (tinea) versicolor. J Am Acad Dermatol. 1996;34(2):287–9.
15. Arendrup MC, Boekhout T, Akova M, Meis JF, Cornely OA, Lortholary O. ESCMID and ECMM joint clinical guidelines for the diagnosis and management of rare invasive yeast infections. Clin Microbiol Infect. 2014;20(S3):76–98.
16. Hald M, Arendrup M, Svejgaard E, Lindskov R, Foged E, Saunte D. Evidence-based Danish guidelines for the treatment of *Malassezia*-related skin diseases. Acta Derm Venereol. 2015;95(1):12–9.
17. Cheong WK, Yeung CK, Torsekar RG, Suh DH, Ungpakorn R, Widaty S, et al. Treatment of seborrhoeic dermatitis in Asia: a consensus guide. Skin Appendage Disord. 2015;1(4):187–96.
18. Commitee for the Drafting of Guidelines for the Clinical Management of Infectious Keratitis. [Guidelines for the clinical management of infectious keratitis]. Nihon Ganka Gakkai Zasshi. 2007;111(10):771–809.
19. Nihon Ganka Gakkai. [Guidelines for the clinical management of infectious keratitis (2nd edition)]. Nihon Ganka Gakkai Zasshi. 2013;117(6):467–509.
20. Rubel D, Thirumoorthy T, Soebaryo RW, Weng SCK, Gabriel TM, Villafuerte LL, et al. Consensus guidelines for the management of atopic dermatitis: an Asia-Pacific perspective. J Dermatol. 2013;40(3):160–71.
21. Verma S, Madhu R. The great Indian epidemic of superficial dermatophytosis: an appraisal. Indian J Dermatol. 2017;62(3):227–36.
22. Behzadi P, Behzadi E, Ranjbar R. Dermatophyte fungi: infections, diagnosis and treatment. SMU Med J. 2014;1:50–62.

23. Sardana K, Khurana A, Garg S, Poojary S. In: Sardana K, Khurana A, Garg S, Poojary S, editors. IADVL manual on management of dermatophytoses. 1st ed. New Delhi: CBS Publishers & Distributors Private Limited; 2018.
24. Shenoy MM, Shenoy MS. Fungal nail disease (Onychomycosis); Challenges and solutions. Arch Med Heal Sci. 2014;2(1):48.
25. Mishra M, Panda P, Tripathy S, Sengupta S, Mishra K. An open randomized comparative study of oral itraconazole pulse and terbinafine pulse in the treatment of onychomycosis. Indian J Dermatol Venereol Leprol. 2005;71(4):262.
26. Velegraki A, Cafarchia C, Gaitanis G, Iatta R, Boekhout T. *Malassezia* infections in humans and animals: pathophysiology, detection, and treatment. PLoS Pathog. 2015;11(1):e1004523.
27. Gupta A, Foley K. Antifungal treatment for pityriasis versicolor. J Fungi. 2015;1(1):13–29.
28. Kagawa S. Clinical efficacy of terbinafine in 629 Japanese patients with dermatomycosis. Clin Exp Dermatol. 1989;14(2):114–5.
29. Köse O. Fluconazole versus itraconazole in the treatment of tinea versicolor. Int J Dermatol. 1995;34(7):498–9.
30. Balwada RP, Jain VK, Dayal S. A double-blind comparison of 2% ketoconazole and 1% clotrimazole in the treatment of pityriasis versicolor. Indian J Dermatol Venereol Leprol. 1996;62(5):298–300.
31. Sankara Rao IV, Rajashekhar N. Oral fluconazole in tinea versicolor. Indian J Dermatol Venereol Leprol. 1997;63(3):166–7.
32. Balachandran C, Thajuddin, Ravikumar BC. Comparative evaluation of single dose regimen with two dose regimen of fluconazole in the treatment of tinea versicolor: a double blind placebo controlled study. Indian J Dermatol Venereol Leprol. 1999;65(1):20–2.
33. Ravikumar BC, Balachandran C, Sabitha L. Single dose itraconazole therapy in tinea versicolor; a double blind, randomised placebo controlled study. Indian J Dermatol Venereol Leprol. 1999;65(3):151–2.
34. Chopra V, Jain VK. Comparative study of topical terbinafine and topical ketoconazole in pityriasis versicolor. Indian J Dermatol Venereol Leprol. 2000;66(6):299–300.
35. Bhogal CS, Singal A, Baruah MC. Comparative efficacy of ketoconazole and fluconazole in the treatment of pityriasis versicolor: a one year follow-up study. J Dermatol. 2001;28(10):535–9.
36. Kokturk A, Kaya T, Ikizoglu G, Bugdayci R, Koca A. Efficacy of three short-term regimens of itraconazole in the treatment of pityriasis versicolor. J Dermatolog Treat. 2002;13(4):185–7.
37. Köse O, Taştan HB, Gür AR, Kurumlu Z. Comparison of a single 400 mg dose versus a 7-day 200 mg daily dose of itraconazole in the treatment of tinea versicolor. J Dermatolog Treat. 2002;13(2):77–9.
38. Aggarwal K, Jain VK, Sangwan S. Comparative study of ketoconazole versus selenium sulphide shampoo in pityriasis versicolor. Indian J Dermatol Venereol Leprol. 2003;69(2):86–7.
39. Rathi SK. Ketoconazole 2% shampoo in pityriasis versicolor: an open trial. Indian J Dermatol Venereol Leprol. 2003;69(2):142–3.
40. Partap R, Kaur I, Chakrabarti A, Kumar B. Single-dose fluconazole versus itraconazole in pityriasis versicolor. Dermatology. 2004;208(1):55–9.
41. Karakaş M, Durdu M, Memişoğlu HR. Oral fluconazole in the treatment of tinea versicolor. J Dermatol. 2005;32(1):19–21.
42. Yazdanpanah MJ, Azizi H, Suizi B. Comparison between fluconazole and ketoconazole effectivity in the treatment of pityriasis versicolor. Mycoses. 2007;50(4):311–3.
43. Dehgan M, Akbari N, Alborzi N, SadaniI S, Keshtkar AA. Single-dose oral fluconazole versus topical clotrimazole in patients with pityriasis versicolor: a double-blind randomized controlled trial. J Dermatol. 2010;37(8):699–702.
44. Shi T-W, Zhang J-A, Tang Y-B, Yu H-X, Li Z-G, Yu J-B. A randomized controlled trial of combination treatment with ketoconazole 2% cream and adapalene 0.1% gel in pityriasis versicolor. J Dermatolog Treat. 2015;26(2):143–6.

45. Sharma S, Das S, Virdi A, Fernandes M, Sahu SK, Kumar Koday N, et al. Re-appraisal of topical 1% voriconazole and 5% natamycin in the treatment of fungal keratitis in a randomised trial. Br J Ophthalmol. 2015;99(9):1190–5.
46. Bunya VY, Hammersmith KM, Rapuano CJ, Ayres BD, Cohen EJ. Topical and oral voriconazole in the treatment of fungal keratitis. Am J Ophthalmol. 2007;143(1):151–3.
47. Thiel MA, Zinkernagel AS, Burhenne J, Kaufmann C, Haefeli WE. Voriconazole concentration in human aqueous humor and plasma during topical or combined topical and systemic administration for fungal keratitis. Antimicrob Agents Chemother. 2007;51(1):239–44.
48. Cretì A, Esposito V, Bocchetti M, Baldi G, De Rosa P, Parrella R, et al. Voriconazole curative treatment for *Acremonium* species keratitis developed in a patient with concomitant *Staphylococcus aureus* corneal infection: a case report. In Vivo. 2006;20(1):169–71.
49. Sponsel W, Chen N, Dang D, Paris G, Graybill J, Najvar LK, et al. Topical voriconazole as a novel treatment for fungal keratitis. Antimicrob Agents Chemother. 2006;50(1):262–8.
50. Ozbek Z, Kang S, Sivalingam J, Rapuano CJ, Cohen EJ, Hammersmith KM. Voriconazole in the management of *Alternaria* keratitis. Cornea. 2006;25(2):242–4.
51. Klont RR, Eggink CA, AJMM R, Wesseling P, Verweij PE. Successful treatment *offusarium* keratitis with cornea transplantation and topical and systemic voriconazole. Clin Infect Dis. 2005;40(12):e110–2.
52. Nulens E, Eggink C, Rijs AJMM, Wesseling P, Verweij PE. Keratitis caused by *Scedosporium apiospermum* successfully treated with a cornea transplant and voriconazole. J Clin Microbiol. 2003;41(5):2261–4.
53. Sharma N, Chacko J, Velpandian T, Titiyal JS, Sinha R, Satpathy G, et al. Comparative evaluation of topical versus intrastromal voriconazole as an adjunct to natamycin in recalcitrant fungal keratitis. Ophthalmology. 2013;120(4):677–81.
54. Loh AR, Hong K, Lee S, Mannis M, Acharya NR. Practice patterns in the management of fungal corneal ulcers. Cornea. 2009;28(8):856–9.
55. Oldenburg CE, Prajna NV, Amza A, Loh A, Acharya NR, Mannis MJ, et al. Evolution of practice patterns for the treatment of fungal keratitis. JAMA Ophthalmol. 2017;135(12):1448.
56. Prajna NV, Krishnan T, Mascarenhas J, Rajaraman R, Prajna L, Srinivasan M, et al. The mycotic ulcer treatment trial: a randomized trial comparing natamycin vs voriconazole. JAMA Ophthalmol. 2013;131(4):422.
57. Rahman MR, Johnson GJ, Husain R, Howlader SA, Minassian DC. Randomised trial of 0.2% chlorhexidine gluconate and 2.5% natamycin for fungal keratitis in Bangladesh. Br J Ophthalmol. 1998;82(8):919–25.
58. Prajna NV, Mascarenhas J, Krishnan T, Reddy PR, Prajna L, Srinivasan M, et al. Comparison of natamycin and voriconazole for the treatment of fungal keratitis. Arch Ophthalmol. 2010;128(6):672–8.
59. Arora R, Gupta D, Goyal J, Kaur R. Voriconazole versus natamycin as primary treatment in fungal corneal ulcers. Clin Exp Ophthalmol. 2011;39(5):434–40.
60. Prajna VN, Lalitha PS, Mascarenhas J, Krishnan T, Srinivasan M, Vaitilingam CM, et al. Natamycin and voriconazole in *Fusarium* and *Aspergillus* keratitis: subgroup analysis of a randomised controlled trial: Table 1. Br J Ophthalmol. 2012;96(11):1440.1–1441.
61. Uddaraju M, Mascarenhas J, Das MR, Radhakrishnan N, Keenan JD, Prajna L, et al. Corneal cross-linking as an adjuvant therapy in the management of recalcitrant deep stromal fungal keratitis: a randomized trial. Am J Ophthalmol. 2015;160(1):131–134.e5.
62. Prajna NV, Krishnan T, Rajaraman R, Patel S, Srinivasan M, Das M, et al. Effect of oral voriconazole on fungal keratitis in the Mycotic Ulcer Treatment Trial II (MUTT II). JAMA Ophthalmol. 2016;134(12):1365.
63. Ansari Z, Miller D, Galor A. Current thoughts in fungal keratitis: diagnosis and treatment. Curr Fungal Infect Rep. 2013;7(3):209–18.

Invasive Candidiasis in Asia

16

Yee-Chun Chen

Key Points

- *Candida* species are the leading fungal pathogens causing severe infections in patients receiving health care or in immunosuppressive status globally.
- *Candida* species are common (>10%) pathogens causing health-care-associated infections.
- Candidemia is the most common form of invasive candidiasis with an incidence of 1.22 episodes per 1000 patients and was up to 11.7 per 1000 ICU patients and mortality rates remain high (40%).
- Intra-abdominal candidiasis is the second most common form of invasive candidiasis while blood cultures are rarely positive.
- The proportion of *Candida tropicalis,* the leading non-*albicans Candida* species, among blood isolates was higher in tropical countries than other Asian countries.
- *C. tropicalis* is the leading fungal pathogen causing bloodstream infection or hepatosplenic fungal infection in patients with hematological malignancies.
- Fluconazole non-susceptibility was common (25%) for *C. tropicalis.*
- Proactive monitoring of fluconazole susceptibility is required in regions where *C. tropicalis* predominates and where fluconazole is used upfront without in vitro susceptibility testing.

Y.-C. Chen (✉)
Division of Infectious Diseases, Department of Internal Medicine, National Taiwan University Hospital, Taipei, Taiwan

Department of Medicine, National Taiwan University, College of Medicine, Taipei, Taiwan

National Institute of Infectious Diseases and Vaccinology, National Health Research Institutes, Miaoli County, Taiwan

A. Chakrabarti (ed.), *Clinical Practice of Medical Mycology in Asia*,
https://doi.org/10.1007/978-981-13-9459-1_16

Candida auris, a recently emerging multidrug-resistant *Candida* species, was first reported from Asia and has caused public health impact globally because of its propensity to be transmitted between patients, develops resistance very fast, and causes high mortality.

Lack of awareness and difficulties with laboratory identification have had a significant impact on outbreak detection and patients' management.

16.1 Benign Colonizers or Big Killers

Candida species are the leading fungal pathogens causing severe infections in patients receiving health care or in immunosuppressive status globally [1–3]. Common *Candida* species causing infections, such as *Candida albicans, Candida parapsilosis, Candida glabrata,* and *Candida tropicalis,* are part of the human microbial flora. *Candida* species cause a spectrum of infections, ranging from superficial candidiasis of the skin and mucosal surfaces to life-threatening invasive candidiasis [3].

Candida can be found at significant levels on mucosal surfaces and the skin, even in healthy hosts, and it is from within their niche in the microbiome that they can cause disease [3]. Of 1910 candidemia episodes evaluated, same *Candida* species from non-blood specimens were identified in 181 patients (9.48%) in the preceding 7 days and in 302 patients (15.8%) in the preceding 30 days [4]. *C. albicans* ranked the top among colonizing/infecting species (23.4%), followed by *C. glabrata* (13.5%), *C. tropicalis* (10.7%), *C. parapsilosis* (9.3%), *C. guilliermondii* (9.5%), *Candida pelliculosa* (7.1%), and *Candida krusei* (5.4%). Of 302 prior colonization/infection, 118 were isolated from urinary tract. Molecular epidemiological studies have shown that the majority of *Candida* blood isolates are similar or identical to prior colonization in the patient's urinary and gastrointestinal tracts [5–7].

16.2 Disease Burdens

Invasive candidiasis mainly occurs in immunocompromised patients, such as those with neutropenia, and in critically ill patients who received intensive care. Invasive infections with *Candida* species continue to represent a major health and economic burden, and are associated with additional mortality and morbidity in already debilitated hospitalized patients [3]. Candidemia is the most common form of invasive candidiasis. According to a recent survey and estimation facilitated by the Leading International Fungal Education (LIFE) portal, the global incidence of invasive candidiasis has been estimated at 750,000 cases annually (2.1 to 21 cases per 100,000 population) [2]. Multistate point-prevalence survey in the USA in 2011 showed that *Candida* species, as a whole, were the leading pathogens causing health-care-associated bloodstream infection (22%) [8]. According to the national surveillance of health-care-associated infections in the intensive care units in 2015, *Candida* species contributed 12% of bloodstream infections in Taiwan and 13% in Korea, and was 31% and 23%, respectively, for urinary tract infection [9].

A large-scale laboratory-based surveillance at 25 hospitals from China, Hong Kong, India, Singapore, Taiwan, and Thailand in 2011 showed that the incidence of candidemia was 1.22 episodes per 1000 discharges and varied among the hospitals (range, 0.16–4.53 per 1000 discharges) and countries (range, 0.25–2.93 per 1000 discharges) [4]. In the same study the incidences of candidemia in ICU was tenfold higher, 11.7 per 1000 ICU admission [4]. The ever-advancing economy with increased access to health care, including more advanced care such as chemotherapy and transplantation, are important considerations throughout Asia, and these factors may likely lead to rise in incidence of candidemia.

The disease burden of candidemia is difficult to quantify because of wide geographic variation and difficult to compare due to difference in patient population [2, 10]. Both decrease and increase in incidence have been reported globally in the past decade [10–12]. According to a recent review, the population-based incidences in Spain (2003–2011) [13], Norway (2003–2012) [14], and Australia (2004–2015) [15] rose. However, the incidence decreased from 14.1 cases and 30.9 cases per 100,000 population in Atlanta and Baltimore, respectively, in 2008 to 9.5 cases and 14.4 cases per 100,000 population, respectively, in 2013 [16]. Thus far, there was no population-based data from Asia. Nevertheless, a recent estimation facilitated by Global Action Fund for Fungal Infections (GAFFI) showed that the prevalence of candidemia was 21 cases per 100,000 in Pakistan [2].

Nevertheless, little is known regarding the reasons of changes in the incidences of invasive candidiasis. The decrease in candidemia incidence in the USA was mainly due to a decline in central-line associated candidemia as 85% of cases had a central venous catheter in place within 2 days prior to the date of their initial culture positive for *Candida* species [16]. A hospital-wide surveillance in a teaching hospital in Taiwan showed that the incidence density of candidemia increased from 0.34 per 1000 patient-days in 2002 to 0.41 per 1000 patient-days in 2010 [17]. In 2010, the hospitalized patients were older, had a higher Charlson comorbidity index, and more underlying disease/status, including chronic pulmonary diseases, moderate-to-severe renal diseases, leukemia, lymphoma, and gastrointestinal malignancies than those seen in 2002. Multivariate analysis identified the following host factors were associated with the occurrence of candidemia: neonate or the elderly, moderate-to-severe renal diseases, leukemia and lymphoma, and gastrointestinal malignancies. The majority of disease-specific incidences of candidemia did not differ between 2002 and 2010 and that for gastrointestinal malignancies decreased from 28.8 per 1000 admission to 12.4 per 1000 admission and metastatic malignancies from 11.9 per 1000 admission to 7.5 per 1000 admission.

Candidemia is associated with an unacceptably high mortality rates in excess of 40% even with the introduction of newer antifungal agents [3, 10, 17, 18] and an associated expenditure of ~$45,000 per case [19]. All-cause mortality of patients with candidemia at 30 days after onset ranged from 29 to 72%, which is very likely that at least in part due to underlying diseases or conditions [10]. A single center study showed that the inhospital mortality rate was >40% for patients with candidemia occurring more than 2 days after admission and was only 33% for those with early infections (within 2 days after admission) [20]. A single center study in Taiwan showed that 30-day mortality of patients with candidemia was 46% in 2002 and 44% in 2010 despite that more patients were treated on the same day of candidemia diagnosis (37% vs. 45%) [17]. As the majority of patients were treated with fluconazole, a fungistatic agent, further improvement was anticipated.

The incidence of invasive candidiasis is underestimated if estimated based on blood culture positive cases. These were assumed to represent about 38% cases of proven or probable invasive candidiasis tested by blood culture techniques, based on a pooled culture positivity rate in patients with proven or probable invasive candidiasis of 0.38 (95% Confidence Interval: 0.29–0.46) [21–23]. Among wide variety of presentation or organ involvement, intra-abdominal candidiasis is the second most common form of invasive candidiasis after candidemia. It is estimated that annual 60,000–100,000 cases of intra-abdominal candidiasis developed globally [2]. Intra-abdominal candidiasis in patients who have had recent abdominal surgery or intra-abdominal events refers to a heterogeneous group of infections that includes intra-abdominal abscess (30–60%), secondary peritonitis after repeated leak (30–40%), infected pancreatic necrosis (5–10%), cholecystitis or cholangitis (5–10%), primary peritonitis (5%) [24, 25]. A true or possible *Candida* infection was observed in 12.2% of 335 patients with acute pancreatitis investigated and *C. tropicalis* was the most common isolate (43.9%) [26]. Unfortunately, blood cultures have poor sensitivity, as *Candida* is rapidly cleared from the blood. Many cases of intra-abdominal candidiasis remain undiagnosed because blood cultures do not detect all cases of candidemia and tissue cultures are not always possible in patients with suspected deep-seated infection [22].

Although rare in occurrence, ocular candidiasis is a potentially severe complication that can lead to visual field defects or blindness if appropriate therapy is delayed. Previous reports have shown that all *Candida* species can cause ocular complications and that ocular involvement occurs in approximately 10–25% of *Candida* infections [27–29]. A recent study in Japan showed that ocular candidiasis were diagnosed in 20 (20%) of 99 candidemia patients examined by ophthalmologists during 2012–2017 [30]. Although *C. parapsilosis* was the most frequent candidemia pathogen, only *C. albicans* infection was significantly associated with ocular candidiasis by multivariate analysis.

16.3 *Candida tropicalis* and Other Common *Candida* Species

C. albicans is the main etiologic *Candida* species associated with health-care-associated invasive candidiasis globally [3, 31]. However, there has been a worrying increase in the number of non-*albicans Candida* species such as *C. glabrata, C. parapsilosis, C. tropicalis, C. krusei* [31], and lastly *C. auris*. These species are more likely to be antifungal resistant and have the potential to cause outbreaks [32]. In particular, resistance to fluconazole is common, which is important as it is the most commonly used antifungal agent for prophylaxis and treatment of *Candida* infections in many parts of the world [33].

Among 1910 non-duplicate blood isolates from 25 hospitals in Asia evaluated, *C. albicans* was most frequently isolated (41%), followed by *C. tropicalis* (25%),

C. glabrata (14%), and *C. parapsilosis* (12%) [4]. Although *C. albicans* was the most common *Candida* species, it accounted for less than 40% of candidemia in 12 of 25 hospitals in this study. The proportion of *C. tropicalis* among blood isolates was higher in hemato-oncology wards than others wards and was more likely to be isolated from tropical countries than other Asian countries. This study showed that both geographic and health-care factors contribute to the variation of species distribution. The proportion of *C. tropicalis* was 25% in Asia, 18% in Latin American, only 8% in Europe, and 5% in Australia (reviewed and summarized in [4]).

There are unique features of *C. tropicalis* infections compared with other *Candida* species. Prior studies have shown that *C. tropicalis* is more likely to be isolated from patients with neutropenia than those non-neutropenia patients or patients with hematological malignancies [3, 34, 35]. In the absence of systemic antifungal prophylaxis, studies have shown *C. tropicalis* is the leading fungal pathogen causing bloodstream infection (51%) or hepatosplenic fungal infection (43%) in patients with hematological malignancies [35, 36]. The time-to-positivity (TTP) of blood cultures of *C. tropicalis* was significantly shorter than that of other species. Almost 40% of the cultures recovered after >3 days for *C. glabrata* compared >40% of the cultures positive <24 h for *C. tropicalis* [37]. Clinically, septic shock and skin emboli are common findings of *C. tropicalis* candidemia [38]. Both short TTP and septic shock are associated with poor prognosis [39]. A recent study showed that *C. tropicalis* is the most common pathogen in persistent candidemia (29.2%) and independently related to 30-day mortality [40].

C. tropicalis, C. albicans, and *C. parapsilosis* isolates are regarded as being susceptible. Primary resistance to azoles is rare in these species. In the past two decades, widespread use of fluconazole and other triazoles coincided with a decreased incidence of infection due to *C. tropicalis* and *C. albicans* and increased incidence of infections due to less susceptible *Candida* species, particularly *C. glabrata* [3, 12]. Nevertheless, more and more azole-resistant clinical isolates of *C. tropicalis* have been detected in Asia and worldwide in recent years. A notable increase in fluconazole non-susceptible *C. tropicalis* causing invasive candidiasis from 11.2 in 2009 to 42.7% in 2014 was reported from 10 hospitals in China [41]. A surveillance study of 861 *Candida* bloodstream isolates collected in 2014 from 13 centers of 7 countries in Asia-Pacific region showed the MIC_{50}/MIC_{90} of *C. tropicalis* isolates were 2 μg/mL and 32 μg/mL, respectively, which were approaching to those for *C. glabrata* (8 μg/mL and 32 μg/mL, respectively) and much higher than those for *C. albicans* (0.064 μg/mL and 0.064 μg/mL, respectively) [4]. Fluconazole susceptibility was 99.7% for *C. albicans*, and 75.8% for *C. tropicalis*, which varied by country, around 60% in Vietnam, 70% in Thailand and Singapore, 80% in Taiwan and Brunei, and 100% in Korea and Philippines. A recent Asian survey demonstrates that antifungal susceptibility testing is performed in 142 (58.9%) of 241 microbiology laboratories affiliated with health-care settings [42]. Thus, antifungal resistance is very likely underestimated and delayed in detection in daily practice in the majority of health-care settings.

In addition, a recent survey in Taiwan identified genetically related *C. tropicalis* isolates from human and environmental samples exhibiting reduced susceptibility to fluconazole [43, 44]. Thus, proactive monitoring of fluconazole susceptibility is required in regions where *C. tropicalis* predominates and where fluconazole is used upfront without in vitro susceptibility testing [45].

16.4 *Candida auris* and Other Rare but Emerging *Candida* Species

Candida auris is a recently identified multi-resistant *Candida* species, an emerging *Candida* species that becomes a global concern [46, 47]. *C. auris* was first reported in Japan in 2009 [48]. The earliest known strain of *C. auris* dates to 1996 in South Korea [49]. Within the past few years *C. auris* has been reported in Europe, Asia, North America, South America, and Africa and has been associated with infections and outbreaks in health-care settings [50–63].

C. auris is different from other pathogenic yeast species and a cause of great concern because of its propensity to be transmitted between patients and causing outbreaks, develops resistance very fast, and causes high mortality. In addition, lack of awareness of this new *Candida* species and difficulties with laboratory identification [64] have had a significant impact on outbreak detection and management, and patient outcomes as summarized in a recent perspective [65]. In addition to molecular identification, MALDI-TOF devices have been recently adopted for identification of *C. auris*. However, only RUO (research use only) but not IVD (in vitro diagnostic) library in both VITEK MS and Bruker MicroFlex MALDI-TOF identification systems can be used to identify the species [66, 67].

The prevalence of *C. auris* in various regions of the world has been difficult to determine because most of the reports are based on outbreaks or individual cases and hence the need for specialized laboratory procedures to differentiate it from other *Candida* species. The incidence rates have varied in different hospitals and among countries. For example, in an 18-month prospective study in intensive care units of an Indian hospital, *C. auris* accounted for 5.3% of candidemia isolates [60].

Before call for international attention to *C. auris*, an increasing number of sporadic cases of invasive infections by rare *Candida* species have been reported from severe immunocompromised patients, or identified as causing pathogens of outbreaks [66]. Increases in susceptible patient populations and advances in identification methods have resulted in the continued recognition of novel yeasts as agents of human infection. Some of these agents are "cryptic species," members of species complexes, and may not be detectable using classical carbohydrate assimilation-based methods of yeast identification. Such species require DNA- or matrix-assisted laser desorption ionization–time of flight mass spectrometry (MALDI-TOF) based methods for correct identification [68]. Many of them are resistant to commonly used systemic antifungal agents and the source of some outbreak strains could be traced to food or other environment [66, 69]. For example, *Pichia kudriavzevii, Issatchenkia orientalis,* and *Candida glycerinogenes* were used for industrial-scale production of glycerol and succinate, also used to make some fermented foods. A recent population genomics shows no distinction between *Candida krusei* and

Pichia kudriavzevii [70]. This case demonstrates that one species has four names. No wonder the contribution of environmental source of these emerging troublesome rare yeasts is underestimated.

According to a recent survey, among 1910 non-duplicate *Candida* blood isolates, the following 11 *Candida* species contributed 6.1%: *Candida guilliermondii*, *Candida krusei*, *Candida famata*, *Candida pelliculosa*, *Candida haemulonii*, *Candida intermedia*, *Candida lusitaniae*, *Candida sake*, *C. dubliniensis*, *Candida pararugosa*, and *Candida catenulate* [4]. Nevertheless, *C. guilliermondii* accounted for 11.7% of *Candida* blood isolates in an Indian hospital. *C. krusei* accounted for 12.2% in the same hospital.

Uncommon candidemia (species other than *C. albicans, C. parapsilosis, C. glabrata, C. tropicalis,* and *C. krusei*) in children in a teaching hospital in Taiwan during 2003–2015 showed that *C. guilliermondii* (31.2%) was most common, followed by *C. lusitaniae* (18.8%), and *C. metapsilosis* (18.8%) [71]. The incidence density of candidemia caused by these uncommon *Candida* species and the proportion to all candidemia episodes increased substantively during the study period. Prior exposure to azoles was uncommon in the 30 days prior to infection, but fluconazole resistant strains were significantly more common (41.3%). Candidemia caused by uncommon *Candida* spp. had poorer response to antifungal treatment, led to longer duration of candidemia (median 4.0 vs. 2.5 days, $p = 0.008$), and had a higher treatment failure rate (56.5% vs. 38.5%, $p = 0.040$) comparing to candidemia caused by *C. albicans*.

16.5 Antifungal Strategy and Optimal Regimen

Although most invasive *Candida* isolates were often susceptible to fluconazole in the past, azole non-susceptibility (including susceptible-dose dependent and resistant) has become a major concern. Cross resistance to other triazoles has been noted for *C. glabrata* and *C. tropicalis*, but not *Candida krusei*. *C. glabrata* that are non-susceptible to azoles are associated with prior use of azoles rather than clonal spread in hospital settings. Antifungal susceptibility testing and search for intravascular lesions or a metastatic focus are often helpful in guiding therapy for patients with breakthrough infection or who fail treatment [72, 73].

Echinocandins are current drug of choice for candidemia [72, 73]. In addition, empiric therapy using a fungicidal agent should be considered for critically ill patients with persistent fever despite antibacterial therapy, multiple risk factors, multiple and heavy colonization of *Candida*, in the absence of an established cause for fever. Patients should be reevaluated at 48–72 h and antifungal therapy can be de-escalated after invasive candidiasis is ruled out by blood cultures and other diagnostic measures. Local epidemiology regarding the incidence of disease and antifungal susceptibility may help to decide antifungal strategy and regimen in selected patient population. Oral fluconazole or other azoles are feasible for prolonged outpatient therapy for infection due to azole-susceptible *Candida* isolates.

C. auris strains are often resistant to one or more commonly used systemic antifungal agents [47]. A large majority of *C. auris* isolates are fluconazole resistant (93%), and amphotericin B and echinocandin resistance rates are approximately 30–40% and 5–10%, respectively. Almost half of isolates are MDR (resistant to two or more antifungal classes), and a small percentage are pan-drug resistant. Though echinocandins revealed best susceptibility result for *C. auris* isolates among the three major antifungal classes, it is recommended to use echinocandins as first-line therapy for empiric treatment of *C. auris* infections. This recommendation may have to be modified as more experience is acquired. Echinocandins have no activity against *C. auris* biofilms, unlike other *Candida* species [74].

In a recent survey conducted in seven Asian countries antifungal susceptibility testing was performed in only 12 (66.7%) of 18 laboratories [42]. This is insufficient to guide selection of an appropriate antifungal agent and inadequate to detect the emerging threat of *C. auris* infections. In addition, since *C. glabrata* and *C. auris* can rapidly develop resistance, susceptibility testing is recommended for all isolates from patients with invasive diseases and should be repeated on persistent isolates obtained during the course of therapy.

16.6 Infection Prevention and Control

In view of the poor outcome and the difficulty in making a timely diagnosis of invasive candidiasis, special efforts through patient education for hyperglycemic control are needed to prevent infection by reducing host factors for acquiring invasive candidiasis [75]. Risk factors associated invasive candidiasis occurring during hospitalization include the use of antibiotics, central venous catheters, surgical procedures, parenteral nutrition, sepsis, severity of illness, neutropenia, renal failure, mechanical ventilation, use of immunosuppressive agents, and *Candida* colonization [3].

In patients with cancer and chemotherapy-induced neutropenia and mucositis, candidemia mainly originate from the gastrointestinal tract. Thus, infections may occur in high-risk patients despite of stringent infection prevention and control measures in the absence of antifungal prophylaxis [17]. On the other hand, critically ill patients acquire the infection from skin flora through intravenous catheter which might be prevented through central-line bloodstream infection prevention care bundle [16]. However, exogenous infections can occur from cross transmission [76, 77]. Furthermore, more and more sporadic cases or outbreaks of severe infection due to rare *Candida* species linked to environmental origin in the community have been reported in the past decade [78, 79].

Among them, *C. auris* is now considered a notorious health-care-associated yeast causing invasive infections with high treatment rate failures due to multidrug resistance [80]. Sporadic cases of *C. auris* have been identified throughout England since August 2013 [51]. An adult critical care unit has been managing an outbreak of *C. auris* that began in April 2015. More than 40 patients were either colonized or infected; approximately 20% had candidemia. The hospital outbreak has been difficult to control, despite enhanced infection control interventions, including regular patient screening, environmental decontamination, and ward closure. A prospective environmental surveillance study in India detected *C. auris* contamination of environmental surfaces and hands of health-care workers [81]. Interventions such as chlorhexidine washing and appropriate use of disinfectants could eradicate *C. auris* from patients and hospital environment. The elements in infection control of this pathogen include hand hygiene and other elements of standard precautions, contact isolation precaution, active surveillance and contact tracing during outbreaks, environmental disinfection, and antifungal stewardship. The major gaps that need to be filled are awareness and more rapid identification and susceptibility testing of *Candida* species. An integrated algorithm was proposed for early detection and institution of effective prevention and to control colonization in response to *C. auris* at the hospital level [65].

16.7 Conclusion

Invasive infections with *Candida* spp. continue to represent a major health and economic burden, increasing both mortality and morbidity in an already vulnerable group of hospital patients. Outbreaks due to multidrug-resistant *C. auris* and increase in cases caused by other uncommon *Candida* species pose a serious challenge regarding identification and therapy, especially in resource-limited countries/regions or health-care settings where modern identification facilities and access to antifungals other than fluconazole are limited.

There are a number of ways in which candidemia management could be improved across many Asian countries: develop and implement diagnostic tools that are more widely available and have shorter turnaround time (for both identification and antifungal susceptibility); improve infection control; perform local epidemiology studies; and improve antifungal treatment, including greater access to echinocandins (particularly in light of recent evidence showing reduced susceptibility to fluconazole in non-*albicans* species in Asia), greater education on appropriate drug selection, and improved antifungal stewardship.

References

1. Brown GD, Denning DW, Gow NAR, Levitz SM, Netea MG, White TC. Hidden Killers: human fungal infections. Sci Transl Med. 2012;4:165rv13.
2. Bongomin F, Gago S, Oladele RO, Denning DW. Global and multi-national prevalence of fungal diseases-estimate precision. J Fungi (Basel). 2017;3:57.
3. Kullberg BJ, Arendrup MC. Invasive candidiasis. New England J Med. 2015;373:1445–56.
4. Tan BH, Chakrabarti A, Li RY, et al. Incidence and species distribution of candidaemia in Asia: a laboratory-based surveillance study. Clin Microbiol Infect. 2015;21:946–3.
5. Chen YC, Chang SC, Tai HM, Hsueh PR, Luh KT. Molecular epidemiology of Candida colonizing critically ill patients in intensive care units. J Formosan Med Assoc. 2001;100(12):791–7.
6. Huang YC, Su LH, Wu TL, Lin TY. Genotyping analysis of colonizing candidal isolates from very-low-birthweight infants in a neonatal intensive care unit. J Hosp Infect. 2004;58(3):200–3.

7. Huang PY, Hung MH, Shie SS, et al. Molecular concordance of concurrent Candida albicans candidemia and candiduria. Diagn Microbiol Infect Dis. 2013;76(3):382–4.
8. Magill SS, Edwards JR, Bamberg B, et al. Multistate point-prevalence survey of health care–associated infections. N Engl J Med. 2014;370:1198–208.
9. Chiang CH, Pan SC, Yang TS, Matsuda K, Kim HB, Choi YH, Hori S, Wang JT, Sheng WH, Chen YC, Chang FY, Chang SC. Healthcare-associated Infections in Intensive Care Units in Taiwan, South Korea, and Japan: recent Trends Based on National Surveillance reports. Antimicrob Resist Infect Control. 2018;7:129.
10. Lamoth F, Lockhart SR, Berkow EL, Calandra T. Changes in the epidemiological landscape of invasive candidiasis. J Antimicrob Chemother. 2018;73(suppl_1):i4–i13.
11. Hobson RP. The global epidemiology of invasive Candida infections—is the tide turning? J Hosp Infect. 2003;55:159–68.
12. Pfaller MA, Diekema DJ. Epidemiology of Invasive Candidiasis: a persistent public health problem. Clin Microbiol Rev. 2007;20:133–63.
13. Puig-Asensio M, Padilla B, Garnacho-Montero J, et al. Epidemiology and predictive factors for early and late mortality in *Candida* bloodstream infections: a population-based surveillance in Spain. Clin Microbiol Infect. 2014;20:O245–54.
14. Hesstvedt L, Gaustad P, Andersen CT, et al. Twenty-two years of candidaemia surveillance: results from a Norwegian national study. Clin Microbiol Infect. 2015;21:938–45.
15. Chapman B, Slavin M, Marriott D, et al. Changing epidemiology of candidaemia in Australia. J Antimicrob Chemother. 2017;72:1103–8.
16. Cleveland AA, Harrison LH, Farley MM, Hollick R, Stein B, Chiller TM, et al. Declining Incidence of candidemia and the shifting epidemiology of *Candida* resistance in two US Metropolitan Areas, 2008–2013: results from Population-Based Surveillance. PLoS One. 2015;10(3):e0120452.
17. Chen PY, Chuang YC, Wang JT, Sheng WH, Yu CJ, Chu CC, Hsueh PR, Chang SC, Chen YC. Comparison of epidemiology and treatment outcome of patients with candidemia at a teaching hospital in Northern Taiwan, in 2002 and 2010. J Microbiol Immunol Infect. 2014;47:95–103.
18. Wisplinghoff H, Bischoff T, Tallent SM, et al. Nosocomial bloodstream infections in US hospitals: analysis of 24,179 cases from a prospective nationwide surveillance study. Clin Infect Dis. 2004;39:309–17.
19. Rentz AM, Halpern MT, Bowden R. The impact of candidemia on length of hospital stay, outcome, and overall cost of illness. Clin Infect Dis. 1998;27:781–8.
20. Moran C, Grussemeyer CA, Spalding JR, Benjamin DJ, Reed SD. Comparison of costs, length of stay, and mortality associated with *Candida glabrata* and *Candida albicans* bloodstream infections. Am J Infect Control. 2010;38:78–80.
21. Avni T, Leibovici L, Paul M. PCR diagnosis of invasive candidiasis: systematic review and meta-analysis. J Clin Microbiol. 2011;49:665–70.
22. Chen P, Chuang Y, Wu U, Sun H, Wang J, Sheng W, et al. Clonality of Fluconazole-Nonsusceptible Candida tropicalis in Bloodstream Infections, Taiwan, 2011–2017. Emerg Infect Dis. 2019;25(9):1668–1675.
23. Berenguer J, Buck M, Witebsky F, Stock F, Pizzo PA, Walsh TJ. Lysis-centrifugation blood cultures in the detection of tissue-proven invasive candidiasis disseminated versus single-organ infection. Diagn Microbiol Infect Dis. 1993;17:103–9.
24. Bassetti M, Marchetti M, Chakrabarti A, et al. A research agenda on the management of intra-abdominal candidiasis: results from a consensus of multinational experts. Intensive Care Med. 2013;39:2092–106.
25. Bassetti M, et al. A multicenter multinational study of abdominal candidiasis: epidemiology, outcomes and predictors of mortality. Intensive Care Med. 2015;41(9):1601–10.
26. Chakrabarti A, Rao P, Tarai B, Rudramurthy S, Wig J. Candida in acute pancreatitis. Surg Today. 2007;37:207–11.
27. Donahue SP, Greven CM, Zuravleff JJ, Eller AW, Nguyen MH, Peacock JE Jr, et al. Intraocular candidiasis in patients with candidemia. Clinical implications derived from a prospective multicenter study. Ophthalmology. 1994;101:1302–9.

28. Oude Lashof AML, Rothova A, Sobel JD, et al. Ocular manifestations of candidemia. Clin Infect Dis. 2011;53:262.
29. Durand ML. Bacterial and fungal endophthalmitis. Clin Microbiol Rev. 2017;30:597–613.
30. Abe M, Kinjo Y, Ueno K, et al. Differences in Ocular Complications Between *Candida albicans* and non-albicans *Candida* Infection analyzed by epidemiology and a mouse ocular candidiasis model. Front Microbiol. 2018;9:2477.
31. Guinea J. Global trends in the distribution of Candida species causing candidemia. Clin Microbiol Infect. 2014;20:5–10.
32. Miceli MH, Diaz JA, Lee SA. Emerging opportunistic yeast infections. Lancet Infect Dis. 2011;11:142–51.
33. Arendrup MC, Dzajic E, Jensen RH, et al. Epidemiological changes with potential implication for antifungal prescription recommendations for fungaemia: data from a nationwide fungaemia surveillance programme. Clin Microbiol Infect. 2013;19:e343–53.
34. Hung CC, Chen YC, Chang SC, Luh KT, Hsieh WC. Nosocomial candidemia in a university hospital in Taiwan. J Formos Med Assoc. 1996;95:19–28.
35. Lai HP, Chen YC, Chang LY, Lu CY, Lee CY, Lin KH, Huang LM. Invasive fungal infection in children with persistent febrile neutropenia. J Formos Med Assoc. 2005;104:174–9.
36. Chen CY, Chen YC, Tang JL, Yao M, Huang SY, Tsai W, Chen YC, Shen MC, Wang CH, Tien HF. Hepatosplenic fungal infection in patients with acute leukemia in Taiwan: incidence, treatment and prognosis. Ann Hematol. 2003;82:1–9.
37. Lortholary O, Renaudat C, Sitbon K, Desnos-Ollivier M, Bretagne S, Dromer F, French Mycoses Study Group. The risk and clinical outcome of candidemia depending on underlying malignancy. Intensive Care Med. 2017;43:652–62.
38. Leung AY, Chim CS, Ho PL, Cheng CC, Yuen KY, Lie AKW, et al. Candida tropicalis fungaemia in adult patients with haematological malignancies: clinical features and risk factors. J Hosp Infect. 2002;50:316–9.
39. Kim SH, Yoon YK, Kim MJ, Sohn JW. Clinical impact of time to positivity for *Candida* species on mortality in patients with candidaemia. J Antimicrob Chemother. 2013;68:2890–7.
40. Kang SJ, Kim SE, Kim UJ, Jang HC, Park KH, Shin JH, Jung SI. Clinical characteristics and risk factors for mortality in adult patients with persistent candidemia. J Infect. 2017;75(3):246–53.
41. Fan X, Xiao M, Liao K, Kudinha T, Wang H, Zhang L, Hou X, Kong F, Xu YC. Notable increasing trend in azole non-susceptible *Candida tropicalis* causing invasive candidiasis in China (August 2009 to July 2014): molecular epidemiology and clinical azole consumption. Front Microbiol. 2017;8:464.
42. Chindamporn A, Chakrabarti A, Li R, Sun PL, Tan BH, Chua M, Wahyuningsih R, Patel A, Liu Z, Chen YC, Chayakulkeeree M. Survey of laboratory practices for diagnosis of fungal infection in seven Asian countries—an Asia Fungal Working Group (AFWG) initiative. Med Mycol. 2018;56:416–25.
43. Tan TY, Hsu LY, Alejandria MM, et al. Antifungal susceptibility of invasive Candida bloodstream isolates from the Asia-Pacific region. Med Mycol J. 2016;54:471–7.
44. Lo HJ, et al. Fruits as the vehicle of drug resistant pathogenic yeasts. J Infect. 2017;75:254–62.
45. Chen P, Chuang Y, Wu U, et al. Clonality of fluconazole-Nonsusceptible Candida tropicalis in bloodstream infections, Taiwan, 2011–2017. Emerg Infect Dis. 2019;25(9):1668–75.
46. Lockhart SR, Etienne KA, Vallabhaneni S, Farooqi J, Chowdhary A, Govender NP, et al. Simultaneous emergence of multidrug-resistant *Candida auris* on 3 continents confirmed by whole-genome sequencing and epidemiological analyses. Clin Infect Dis. 2017;64:134–40.
47. Clancy CJ, Nguyen MH. Emergence of *Candida auris*: an international call to arms. Clin Infect Dis. 2017;64:141–3.
48. Satoh K, Makimura K, Hasumi Y, Nishiyama Y, Uchida K, Yamaguchi H. *Candida auris* sp. nov., a novel ascomycetous yeast isolated from the external ear canal of an inpatient in a Japanese hospital. Microbiol Immunol. 2009;53:41–4.
49. Lee WG, Shin JH, Uh Y, Kang MG, Kim SH, Park KH, et al. First three reported cases of nosocomial fungemia caused by *Candida auris*. J Clin Microbiol. 2011;49:3139–42.

50. Centers for Disease Control and Prevention. Clinical alert to US healthcare facilities: global Emergence of Invasive Infections Caused by the Multidrug-Resistant Yeast *Candida auris*. Atlanta: CDC; 2017.
51. Public Health England. Research and analysis: Candida auris identified in England. Public Health England; 2017. https://www.gov.uk/government/publications/candida-auris-emergence-in-england/candida-auris-identified-in-England. Accessed 25 Sept 2017.
52. Public Health England. Guidance for the laboratory investigation, management and infection prevention and control for cases of *Candida auris*. London: Public Health England; 2017.
53. Chakrabarti A, Sood P, Rudramurthy SM, Chen S, Kaur H, Capoor M, et al. Incidence, characteristics and outcome of ICU-acquired candidemia in India. Intensive Care Med. 2015;41:285–95.
54. Chowdhary A, Voss A, Meis JF. Multidrug-resistant *Candida auris*: 'new kid on the block' in hospital-associated infections? J Hosp Infect. 2016;94:209–12.
55. Navalkele BD, Revankar S, Chandrasekar P. *Candida auris*: a worrisome, globally emerging pathogen. Expert Rev Anti Infect Ther. 2017;15(9):819–27.
56. Chowdhary A, Anil Kumar V, Sharma C, Prakash A, Agarwal K, Babu R, et al. Multidrug-resistant endemic clonal strain of *Candida auris* in India. Eur J Clin Microbiol Infect Dis. 2014;33:919–26.
57. Schelenz S, Hagen F, Rhodes JL, Abdolrasouli A, Chowdhary A, Hall A, et al. First hospital outbreak of the globally emerging *Candida auris* in a European hospital. Antimicrob Resist Infect Control. 2016;5:35.
58. Vallabhaneni S, Kallen A, Tsay S, Chow N, Welsh R, Kerins J, et al. Investigation of the first seven reported cases of *Candida auris*, a globally emerging invasive, multidrug-resistant fungus—United States, May 2013–August 2016. MMWR Morb Mortal Wkly Rep. 2016;65:1234–7.
59. Calvo B, Melo AS, Perozo-Mena A, Hernandez M, Francisco EC, Hagen F, et al. First report of *Candida auris* in America: clinical and microbiological aspects of 18 episodes of candidemia. J Infect. 2016;73:369–74.
60. Rudramurthy SM, Chakrabarti A, Paul RA, Sood P, Kaur H, Capoor MR, et al. *Candida auris* candidaemia in Indian ICUs: analysis of risk factors. J Antimicrob Chemother. 2017;72:1794–801.
61. Tsay S, Welsh RM, Adams EH, Chow NA, Gade L, Berkow EL, et al. Notes from the field: ongoing transmission of *Candida auris* in health care facilities—United States, June 2016–May 2017. MMWR Morb Mortal Wkly Rep. 2017;66:514–5.
62. Chowdhary A, Sharma C, Duggal S, Agarwal K, Prakash A, Singh PK, et al. New clonal strain of *Candida auris*, Delhi, India. Emerg Infect Dis. 2013;19:1670–3.
63. Emara M, Ahmad S, Khan Z, Joseph L, Al-Obaid I, Purohit P, et al. *Candida auris* candidemia in Kuwait, 2014. Emerg Infect Dis. 2015;21:1091–2.
64. Kathuria S, Singh PK, Sharma C, Prakash A, Masih A, Kumar A, et al. Multidrug-resistant *Candida auris* misidentified as candida haemulonii: characterization by matrix-assisted laser desorption ionization-time of flight mass spectrometry and DNA sequencing and its antifungal susceptibility profile variability by Vitek 2, CLSI Broth Microdilution, and Etest Method. J Clin Microbiol. 2015;53:1823–30.
65. Lu P-L, Liu W-L, Lo H-J, Wang F-D, Ko W-C, Ho M-W, Liu C-E, Chen Y-H, Chen Y-C, Chuang Y-C, Chang S-C. Are we ready for the global emergence of multidrug-resistant *Candida auris* in Taiwan? J Formos Med Assoc. 2018;117:462–70.
66. Florio W, Tavanti A, Ghelardi E, Lupetti A. MALDI-TOF MS applications to the detection of antifungal resistance: state of the art and future perspectives. Front Microbiol. 2018;9:2577.
67. Arastehfar A, Fang W, Badali H, Vaezi A, Jiang W, Liao W, Pan W, Hagen F, Boekhout T. Low-cost Tetraplex PCR for the global spreading multi-drug resistant fungus, *Candida auris* and its phylogenetic relatives. Front Microbiol. 2018;9:1119.

68. Brandt ME, Lockhart SR. Recent taxonomic developments with *Candida* and other opportunistic yeasts. Curr Fungal Infect Rep. 2012;6(3):170–7.
69. Cheng JW, Liao K, Kudinha T, Yu SY, Xiao M, Wang H, Kong F, Xu YC. Molecular epidemiology and azole resistance mechanism study of *Candida guilliermondii* from a Chinese surveillance system. Sci Rep. 2017;7:907.
70. Douglass AP, Offei B, Braun-Galleani S, et al. Population genomics shows no distinction between pathogenic Candida krusei and environmental Pichia kudriavzevii: One species, four names. PLoS Pathog. 2018;14:e1007138.
71. Tsai MH, Hsu JF, Yang LY, et al. Candidemia due to uncommon Candida species in children: new threat and impacts on outcomes. Sci Rep. 2018;8:15239.
72. Pappas PG, Kauffman CA, Andes DR, et al. Clinical practice guideline for the management of candidiasis: 2016 update by the Infectious Diseases Society of America. Clin Infect Dis. 2016;62:e1–50.
73. Kung HC, Huang PY, Chen WT, et al. 2016 guidelines for the use of antifungal agents in patients with invasive fungal diseases in Taiwan. J Microbiol Immunol Infect. 2018;51:287–301.
74. Sherry L, Ramage G, Kean R, Borman A, Johnson EM, Richardson MD, et al. Biofilm-forming capability of highly virulent, multidrug-resistant Candida auris. Emerg Infect Dis. 2017;23:328–31.
75. Kung HC, Wang JL, Chang SC, Wang JT, Sun HY, Hsueh PR, Chen YC. Community-onset candidemia at a university hospital, 1995 to 2005. J Microbiol Immunol Infect. 2007;40:355–63.
76. Binelli CA, Moretti ML, Assis RS, et al. Investigation of the possible association between nosocomial candiduria and candidaemia. Clin Microbiol Infect. 2006;12(6):538–43.
77. da Silva CM, de Carvalho Parahym AM, Leao MP, de Oliveira NT, de Jesus Machado Amorim R, Neves RP. Fungemia by *Candida pelliculosa (Pichia anomala)* in a neonatal intensive care unit: a possible clonal origin. Mycopathologia. 2013;175(1–2):175–9.
78. Berger C, Frei R, Gratwohl A, Scheidegger C. Bottled lemon juice—a cryptic source of invasive Candida infections in the immunocompromised host. J Infect Dis. 1988;158:654–5.
79. Bougnoux ME, Brun S, Zahar JR. Healthcare-associated fungal outbreaks: new and uncommon species, New molecular tools for investigation and prevention. Antimicrob Resist Infect Control. 2018;7:45.
80. Arendrup MC, Patterson TF. Multidrug-resistant *Candida*: epidemiology, molecular mechanisms, and treatment. J Infect Dis. 2017;216(suppl_3):S445–51.
81. Biswal M, Rudramurthy SM, Jain N, et al. Controlling a possible outbreak of *Candida auris* infection: lessons learnt from multiple interventions. J Hosp Infect. 2017;97:363–70.

Invasive Aspergillosis in Asia

17

Ban-Hock Tan

Key Points

- Neutropenia and steroids are the main risk factors for IA in Asia, as in the rest of the world.
- There are subtle shifts in the epidemiology of IA, and clinicians should be on the lookout for IA, and consider it in new categories of at risks persons, e.g., those with myeloma, those with COPD, those with severe liver disease, post-H1N1 influenza, etc.
- Sino-orbital aspergillosis is a distinct entity in South Asian countries.
- Galactomannan is a crucial tool in IA diagnosis.
- HRCT helps in suspecting pulmonary aspergillosis in neutropenic patients.
- Use of a clinical algorithm may improve the diagnosis of pulmonary aspergillosis in COPD patients but requires further validation.
- There is a need to improve the capabilities of diagnostic mycology laboratories in Asian countries, especially incorporation of biomarker tests.
- For a variety of reasons, e.g., cost, Asian physicians may not be able to use their antifungal of choice.
- Therapeutic drug monitoring is essential in azole especially voriconazole therapy.

17.1 Introduction

Invasive aspergillosis (IA) is the commonest invasive mold infection (IMI) in Asia [1]. Its diagnosis and management have long been a challenge [2]. From the turn of this century, however, new diagnostic modalities and effective antifungals led to a

B.-H. Tan (✉)
Department of Infectious Diseases, Singapore General Hospital, Singapore, Singapore
e-mail: tan.ban.hock@singhealth.com.sg

A. Chakrabarti (ed.), *Clinical Practice of Medical Mycology in Asia*,
https://doi.org/10.1007/978-981-13-9459-1_17

surge of interest in, and hence a burgeoning of research papers on, IA. This, in turn, spawned international collaborations that have yielded diagnostic criteria and treatment guidelines [2–7]. For the clinician, the approach to IA has been streamlined to a great extent.

As many publications already describe the clinical features, diagnosis, and management of IA, this chapter will point out features of IA that Asian practitioners will find clinically useful, with literature drawn mainly from Asian centers.

17.2 Understanding the Risk Factors for IA

17.2.1 Clinical Overview of Risk Factors

The diagnosis of IA cannot be made at the bedside without an understanding of the conditions that predispose to it. The risk factors for IA in much of Asia are similar to those in other parts of the world [1]. The Asiamold study, a study of IMIs at five tertiary centers in Asia, found that 70% of IMIs were caused by IA. In keeping with the established literature, neutropenia and steroid exposure were the common host factors [1, 8]. Of note, acute myeloid leukemia (AML), well-known as a major underlying condition in IA, was found in only 19% of Asiamold subjects [1]. However, on the whole, 42% of the subjects had an underlying hematologic malignancy [1]. The relative decline in AML was attributed by the authors to the use of antifungal prophylaxis. This subtle shift in epidemiology in some of Asia's leading centers mirrors that of the west, where IA is increasingly recognized in patients with myeloma and lymphoma, likely related to new therapies [9, 10].

Interestingly, diabetes mellitus (DM) was an underlying condition in 30% of Asiamold subjects [1]. DM has featured as an underlying condition in several Asian papers on IA [11, 12]. The role of DM is difficult to tease out but there is the possibility that the presence of two or more risk factors/predisposing conditions "may precipitate the occurrence" of IMI [8]. Keeping in mind the possibility that DM may be a risk factor for IA may help when faced with diagnostic problems [13].

17.2.2 IA in "New" Host Categories

The classical immunocompromised hosts at risk for IA are febrile neutropenics, hematopoietic stem cell transplant (HSCT) recipients, solid organ transplant (SOT) recipients, and patients with chronic granulomatous disease. However, more recent data suggest that IA is a problem also in patients with chronic obstructive pulmonary disease (COPD), acute on chronic liver failure (ACLF), and in those with severe influenza.

These "new" categories of hosts potentially susceptible to IA have received much attention from Asian researchers.

17.2.2.1 COPD

The reasons for the association between COPD and IA are complex. We inhale *Aspergillus* conidia daily, and they do reach the deepest parts of the lungs [14]. Infection, however, is rare, as long as the respiratory tract is anatomically and functionally normal, and the immune response unimpaired. In COPD, there is damage to the respiratory mucosa and to the cilia, as well as chronic mucus production. This leads to chronic obstruction and reduced mucociliary clearance. As infection with *Aspergillus* sets in, chronic steroid therapy prevents adequate control of fungal proliferation [14]. In China, the smoking rate among those above the age of 15 is >40% [15]. Perhaps because of this, Chinese authors have contributed much to our understanding of IA in COPD.

The true incidence of IA in COPD in Asia is not clear. Investigators from Guangzhou found IA in 3.9% of patients admitted for acute exacerbation of COPD [16]. Among COPD patients admitted to an ICU in Beijing, however, the incidence of IA was much higher (23%) [17].

The Bulpa criteria for the diagnosis of IA in COPD provided standardized definitions useful for both clinicians and researchers [4]. However, its adoption has not been universal, and investigators still use other criteria, e.g., the EORTC/MSG criteria, for the diagnosis of IA in COPD, though the patients are not ideal hosts by these criteria. One Chinese group compared the utility of the different published criteria for IA diagnosis in COPD and found that the Bulpa criteria gave the highest "diagnostic rate" [18].

IA complicating COPD was associated with worsening radiological infiltrates, the need for mechanical ventilation, a longer hospital stay, and a higher mortality [16]. Among COPD patients admitted to an ICU, pre-ICU factors that independently predicted IA were receipt of >3 antibiotics, cumulative steroid dose >350 mg (of prednisolone or equivalent), and an APACHE score >18 [17]. The temperature and white cell count were also higher in those with IA than those without. During bronchoscopy, COPD patients with IA tended to have bronchospasm and plague formation. Radiologically, COPD patients with IA tended to have nodules on Day 1 of ICU admission, which progressed to consolidation by day 7 [17]. Taking together the features commoner in COPD patients with IA than those without, He at al proposed a diagnostic algorithm (Table 17.1) [17].

The algorithm of He et al. is useful as it suggests when physicians managing COPD patients in the ICU should start ordering tests for IA. It also emphasizes the need to consider *Aspergillus* tracheobronchitis as it does not wait for chest imaging to show opacification. However, a few of the criteria are subjective (e.g., "dry" rales, and sputum "ropiness") and others are inadequately defined (e.g., period over which total steroid dose should be calculated). Further refinement of the algorithm is needed for widespread uptake.

The utility of GM in the setting of COPD was investigated by He et al., who systematically performed serum GM assays on the first and fourth ICU days of critically ill COPD patients [19]. Using the 2002 rather than the 2008 EORTC definitions of IA, He et al. appropriately did not use GM, their study variable, as a

Table 17.1 When to suspect IA in COPD patients (Modified from He et al., Crit Care 2011;15:R5)

1. Host factors
>3 antibiotics
Receipt of steroids (prednisolone equivalent >350 mg)
APACHE ≥18
2. Clinical symptoms/signs
Temp >38.5 °C
Wheeze not responsive to steroids/antibiotics
Rales not responsive to steroids/antibiotics
3. Laboratory findings
WBC > 20 × 10^9/L
CCT < 40 ml/min
4. Chest X-ray
Any of patchiness, consolidation or nodules
5. At or during bronchoscopy
Bronchospasm
Ropiness of sputum
Plug formation
Pseudomembrane formation

ICU patients with COPD fulfilling 1, 2, and 3 should have a lower respiratory tract specimen sent for fungal smear and culture, a serum GM, and a bronchoscopy
ICU patients with COPD who also fulfil 4 and 5 are said to have "possible" IA; those with possible IA who have a positive culture for Aspergillus or a positive serum GM are said to have "probable" IA

criterion for diagnosis. They found that two consecutive positives gave positive and negative predictive values of 89% and 85% respectively. Further, a positive lower respiratory culture for *Aspergillus* in association with a positive GM portended a high mortality (73–83%) [19].

The role of bronchoalveolar lavage (BAL) has also been emphasized by Chinese authors. The diagnostic algorithm of He et al. (Table 17.1) leads to a bronchoscopy, which, the authors stressed, should be done early. Zhang et al. evaluated the role of GM in BAL fluid (a criterion not used by Bulpa et al) and found that at a cut-off of 1.25, the test had a sensitivity of 91% and a specificity of 96% [20].

17.2.2.2 IA in Decompensated Liver Disease

Multiple reports document the association between IA and liver disease. An early report described IA complicating acute liver failure [21]. IA is also known to complicate alcoholic hepatitis [22]. The predisposition to invasive fungal infection results from a variety of immune defects present in severe liver disease, well reviewed by Lipke et al. [23]. These include defects in neutrophil and macrophage function, lymphocyte activation, and opsonization of certain organisms.

IA in patients with decompensated liver disease has also been recognized in Asia [24–26]. Chen et al. found 39 (5.0%) patients with IA out of 787 with acute on chronic liver failure (ACLF). Risk factors for IA were age, encephalopathy, and steroid use [25]. Thirty-seven of the 39 died. Zhang et al. found 55 (5.1%) cases of IA in a cohort of 1077 patients with various categories of liver failure [26]. Risk factors for IA were hepatorenal syndrome, use of antibiotics for >5 days, and use of steroid for >7 days. They emphasized the need to consider IA as a diagnosis should patients with such risk factors develop respiratory symptoms [26].

Gao et al. determined that the main risk factor for death among ACLF patients developing IA was a CLIF-SOFA score >2 [27]. They also noted that procalcitonin and white cell count did not change much as IA developed in their cohort of ACLF patients. They treated IA in ACLF with voriconazole and found that standard dosing led to very high voriconazole levels. With the help of therapeutic drug monitoring (TDM), they were able to recommend a loading dose of 200 mg twice a day followed by a maintenance dose of 100 mg once a day [27]. The study shows TDM is mandatory while using voriconazole in such patients.

17.2.2.3 Aspergillus Complicating Influenza

Despite the recent flurry of publications on this topic, the association has been intermittently reported for a long time [28–32]. A 1952 report described a case of pulmonary aspergillosis (proven on autopsy) following "post-influenzal bronchopneumonia" [33]. Of scattered reports that followed, three were from Japan [34–36]. From these and the more recent reports, it can be seen that IA complicates influenza in the immunocompromised as well as those who were previously healthy [29, 30]. One literature review found that only a third of the reported cases had an underlying condition classically associated with IA [29]. IA may complicate influenza A and B [29, 37, 38].

The mechanisms by which influenza predisposes a patient to IA are not clear. Researchers in Barcelona noted that an increase in environmental spore counts was associated with an increase in the diagnosis of IA about 4–6 weeks later [28]. An increase in the circulation of certain viruses (e.g., influenza and adenovirus) was also associated with an increase in the diagnosis of IA. During periods of circulating viruses, a lower environmental spore count was required for IA to occur [28]. An almost similar trend was noted in southern Taiwan. In the Taiwanese experience, persistent high ambient levels of particulate matter 2.5 μm ($PM_{2.5}$) over a 2-month period were associated with an increase in the number of cases of influenza and IA [39]. Although the links between environmental spore counts and influenza, and between influenza and IA still need to be better understood, it might appear that viruses (and influenza in particular) enhanced one's susceptibility to IA. In support of such a hypothesis are reports suggesting that influenza may reduce alveolar macrophage activity or increase IL-10 levels, which, in turn, inhibit natural killer cells. Moreover, steroid use in severe influenza (which occurs intermittently) also make the patients susceptible for IA [40, 41].

17.2.2.4 Sino-Orbital/Sino-Orbital-Cerebral Aspergillosis

Aspergillus sinusitis with extension to the orbit and cranial cavity is a dreaded but well-recognized condition in classical immunocompromised hosts [42]. As a manifestation of IA in the apparently immunocompetent, however, it was once reported almost exclusively from the Middle East, South Asia and Sudan [43–49].

This condition has been linked by some authors to high spore counts [48, 49]. Other authors have speculated that "dust and sand storms in the summer months" likely contain large numbers of Aspergillus conidia, which can "easily settle" in the "injured nasal mucosae" of young men working outdoors [46]. In a study on rural population of north India, fungal rhinosinusitis (FRS) was noted in 8.1% of chronic rhinosinusitis (CRS) cases (1.4% of adult of the villages suffered from CRS), and *Aspergillus* species was the etiological agent in majority of the cases. Wheat thrashing in the winter months releases large number of spores in the air and may be linked with high number of FRS cases in the population [50].

Young males working in agricultural settings are the archetypal patients. Common presenting symptoms and signs include the orbital apex syndrome, the cavernous sinus syndrome, proptosis with extraocular palsies, cheek swelling, and visual loss. Symptoms of a mass lesion in the brain such as headache, vomiting, an altered sensorium, and seizures may also be part of the presentation [43–46, 49]. Patients might have had repeated nasal polypectomies performed previously [43, 44].

The condition occurs in immunocompetent persons, though DM appears as a common underlying condition. As a clinical definition of invasive mold sinusitis akin to the EORTC/MSG criteria does not exist, Asiamold investigators modified the EORTC criteria by allowing DM as a host factor for Indian patients with sinusitis [1]. With this, the authors were able to include eight of their 17 patients with sino-orbito-cranial aspergillosis. An Indian series found that an invasive fungal infection (IFI) was among the top three causes of cavernous sinus syndrome, and that DM was "positively associated" with a fungal etiology of the syndrome [51].

More recently, investigators from other Asian countries as well have described IA of the sinuses, with extension into the orbit, or cranial cavity, or both. Case reports/series hail from Japan, Korea, Malaysia, Taiwan, and Thailand [52–56]. In these reports, DM is a commonly identified underlying condition. The Japanese series found that late diagnosis was common, and emphasized the importance of a biopsy [52]. In addition, they stressed the importance of stains (e.g., PAS) that could demonstrate the hyphae when such biopsies were performed [52]. A warning on the importance of an accurate diagnosis comes from the Korean series, which described three diabetics presenting with eye pain, headache, and impairment of vision and/or extraocular movement [53]. Visual outcome was poor in those who had received steroids. The authors emphasized the need for surgical intervention, and advised repeated biopsies before commencing steroids patients with such a presentation, especially if they were diabetic [53].

17.3 Diagnosis

17.3.1 Galactomannan (GM)

As mentioned, the diagnosis of IA has been streamlined by the "diagnostic criteria" established internationally. The use of the GM assay is central to these definitions.

Unfortunately, the GM assay is not widely available in Asia. In a recent survey conducted by the Asia Fungal Working Group (AFWG), only 22.8% of 241 laboratories offered this test [57]. Yet 60% of physicians who participated in a survey of physicians had access to this test, suggesting that they sent it out to a laboratory in a different hospital or, perhaps, a different city [58]. Perhaps because of lack of access to GM, and possibly because of a slower turnaround time, 74% of physicians who participated in the survey used the empiric approach in persistent febrile neutropenia.

Nevertheless Asian investigators working with the assay have pointed out its uses and pitfalls. Taiwanese investigators speculated that the more widespread use of the GM assay enabled IA to be diagnosed more frequently, possibly contributing to the observed rise in the incidence of IA over the years [59]. By interrogating their national health insurance database, they found that the incidence of invasive pulmonary aspergillosis (IPA) rose from 0.94 to 2.06 per million patient-years from 2002 to 2011. This appeared to correlate with a rise in the use of the GM assay.

In an early study, Tan et al. randomized febrile neutropenics into two arms—an empirical antifungal therapy arm versus a GM-guided preemptive therapy arm. Although the study had to be stopped prematurely, the investigators found that the GM-guided preemptive strategy was safe [60]. Such an approach, termed "tailored" or "diagnosis-driven," has also been employed elsewhere [61–63]. As is well-known, the GM assay may be associated with false-positives. This has received the attention of Asian investigators too [64–66].

In a cohort of HSCT patients, Kimura et al. noted that the cumulative 1-year incidence of IA was 10.1%, but that of a positive GM test was 48% [65]. Japanese investigators have also noticed that patients with rheumatoid arthritis tended to have an elevated GM value [66]. Out of 340 patients, 62 (18.2%) had an elevated GM value. Fifty-six (90.3%) of the 62 underwent repeat testing a few months later, and an elevated value persisted in 50 (89.3%) of them. A positive value correlated with globulin levels. No patient was diagnosed with IA in the course of the study.

Most interestingly, false-positives have been used as an aid in the diagnosis of non-*Aspergillus* fungal infections. Penicillium, for example, has long been known to be a genus that would cross-react with the GM assay to produce a false-positive result. This has been used by at least one Chinese group to help with the diagnosis of *Talaromyces marneffei* infection [67]. These investigators found that in patients with AIDS, GM had sensitivity and specificity of 95.8% and 90.9%, respectively for the diagnosis of talaromycosis (penicilliosis).

17.3.2 Beta-D-Glucan (BDG)

This test is even less readily available in Asia, being offered by only 10% of the laboratories surveyed by the AFWG [57]. The cost of the test and the tendency for false-positives are the main reasons for not making the test available (unpublished observations). The data for using BDG appear less robust than that for GM. In the 2018 ESCMID guidelines on Aspergillosis, GM received an A1 rating as a screening tool in HSCT patients not on mold-active prophylaxis, and an A2 rating as a diagnostic tool in febrile neutropenics. BDG, on the other hand, received a B2 for both of these purposes [5].

A novel use of the BDG and GM assays was attempted by Thai investigators, who studied their utility in the diagnosis of fungal peritonitis in patients undergoing peritoneal dialysis. The BDG assay tended to be falsely-positive, yielding positive results even in cases of gram-negative peritonitis. However, they noted that a higher cut-off BDG value, and a concomitantly positive GM, reduced the rate of false-positives [68].

17.3.3 CT Scans

CT scans are critical in the diagnosis of IA. They are the only acceptable "clinical" criterion in the EORTC/MSG guideline [7]. The 2018 ESCMID guideline emphasizes the importance of integrating clinical, microbiological, and radiological features to achieve a diagnosis [5].

Useful clinical tips on CT features of IA have been highlighted by Asian authors. Park et al. noted that, compared with neutropenic hosts, SOT recipients with IPA tended to have a wide variety of CT signs [69]. The halo sign, for example, was uncommon in such hosts. A Korean review of the literature yielded a long list of conditions reported to show the halo sign [70]. It was the clinical context that gave a clue to the diagnosis [70]. Girmenia et al. pointed out that sometimes, a second CT was needed for radiological features fitting the EORTC/MSG criteria to develop [63]. In the Asiamold study, a wide range of CT features was described in proven/probable IPA cases. This led the authors to conclude that IMI "should not be ruled out in patients with a suspected infection whose chest features on CT did not fit the EORTC/MSG criteria" [1]. In this respect, it is worth remembering that the EORTC/MSG criteria were developed for research purposes—in particular, to permit standardized enrolment into studies [7].

Tuberculosis (TB) is a major problem in much of Asia. TB affects immunocompetent and immunocompromised persons. Korean investigators have reported a series of SOT recipients with TB that radiologically mimicked IPA [71]. Hence, while the chest CT is indispensable in the clinical diagnosis of IPA, appreciating the caveats and exceptions will enhance one's bedside acumen.

17.4 Treatment

17.4.1 General Comments

The development of new diagnostic tools, such as the GM assay, and the introduction of new antifungals, have revolutionized the management of invasive fungal infection (IFI) in the immunocompromised host.

Prophylaxis against IFIs in the hematology setting is well-studied. Posaconazole (POS) was better than comparators in protecting against an IFI (including IA) in patients with AML and high-risk myelodysplastic syndrome (MDS) [72]. It also protected HSCT recipients with graft-versus-host disease from an IFI [73]. One category of patients left out by these landmark studies are those undergoing conditioning during an HSCT. One large study comparing voriconazole (VCZ) against fluconazole did enrol such patients but they were a small minority [74]. Here Chinese investigators have stepped in, suggesting that micafungin was non-inferior to itraconazole [75]. In the AFWG survey of clinicians, 59% of respondents used antifungal prophylaxis in allo-HSCT, and 43% in AML/MDS [58]. Antifungal prophylaxis was more commonly employed in India, Singapore, and Taiwan. The Singapore group has reported that the introduction of posaconazole in their AML population led to a remarkable reduction in IFI [76].

As mentioned above, in patients with hematological malignancies with febrile neutropenia, a preemptive or diagnosis-driven approach is an alternative to an empirical antifungal approach to prolonged febrile neutropenia. Clinicians preferring the empirical approach also have more options—caspofungin proved to be as effective as and was better tolerated than liposomal amphotericin [21]. In this setting, Korean investigators have compared micafungin with itraconazole and shown both drugs to be equivalent, with micafungin associated with a shorter duration of fever [77].

Where the treatment of IA is concerned, the new-generation azoles have proved their worth. An Austrian study suggested that VCZ helped reduce mortality in IA, a finding that Asiamold investigators could agree with [1, 78]. However, Asian clinicians face many barriers to using effective antifungals of choice. In the AFWG survey, a large proportion of respondents could not use the drug of choice because the patient "could not afford" it [58]. This was most marked in India, with 93% of respondents selecting this option. On the other hand, physicians from Indonesia, China, and the Philippines tended to select "drug not available in country" as a likely reason for not using a guideline-recommended antifungal [58].

These factors might explain some of the findings of the Asiamold study. Here amphotericin deoxycholate (amD) was the most commonly used drug for empirical therapy if a suspected IMI [1]. However, there were wide variations in different countries—it was not used at all in the period under study in both the Beijing and Singapore centers [1].

Similarly cost and local health-care economics may explain the differences between certain Asian and western guidelines. The 2016 Taiwanese guideline on fungal infections still listed amD as an alternative to VCZ in the treatment of IA though it is omitted from the 2018 ESCMID guideline [79].

17.4.2 Therapeutic Drug Monitoring (TDM)

TDM for VCZ, POS, and itraconazole (ITC) is recommended internationally [5, 80]. The main reasons are the inter- and intra-individual variability in drug levels, as well as the likelihood of drug–drug interactions [81, 82].

VCZ is metabolized in the liver via the cytochrome p450 pathway by the isoenzymes 2C19, 3A4, and 2C9. The isoenzyme 2C19 plays a major role but also exhibits great polymorphism [83]. Most relevant to Asia is the fact that >15% of Asians are poor metabolizers [84]. Hence, azole TDM appears to be a crucial service in Asia. Yet TDM is offered by few laboratories in Asia [57].

Nevertheless, it was a Korean center that published the first randomized controlled trial on VCZ TDM [85]. After excluding poor metabolizers, they demonstrated that TDM reduced the discontinuation rate due to adverse drug events, and also increased the likelihood of treatment success.

In patients with hepatic impairment, TDM allows for dosing that will minimize toxicity [27]. Nevertheless, VRC is known to cause hepatotoxicity, and some authors advise against its use in patients with severe liver disease, unless benefits clearly outweigh risks [86]. Establishing a diagnosis of IA is therefore essential in such circumstances.

17.5 Conclusions

In the advanced centers of Asia, awareness of IA and access to essential diagnostic tools are not a problem. Case reports and series suggest that it is present elsewhere too, and the lack of access to diagnostic testing may explain the relative lack of formal studies on IA. Much work needs to be done to further mycology education in Asia.

References

1. Rotjanapan P, Chen Y, Chakrabarti A, et al. Epidemiology and clinical characteristics of invasive mould infections: a multicenter, retrospective analysis in five Asian countries. Med Mycol. 2017;56(2):186–96.
2. Patterson TF, Thompson GR III, Denning DW, et al. Practice guidelines for the diagnosis and management of aspergillosis: 2016 update by the Infectious Diseases Society of America. Clin Infect Dis. 2016;63(4):e1–e60.
3. Blot SI, Taccone FS, Van den Abeele A-M, et al. A clinical algorithm to diagnose invasive pulmonary aspergillosis in critically ill patients. Am J Respir Crit Care Med. 2012;186(1):56–64.
4. Bulpa P, Dive A, Sibille Y. Invasive pulmonary aspergillosis in patients with chronic obstructive pulmonary disease. Eur Respir J. 2007;30(4):782–800.
5. Ullmann AJ, Aguado JM, Arikan-Akdagli S, et al. Diagnosis and management of Aspergillus diseases: executive summary of the 2017 ESCMID-ECMM-ERS guideline. Clin Microbiol Infect. 2018;24:e1–e38.
6. Blyth C, Gilroy N, Guy S, et al. Consensus guidelines for the treatment of invasive mould infections in haematological malignancy and haemopoietic stem cell transplantation, 2014. Intern Med J. 2014;44(12b):1333–49.
7. De Pauw B, Walsh TJ, Donnelly JP, et al. Revised definitions of invasive fungal disease from the European organization for research and treatment of cancer/invasive fungal infections cooperative group and the national institute of allergy and infectious diseases mycoses study group (EORTC/MSG) consensus group. Clin Infect Dis. 2008;46(12):1813–21.
8. Herbrecht R, Bories P, Moulin JC, Ledoux MP, Letscher-Bru V. Risk stratification for invasive aspergillosis in immunocompromised patients. Ann NY Acad Sci. 2012;1272(1):23–30.
9. Nucci M, Nouér SA, Grazziutti M, Kumar NS, Barlogie B, Anaissie E. Probable invasive aspergillosis without prespecified radiologic findings: proposal for inclusion of a new cat-

egory of aspergillosis and implications for studying novel therapies. Clin Infect Dis. 2010;51(11):1273–80.

10. Ghez D, Calleja A, Protin C, et al. Early-onset invasive aspergillosis and other fungal infections in patients treated with ibrutinib. Blood. 2018;131(17):1955–9.
11. Kiertiburanakul S, Thibbadee C, Santanirand P. Invasive aspergillosis in a tertiary-care hospital in Thailand. J Med Assoc Thai. 2007;90(5):895.
12. Dai Z, Zhao H, Cai S, Lv Y, Tong W. Invasive pulmonary aspergillosis in non-neutropenic patients with and without underlying disease: a single-Centre retrospective analysis of 52 subjects. Respirology. 2013;18(2):323–31.
13. Norlinah MI, Ngow H, Hamidon B. Angioinvasive cerebral aspergillosis presenting as acute ischaemic stroke in a patient with diabetes mellitus. Singap Med J. 2007;48(1):e1–4.
14. Arribi A. How should we approach Aspergillus in lung secretions of patients with COPD? Rev Esp Quimioter. 2016;29(4):175–82.
15. World Health Organisation. Prevalence of tobacco smoking. http://gamapserver.who.int/gho/interactive_charts/tobacco/use/atlas.html. Accessed 9 Sept.
16. Xu H, Li L, Huang WJ, Wang LX, Li WF, Yuan WF. Invasive pulmonary aspergillosis in patients with chronic obstructive pulmonary disease: a case control study from China. Clin Microbiol Infect. 2012;18(4):403–8.
17. He H, Ding L, Sun B, Li F, Zhan Q. Role of galactomannan determinations in bronchoalveolar lavage fluid samples from critically ill patients with chronic obstructive pulmonary disease for the diagnosis of invasive pulmonary aspergillosis: a prospective study. Crit Care. 2012;16(4):R138.
18. Huang L, He H, Jin J, Zhan QI. Bulpa criteria suitable for the diagnosis of probable invasive pulmonary aspergillosis in critically ill patients with chronic obstructive pulmonary disease? A comparative study with EORTC/MSG and ICU criteria. BMC Infect Dis. 2017;17(1):209.
19. He H, Ding L, Chang S, Li F, Zhan Q. Value of consecutive galactomannan determinations for the diagnosis and prognosis of invasive pulmonary aspergillosis in critically ill chronic obstructive pulmonary disease. Med Mycol. 2011;49(4):345–51.
20. Zhang X-B, Chen G-P, Lin Q-C, Lin X, Zhang H-Y, Wang J-H. Bronchoalveolar lavage fluid galactomannan detection for diagnosis of invasive pulmonary aspergillosis in chronic obstructive pulmonary disease. Med Mycol. 2013;51(7):688–95.
21. Walsh TJ, Hamilton SR. Disseminated aspergillosis complicating hepatic failure. Arch Intern Med. 1983;143(6):1189–91.
22. Gustot T, Maillart E, Bocci M, et al. Invasive aspergillosis in patients with severe alcoholic hepatitis. J Hepatol. 2014;60(2):267–74.
23. Lipke AB, Mihas AA. Non-decompensated cirrhosis as a risk factor for invasive aspergillosis: a case report and review of the immune dysfunction of cirrhosis. Am J Med Sci. 2007;334(4):314–6.
24. Tang H-J, Liu W-L, Chang TC, et al. Multiple brain abscesses due to Aspergillus fumigatus in a patient with liver cirrhosis: a case report. Medicine. 2016;95(9):e2813.
25. Chen J, Yang Q, Huang J, Li L. Risk factors for invasive pulmonary aspergillosis and hospital mortality in acute-on-chronic liver failure patients: a retrospective-cohort study. Int J Med Sci. 2013;10(12):1625.
26. Zhang X, Yang M, Hu J, Zhao H, Li L. Epidemiology of invasive pulmonary aspergillosis in patients with liver failure: clinical presentation, risk factors, and outcomes. J Int Med Res. 2018;46(2):819–27.
27. Gao J, Zhang Q, Wu Y, et al. Improving survival of acute-on-chronic liver failure patients complicated with invasive pulmonary aspergillosis. Sci Rep. 2018;8(1):876.
28. Garcia-Vidal C, Barba P, Arnan M, et al. Invasive aspergillosis complicating pandemic influenza A (H1N1) infection in severely immunocompromised patients. Clin Infect Dis. 2011;53(6):e16–e9.
29. Crum-Cianflone NF. Invasive aspergillosis associated with severe influenza infections. Open Forum Infect Dis. 2016;3(3):ofw171.

30. Adalja AA, Sappington PL, Harris SP, et al. Isolation of Aspergillus in three 2009 H1N1 influenza patients. Influenza Other Respir Viruses. 2011;5(4):225–9.
31. van de Veerdonk FL, Kolwijck E, Lestrade PP, et al. Influenza-associated aspergillosis in critically ill patients. Am J Respir Crit Care Med. 2017;196(4):524–7.
32. Shah MM, Hsiao EI, Kirsch CM, Gohil A, Narasimhan S, Stevens DA. Invasive pulmonary aspergillosis and influenza co-infection in immunocompetent hosts: case reports and review of the literature. Diagn Microbiol Infect Dis. 2018;91:147.
33. Abbott J, Fernando H, Gurling K, Meade B. Pulmonary aspergillosis following post-influenzal bronchopneumonia treated with antibiotics. Br Med J. 1952;1(4757):523.
34. Kobayashi O, Sekiya M, Saitoh H. A case of invasive broncho-pulmonary aspergillosis associated with influenza A (H3N2) infection. Nihon Kyobu Shikkan Gakkai Zasshi. 1992;30(7):1338–44.
35. Funabiki Y, Ishii K, Kusaka S, et al. Aspergillosis following influenza A infection. Nihon Ronen Igakkai Zasshi. 1999;36(4):274–8.
36. Matsushima H, Takayanagi N, Ubukata M, Sugita Y, Kanazawa M, Kawabata Y. Invasive pulmonary aspergillosis following influenza A infection. Nihon Kokyuki Gakkai zasshi. 2001;39(9):672–7.
37. Nulens EF, Bourgeois MJ, Reynders MB. Post-influenza aspergillosis, do not underestimate influenza B. Infect Drug Resist. 2017;10:61.
38. Sim Jean WL, Tan BH. Influencing aspergillus: a case report of IPA complicating influenza B pneumonia. Asia Fungal Working Group Newsletter. 2016;4.
39. Yu W-L, Liu W-L, Chan K-S, et al. High-level ambient particulate matter before influenza attack with increased incidence of Aspergillus antigenemia in Southern Taiwan, 2016. J Microbiol Immunol Infect. 2018;51(1):141–7.
40. Astry CL, Jakab GJ. Influenza virus-induced immune complexes suppress alveolar macrophage phagocytosis. J Virol. 1984;50(2):287–92.
41. Barthelemy A, Ivanov S, Fontaine J, et al. Influenza A virus-induced release of interleukin-10 inhibits the anti-microbial activities of invariant natural killer T cells during invasive pneumococcal superinfection. Mucosal Immunol. 2017;10(2):460.
42. Chen C-Y, Sheng W-H, Cheng A, et al. Invasive fungal sinusitis in patients with hematological malignancy: 15 years experience in a single university hospital in Taiwan. BMC Infect Dis. 2011;11(1):250.
43. Mohandas S, Ahuja G, Sood V, Virmani V. Aspergillosis of the central nervous system. J Neurol Sci. 1978;38(2):229–33.
44. Rao GSP, Mann S, Talwar P, Arora M. Primary mycotic infection of paranasal sinuses. Mycopathologia. 1984;84(2–3):73–6.
45. Das T, Vyas P, Sharma S. Aspergillus terreus postoperative endophthalmitis. Br J Ophthalmol. 1993;77(6):386.
46. Panda NK, Sharma SC, Chakrabartu A, Mann S. Paranasal sinus mycoses in North India: Nebenhöhlen-Mykosen in Nordinien. Mycoses. 1998;41(7–8):281–6.
47. Siddiqui AA, Shah AA, Bashir SH. Craniocerebral aspergillosis of sinonasal origin in immunocompetent patients: clinical spectrum and outcome in 25 cases. Neurosurgery. 2004;55(3):602–13.
48. Shankar S, Mahadevan A, Sundaram C, et al. Pathobiology of fungal infections of the central nervous system with special reference to the Indian scenario. Neurol India. 2007;55(3):198.
49. Murthy J, Sundaram C, Prasad V, Purohit A, Rammurti S, Laxmi V. Sinocranial aspergillosis: a form of central nervous system aspergillosis in South India. Mycoses. 2001;44(5):141–5.
50. Chakrabarti A, Rudramurthy SM, Panda N, Das A, Singh A. Epidemiology of chronic fungal rhinosinusitis in rural India. Mycoses. 2015;58(5):294–302.
51. Bhatkar S, Goyal M, Takkar A, et al. Cavernous sinus syndrome: a prospective study of 73 cases at a tertiary care centre in Northern India. Clin Neurol Neurosurg. 2017;155:63–9.
52. Kawakami H, Mochizuki K, Ishida K, Ohkusu K. Seven cases of localized invasive sino-orbital aspergillosis. Jpn J Ophthalmol. 2017;61(2):179–88.

53. Yoon JS, Park HK, Cho NH, Lee SY. Outcomes of three patients with intracranially invasive sino-orbital aspergillosis. Ophthalmic Plast Reconstr Surg. 2007;23(5):400–6.
54. Goh L, Shakri E, Ong H, et al. A seven-year retrospective analysis of the clinicopathological and mycological manifestations of fungal rhinosinusitis in a single-centre tropical climate hospital. J Laryngol Otol. 2017;131(9):813–6.
55. Chang Y-M, Chang Y-H, Chien K-H, et al. Orbital apex syndrome secondary to aspergilloma masquerading as a paranasal sinus tumor: a case report and literature review. Medicine. 2018;97(30):e11650.
56. Sungkanuparph S, Sathapatayavongs B, Kunachak S, Luxameechanporn T, Cheewaruangroj W. Treatment of invasive fungal sinusitis with liposomal amphotericin B: a report of four cases. J Med Assoc Thai. 2001;84(4):593–601.
57. Chindamporn A, Chakrabarti A, Li R, et al. Survey of laboratory practices for diagnosis of fungal infection in seven Asian countries: an Asia Fungal Working Group (AFWG) initiative. Med Mycol. 2017;56(4):416–25.
58. Tan BH, Chakrabarti A, Patel A, Chua MMM, Sun P-L, Liu Z, Rotjanapan P, Li R, Wahyuningsih R, Chayakulkeeree M, Chen Y-C, on behalf of the Asia Fungal Working Group (AFWG). Clinicians' challenges in managing patients with invasive fungal diseases in seven Asian countries: an Asia Fungal Working Group (AFWG) survey. (under publication).
59. Sun K-S, Tsai C-F, Chen SC-C, Chen Y-Y, Huang W-C. Galactomannan testing and the incidence of invasive pulmonary aspergillosis: a 10-year Nationwide population-based study in Taiwan. PLoS One. 2016;11(2):e0149964.
60. Tan BH, Low JGH, Chlebicka NL, et al. Galactomannan-guided preemptive vs. empirical antifungals in the persistently febrile neutropenic patient: a prospective randomized study. Int J Infect Dis. 2011;15(5):e350–e6.
61. Morrissey CO, Chen SC, Sorrell TC, et al. Galactomannan and PCR versus culture and histology for directing use of antifungal treatment for invasive aspergillosis in high-risk haematology patients: a randomised controlled trial. Lancet Infect Dis. 2013;13(6):519–28.
62. Aguilar-Guisado M, Martín-Peña A, Espigado I, de Pipaon MRP, de la Cruz F. Universal antifungal therapy is not needed in persistent febrile neutropenia: a tailored diagnostic and therapeutic approach. Haematologica. 2011;97(3):464–71.
63. Girmenia C, Micozzi A, Gentile G, et al. Clinically driven diagnostic antifungal approach in neutropenic patients: a prospective feasibility study. J Clin Oncol. 2009;28(4):667–74.
64. Ng T-Y, Kang M-L, Tan B-H, CC-L N. Case report: enteral nutritional supplement as a likely cause of false-positive galactomannan testing. Med Mycol Case Rep. 2014;3:11–3.
65. Kimura S-i, Akahoshi Y, Nakano H, et al. False-positive Aspergillus galactomannan and its kinetics in allogeneic hematopoietic stem cell transplantation. J Infect. 2015;70(5):520–40.
66. Horie M, Tamiya H, Goto Y, et al. Nonspecific elevation of serum Aspergillus galactomannan antigen levels in patients with rheumatoid arthritis. Respir Investig. 2016;54(1):44–9.
67. Zheng J, Gui X, Cao Q, et al. A clinical study of acquired immunodeficiency syndrome associated Penicillium marneffei infection from a non-endemic area in China. PLoS One. 2015;10(6):e0130376.
68. Worasilchai N, Leelahavanichkul A, Kanjanabuch T, et al. (1→3)-β-d-glucan and galactomannan testing for the diagnosis of fungal peritonitis in peritoneal dialysis patients, a pilot study. Med Mycol. 2015;53(4):338–46.
69. Park S, Kim SH, Choi SH, et al. Clinical and radiological features of invasive pulmonary aspergillosis in transplant recipients and neutropenic patients. Transpl Infect Dis. 2010;12(4):309–15.
70. Lee Y, Choi Y, Lee K, Jeon S, Park C, Heo J. CT halo sign: the spectrum of pulmonary diseases. Br J Radiol. 2005;78(933):862–5.
71. Kim S-H, Kim MY, Hong SI, et al. Invasive pulmonary aspergillosis-mimicking tuberculosis. Clin Infect Dis. 2015;61(1):9–17.
72. Cornely OA, Maertens J, Winston DJ, et al. Posaconazole vs. fluconazole or itraconazole prophylaxis in patients with neutropenia. N Engl J Med. 2007;356(4):348–59.

73. Ullmann AJ, Lipton JH, Vesole DH, et al. Posaconazole or fluconazole for prophylaxis in severe graft-versus-host disease. N Engl J Med. 2007;356(4):335–47.
74. Wingard JR, Carter SL, Walsh TJ, et al. Randomized double-blind trial of fluconazole versus voriconazole for prevention of invasive fungal infection (IFI) after allo hematopoietic cell transplantation (HCT). Blood. 2010;116(24):5111–8.
75. Huang X, Chen H, Han M, et al. Multicenter, randomized, open-label study comparing the efficacy and safety of micafungin versus itraconazole for prophylaxis of invasive fungal infections in patients undergoing hematopoietic stem cell transplant. Biol Blood Marrow Transplant. 2012;18(10):1509–16.
76. Wong G-C, Halim NAA, Tan B-H. Antifungal prophylaxis with posaconazole is effective in preventing invasive fungal infections in acute myeloid leukemia patients during induction and salvage chemotherapy. Clin Infect Dis. 2015;61(8):1351–2.
77. Jeong SH, Kim DY, Jang JH, et al. Efficacy and safety of micafungin versus intravenous itraconazole as empirical antifungal therapy for febrile neutropenic patients with hematological malignancies: a randomized, controlled, prospective, multicenter study. Ann Hematol. 2016;95(2):337–44.
78. Perkhofer S, Lass-Flörl C, Hell M, et al. The Nationwide Austrian Aspergillus registry: a prospective data collection on epidemiology, therapy and outcome of invasive mould infections in immunocompromised and/or immunosuppressed patients. Int J Antimicrob Agents. 2010;36(6):531–6.
79. Kung H-C, Huang P-Y, Chen W-T, et al. 2016 guidelines for the use of antifungal agents in patients with invasive fungal diseases in Taiwan. J Microbiol Immunol Infect. 2017;51(1):1–17.
80. Ashbee HR, Barnes RA, Johnson EM, Richardson MD, Gorton R, Hope WW. Therapeutic drug monitoring (TDM) of antifungal agents: guidelines from the British Society for Medical Mycology. J Antimicrob Chemother. 2013;69(5):1162–76.
81. Pascual A, Calandra T, Bolay S, Buclin T, Bille J, Marchetti O. Voriconazole therapeutic drug monitoring in patients with invasive mycoses improves efficacy and safety outcomes. Clin Infect Dis. 2008;46(2):201–11.
82. Dekkers BG, Bakker M, van der Elst KC, et al. Therapeutic drug monitoring of posaconazole: an update. Curr Fungal Infect Rep. 2016;10(2):51–61.
83. Trifilio S, Ortiz R, Pennick G, et al. Voriconazole therapeutic drug monitoring in allogeneic hematopoietic stem cell transplant recipients. Bone Marrow Transplant. 2005;35(5):509.
84. Shimizu T, Ochiai H, Åsell F, et al. Bioinformatics research on inter-racial difference in drug metabolism I. analysis on frequencies of mutant alleles and poor metabolizers on CYP2D6 and CYP2C19. Drug Metab Pharmacokinet. 2003;18(1):48–70.
85. Park WB, Kim N-H, Kim K-H, et al. The effect of therapeutic drug monitoring on safety and efficacy of voriconazole in invasive fungal infections: a randomized controlled trial. Clin Infect Dis. 2012;55(8):1080–7.
86. Mihăilă R-G. Voriconazole and the liver. World J Hepatol. 2015;7(14):1828.

Cryptococcosis in Asia

18

O. C. Abraham

18.1 Introduction

Human cryptococcosis is caused by encapsulated basidiomycetous yeast *Cryptococcus neoformans*, and less frequently by *C. gatti*. Both species are ubiquitously distributed in the environment, and can be isolated from the bark of a wide variety of tree species; and from other organic matter, notably, bird feces. They are typically opportunistic pathogens. Primary infection, acquired by inhalation, is most often asymptomatic. This is followed by hematogenous dissemination, which occurs primarily in hosts with defective cell-mediated immune responses (e.g., HIV infection, solid organ and stem cell transplant recipients, etc.). Cryptococcal meningitis (CM), the commonest clinical manifestation of cryptococcosis, is potentially fatal, accounting for 15% of AIDS-associated deaths.

18.2 Epidemiology: Global and Asian

Rajasingham et al. estimated that there were 223,100 (95% CI 150,600–282,400) incident cases, and 181,000 (95% CI 119,400–234,300) deaths due to CM globally in 2014 [1]. Sub-Saharan Africa had the highest burden, accounting for 73% of these cases and 75% of the deaths.

An earlier study had estimated an yearly incidence of 120,000 cases and 66,000 deaths due to CM in South and Southeast Asia [2].

The average global cryptococcal antigenemia prevalence is estimated to be 6.0% (95% CI 5.8–6.2) among PLHIV with CD4+ T-lymphocyte counts <100 cells/mm^3.

O. C. Abraham (✉)
Department of Medicine and Infectious Diseases, Christian Medical College, Vellore, Tamil Nadu, India
e-mail: ocabraham@cmcvellore.ac.in

A. Chakrabarti (ed.), *Clinical Practice of Medical Mycology in Asia*,
https://doi.org/10.1007/978-981-13-9459-1_18

Table 18.1 Prevalence of cryptococcal antigenemia in Asian PLHIV

Country	Prevalence (95% CI) (%)	Population	Reference
India	8 (4–12)	Age > 18 years CD4 < 100	Kadam, Indian J Med Microbiol 2017 [3]
India	3 (NA)	ART naïve adults CD4 < 100	Anuradha, J Assoc Physicians India 2017 [4]
Vietnam	6 (3–11)	ART naïve CD4 < 100	Smith, PLoS ONE 2013 [5]
Thailand	11 (NA)	Women initiating ART CD4 < 100	Kwan, J Int Assoc Provid AIDS Care 2014 [6]
Thailand	13 (NA)	PLHIV with ARI	Harris, Clin Infect Dis 2012 [7]
Thailand	13 (NA)	PLHIV with ARI	Lindsley, Clin Infect Dis 2011
Thailand	9.2 (NA)	ART naïve	Pongsai, J Infect 2010 [8]

NA not available

The above table summarizes the reported CrAg prevalence among PLHIV in various Asian countries, which is above the global average (Table 18.1).

18.3 Clinical Features

The vast majority of patients with cryptococcosis and CM are immunocompromised due to AIDS, solid organ or stem cell transplantation, long-term steroid use, cirrhosis liver, etc. [9]. Neutralizing anti-interferon-γ autoantibody (nAIGA) associated immunodeficiency is emerging as an important predisposing condition for cryptococcosis in Southeast Asia [10]. CM can also occur in patients with no known causes for immunodeficiency. CM presents as subacute meningo-encephalitis. Common presenting symptoms include headache, fever, and malaise with duration of 7–14 days. Signs of meningeal irritation like neck stiffness and Kernig's sign are uncommonly present among PLHIV with CM. Severe manifestations include coma, which can end fatally. The case fatality rate can be as high as 40–60% despite antifungal treatment in resource-limited settings. Disseminated cryptococcosis can involve virtually any organ system—skin, reticulo-endothelial system, lungs, bones, prostate in men, fungemia, etc. Of these skin manifestations are the most common. Skin involvement (Fig. 18.1) can present as umbilicated papules, nodules, ulcers, and cellulitis (particularly among transplant recipients.)

18.4 Laboratory Diagnosis [9, 11, 12]

Mycological evidence of infection is essential for planning antifungal treatment. Laboratory methods include direct smear, antigen detection, and culture of CSF, blood, bone marrow, biopsy specimens, etc.

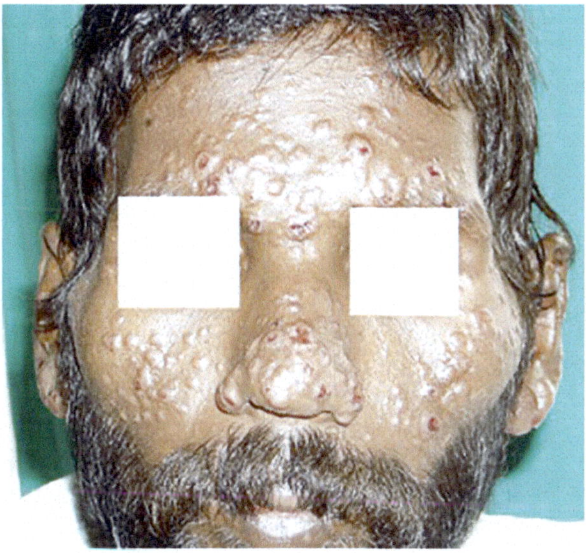

Fig. 18.1 Typical skin lesions in disseminated cryptococcosis among PLHIV - umbilicated papules, some with ulceration

Table 18.2 Comparison of diagnostic tests for CM

Test	Sensitivity	Specificity	Turnaround time	Cost
Culture	Gold standard	Gold standard	Slow	++
India ink smear	86%	100%	Rapid	+
CrAg LFA	99%	99%	Rapid	++

1. Culture is considered the "gold standard" for the diagnosis of CM. The major drawbacks of culture include the need for laboratory infrastructure, skilled personnel, and the turnaround time of up to 4 weeks.
2. India ink smear is quick, easy to perform, inexpensive, and is fairly accurate (sensitivity 86%). However, it may be falsely negative, especially in early stages of CM, when the fungal burden in the CSF is low.
3. Cryptococcal antigen (CrAg): The availability of CrAg lateral flow assay (LFA) has revolutionized the diagnosis of CM in resource-limited setting. This is an immunochromatographic dipstick test, which detects the presence of cryptococcal polysaccharide capsular antigen in serum, plasma, or CSF. This test is very accurate (high sensitivity and specificity), inexpensive, easy to perform, does not need sophisticated laboratory, and has a rapid turnaround time. All these advantages make this test ideal for use as a point-of-care test in resource-limited settings (Table 18.2) [12].

18.5 Treatment

Antifungal treatment: Antifungal treatment in HIV-associated CM is divided into three phases—induction, consolidation, and maintenance [13].

1. Induction: Combination of amphotericin B deoxycholate (1 mg/kg/day i.v.) with flucytosine (25 mg/kg Q6H p.o.) for 7 days (both potent fungicidal drugs), followed by fluconazole (1200 mg/day p.o.) for 7 more days has been shown to have the lowest mortality rate in comparison to amphotericin B with fluconazole and flucytosine with fluconazole in the recently published ACTA trial [14]. This regimen is the preferred treatment option recommended by WHO. The beneficial effect of this regimen is correlated with better clearance of the cryptococcal burden when compared to the other regimes. If flucytosine is not available, amphotericin B with fluconazole for 14 days can be used.

   Both amphotericin B (thrombophlebits, infusion-related toxicities like fever and rigors, hypokalemia, nephrotoxicity, anemia) and flucytosine (bone marrow suppression) are associated with significant toxicity. Using a central venous catheter or rotating the peripheral venous access site every 3 days can reduce thrombophlebitis. Pre-hydration (1 L 0.9% NaCl), potassium supplementation, and frequent monitoring of potassium, creatinine, and hemoglobin are recommended to reduce the incidence of toxicity [13].
2. Consolidation: Fluconazole 800 mg/day p.o. for 8 weeks is recommended [13].
3. Maintenance phase (secondary prophylaxis) of antifungal treatment (fluconazole 200 mg/day p.o.) is continued for at least 1 year on antifungals and antiretroviral treatment (ART), and there is evidence of sustained immunological recovery (CD4+ T-lymphocyte count >200 cells/mm^3 for 12 months) (Table 18.3) [13].

Management of raised intracranial pressure (ICP) [13, 15]: Raised ICP is a common complication, occurring in up to 80% of patients with HIV-associated CM. Raised ICP contributes to increased morbidity and mortality. Elevated ICP is most often characterized by headaches, vomiting, papilledema, reduction of visual acuity, cranial nerve palsy (most commonly cranial nerve VI), confusion, altered mental status, and coma. ICP may be elevated even in the absence of symptoms. Studies have shown that reduction of ICP is associated with improved survival. Therefore, measurement of ICP at the time of initial lumbar puncture (LP) is an

Table 18.3 Antifungal treatment of HIV-associated CM

Phase	Drugs	Duration	Comments
Induction	Ampho B 1 mg/kg/day i.v. + FC 25 mg/kg Q6H p.o. × 7 days, followed by FLU 1200 mg/day p.o. × 7 days	14 days	• Use central venous catheter or rotate infusion site • Monitor Hb, creat, K+ • Pre-hydration: 1 L 0.9% NaCl with 20 mEq KCl daily
Consolidation	FLU 800 mg/day p.o.	8 weeks	
Maintenance	FLU 200 mg/day p.o.	Till immunological recovery	

Ampho B amphotericin B, *FC* flucytosine, *FLU* fluconazole, *Hb* hemoglobin, *creat* creatinine essential part of management of patients with CM. Aggressive reduction of ICP should be done by draining adequate amount of CSF (approximately 20 mL) to lower the pressure to <20 cm CSF (therapeutic LP). Persistent or recurrent symptoms of raised ICP during the initial induction phase of antifungal treatment require daily therapeutic LPs till resolution of symptoms. There are no published studies evaluating the optimal frequency of therapeutic LPs or volume CSF to be drained. Hence, the decision has to be guided by clinical features.

There is no role for drugs like frusemide, acetazolamide, mannitol, or dexamethasone in the management of raised ICP in patients with CM. A randomized trial (which included patients from Vietnam, Thailand, Indonesia, Laos, Uganda, and Malawi) evaluating the role of adjunctive dexamethasone in management of HIV-associated CM showed no benefit, but increased harm in dexamethasone treated patients [16].

Assessing treatment response is by clinical criteria. Adequate response is indicated by resolution of headache, altered mental status, other neurological symptoms, and fever. There is no role for routine LP at the end of induction phase of antifungals to document CSF sterilization in patients who have substantial clinical improvement. Randomized trials have shown that only about 60% of patients have negative cultures at the end of induction therapy. Serial estimation CrAg has also no role in assessment of therapeutic response [13].

Antiretroviral treatment: ART dramatically reduces morbidity and mortality due to HIV infection, and should be started in all ART naïve PLHIV presenting with CM. The COAT trial [17] done in Uganda showed that early ART (started within 2 weeks of the diagnosis of CM) was associated with higher mortality when compared to deferred (5 weeks) ART. A subsequent Cochrane review also concluded that early ART initiation increased mortality compared to delayed ART (RR 1.42, 95% CI 1.02–1.97) [18]. Based on these, WHO recommends initiating ART 4–6 weeks after starting the induction regimen of antifungals.

Cryptococcal immune reconstitution inflammatory syndrome (C-IRIS) can occur in up to 50% patients [19] and typically occurs within 12 weeks of ART initiation, but may occur as late as 1 year following the initial diagnosis. The paradoxical form of C-IRIS presents as a worsening or recurrent meningeal or CNS disease, or at a new anatomic site (e.g., lymph node, lung). Patients present with fever and headache. CSF analysis typically reveals elevated WBC counts, low titers of CrAg and negative culture. Risk factors for C-IRIS include low CD4+ T-lymphocyte counts, very high plasma HIV load, and early initiation of ART. Management of C-IRIS includes continuation of ART and antifungals (consider restarting induction treatment) and a short course of steroids [13].

18.6 Prevention [13]

The best way to prevent CM in PLHIV is early initiation of ART. In patients presenting late (CD4+ T-lymphocyte count <100 cells/mm^3), screening for CrAg and preemptive fluconazole treatment (similar to the induction, consolidation, and maintenance phase of definitive treatment) is recommended for those who test positive. Patients should also be carefully evaluated for clinical features suggestive of CM if the CrAg is positive, and if LP confirms the diagnosis, they should be managed as CM. ART can be initiated after 2 weeks of preemptive antifungal treatment if there is no evidence of CM.

18.7 Conclusions

South and Southeast Asian countries have substantial burden of morbidity and mortality due to HIV-associated CM. The availability of CrAg LFA has been a major advance in the diagnosis of CM. Combination of amphotericin B with flucytosine is the preferred initial treatment due to its ability to sterilize the CSF faster and survival benefit. Screening using CrAg LFA followed by preemptive antifungal treatment is now recommended for all PLHIV with CD4 cell counts below 100 cells/ mm^3 at presentation.

References

1. Rajasingham R, Smith RM, Park BJ, Jarvis JN, Govender NP, Chiller TM, Denning DW, Loyse A, Boulware DR. Global burden of disease of HIV-associated cryptococcal meningitis: an updated analysis. Lancet Infect Dis. 2017;17(8):873–81. https://doi.org/10.1016/S1473-3099(17)30243-8.
2. Park BJ, Wannemuehler KA, Marston BJ, Govender N, Pappas PG, Chiller TM. Estimation of the current global burden of cryptococcal meningitis among persons living with HIV/AIDS. AIDS. 2009;23(4):525–30.
3. Kadam D, Chandanwale A, Bharadwaj R, Nevrekar N, Joshi S, Patil S, Gupte N, Sangle S, Chopade K, Kulkarni V, Balasubramanian U, Suryavanshi N, Jain D, Kanade S, Dharmashale S, Kagal A, Gupta A, Mave V. High prevalence of cryptococcal antigenaemia amongst asymptomatic advanced HIV patients in Pune, India. Indian J Med Microbiol. 2017;35(1):105–8.
4. Anuradha S, Abhaya Narayana H, Dewan R, Kaur R, Rajeshwari K. Asymptomatic cryptococcal antigenemia in people living with HIV (PLHIV) with severe immunosuppression: is routine CrAg screening indicated in India? J Assoc Physicians India. 2017;65(4):14–7.
5. Smith RM, Nguyen TA, Ha HT, Thang PH, Thuy C, Lien TX, Bui HT, Le TH, Struminger B, McConnell MS, Fanfair RN, Park BJ, Harris JR. Prevalence of cryptococcal antigenemia and cost-effectiveness of a cryptococcal antigen screening program—Vietnam. PLoS One. 2013;8(4):e62213.
6. Kwan CK, Leelawiwat W, Intalapaporn P, Anekthananon T, Raengsakulrach B, Peters PJ, McNicholl JM, Park BJ, McConnell MS, Weidle PJ. Utility of cryptococcal antigen screening and evolution of asymptomatic cryptococcal antigenemia among HIV-infected women starting antiretroviral therapy in Thailand. J Int Assoc Provid AIDS Care. 2014;13(5):434–7.
7. Harris JR, Lindsley MD, Henchaichon S, Poonwan N, Naorat S, Prapasiri P, Chantra S, Ruamcharoen F, Chang LS, Chittaganpitch M, Mehta N, Peruski L, Maloney SA, Park BJ, Baggett HC. High prevalence of cryptococcal infection among HIV-infected patients hospitalized with pneumonia in Thailand. Clin Infect Dis. 2012;54(5):e43–50.
8. Pongsai P, Atamasirikul K, Sungkanuparph S. The role of serum cryptococcal antigen screening for the early diagnosis of cryptococcosis in HIV-infected patients with different ranges of CD4 cell counts. J Infect. 2010;60(6):474–7.

9. Williamson PR, Jarvis JN, Panackal AA, Fisher MC, Molloy SF, Loyse A, Harrison TS. Cryptococcal meningitis: epidemiology, immunology, diagnosis and therapy. Nat Rev Neurol. 2017;13(1):13–24.
10. Browne SK, Burbelo PD, Chetchotisakd P, Suputtamongkol Y, Kiertiburanakul S, Shaw PA, Kirk JL, Jutivorakool K, Zaman R, Ding L, Hsu AP, Patel SY, Olivier KN, Lulitanond V, Mootsikapun P, Anunnatsiri S, Angkasekwinai N, Sathapatayavongs B, Hsueh PR, Shieh CC, Brown MR, Thongnoppakhun W, Claypool R, Sampaio EP, Thepthai C, Waywa D, Dacombe C, Reizes Y, Zelazny AM, Saleeb P, Rosen LB, Mo A, Iadarola M, Holland SM. Adult-onset immunodeficiency in Thailand and Taiwan. N Engl J Med. 2012;367(8):725–34.
11. Greene G, Sriruttan C, Le T, Chiller T, Govender NP. Looking for fungi in all the right places: screening for cryptococcal disease and other AIDS-related mycoses among patients with advanced HIV disease. Curr Opin HIV AIDS. 2017;12(2):139–47.
12. Rajasingham R, Wake RM, Beyene T, Katende A, Letang E, Boulware DR. Cryptococcal meningitis diagnostics and screening in the era of point-of-care laboratory testing. J Clin Microbiol. 2019;57(1):e01238-18.
13. Guidelines on the diagnosis, prevention and management of cryptococcal disease in HIV-infected adults, adolescents and children: supplement to the 2016 consolidated guidelines on the use of antiretroviral drugs for treating and preventing HIV infection. Geneva: World Health Organization; 2018.
14. Molloy SF, Kanyama C, Heyderman RS, Loyse A, Kouanfack C, Chanda D, Mfinanga S, Temfack E, Lakhi S, Lesikari S, Chan AK, Stone N, Kalata N, Karunaharan N, Gaskell K, Peirse M, Ellis J, Chawinga C, Lontsi S, Ndong JG, Bright P, Lupiya D, Chen T, Bradley J, Adams J, van der Horst C, van Oosterhout JJ, Sini V, Mapoure YN, Mwaba P, Bicanic T, Lalloo DG, Wang D, Hosseinipour MC, Lortholary O, Jaffar S, Harrison TS, Trial Study Team ACTA. Antifungal combinations for treatment of cryptococcal meningitis in Africa. N Engl J Med. 2018;378(11):1004–17.
15. Oladele RO, Bongomin F, Gago S, Denning DW. HIV-associated cryptococcal disease in resource-limited settings: a case for "prevention is better than cure"? J Fungi (Basel). 2017;3(4).
16. Beardsley J, Wolbers M, Kibengo FM, Ggayi AB, Kamali A, Cuc NT, Binh TQ, Chau NV, Farrar J, Merson L, Phuong L, Thwaites G, Van Kinh N, Thuy PT, Chierakul W, Siriboon S, Thiansukhon E, Onsanit S, Supphamongkholchaikul W, Chan AK, Heyderman R, Mwinjiwa E, van Oosterhout JJ, Imran D, Basri H, Mayxay M, Dance D, Phimmasone P, Rattanavong S, Lalloo DG, Day JN, Investigators CD. Adjunctive dexamethasone in HIV-associated cryptococcal meningitis. N Engl J Med. 2016;374(6):542–54.
17. Boulware DR, Meya DB, Muzoora C, Rolfes MA, Huppler Hullsiek K, Musubire A, Taseera K, Nabeta HW, Schutz C, Williams DA, Rajasingham R, Rhein J, Thienemann F, Lo MW, Nielsen K, Bergemann TL, Kambugu A, Manabe YC, Janoff EN, Bohjanen PR, Meintjes G, Trial Team COAT. Timing of antiretroviral therapy after diagnosis of cryptococcal meningitis. N Engl J Med. 2014;370(26):2487–98.
18. Eshun-Wilson I, Okwen MP, Richardson M, Bicanic T. Early versus delayed antiretroviral treatment in HIV-positive people with cryptococcal meningitis. Cochrane Database Syst Rev. 2018,7.CD009012.
19. Haddow LJ, Colebunders R, Meintjes G, Lawn SD, Elliott JH, Manabe YC, Bohjanen PR, Sungkanuparph S, Easterbrook PJ, French MA, Boulware DR, International Network for the Study of HIV-associated IRIS (INSHI). Cryptococcal immune reconstitution inflammatory syndrome in HIV-1-infected individuals: proposed clinical case definitions. Lancet Infect Dis. 2010;10(11):791–802.

Mucormycosis in Asia

19

Arunaloke Chakrabarti

Key Points

- The prevalence of mucormycosis is very high in Asian countries especially in uncontrolled diabetic patients of China and India. The prevalence of diabetes is also very high in those two countries.
- Though the disease is also prevalent in patients with hematological malignancies under chemotherapy and transplant recipients, large number of cases in diabetics overshadow those risk factors.
- In a recent prospective multicenter study from Indian ICUs, mucormycosis reported in 24% of all invasive mold infections.
- Isolated renal mucormycosis in apparently healthy hosts is an intriguing disease in China and India.
- Isolated renal mucormycosis may be suspected in patients with fever, flank pain, hematuria/anuria with imaging shows enlarged kidney with hypo-echoic shadow and cortical rim sign.
- Spectrum of *Mucorales* causing the disease is also wide and many new agents have been reported causing mucormycosis from this part of the world.
- Identification of the agent is important, as susceptibility varies among the strains and species.
- Rhino-cerebral and cutaneous mucormycosis are easier to diagnose due to ease of sampling.
- The diagnosis of pulmonary mucormycosis may improve with imaging guided needle biopsy and endobronchial ultrasound bronchoscocpy (EBUS) techniques.
- The diagnosis of gastrointestinal mucormycosis is most difficult, more so when the lesion is in lower gut. The disease may be suspected in premature baby with shock, metabolic acidosis, and abdominal distension. In other patients, when the patient presents with fever, abdominal distension, and gastrointestinal bleed.

A. Chakrabarti (✉)
Department of Medical Microbiology, Postgraduate Institute of Medical Education and Research (PGIMER), Chandigarh, India

A. Chakrabarti (ed.), *Clinical Practice of Medical Mycology in Asia*,
https://doi.org/10.1007/978-981-13-9459-1_19

- In the laboratory, tissue should not be ground as the fungus is very friable. Despite all precaution, culture fails in nearly 50% cases. Molecular techniques or MALDI-TOF may be utilized to identify the fungus. If not available in local laboratory, send the sample to reference laboratory.
- Multi-modality management at the earliest is essential, as the disease is also called "Fungal emergency." The management includes surgery, antifungal drug, minimizing immunosuppression/controlling diabetes, and if required immune-potentiation.
- Aggressive and extensive debridement is essential.
- Lipid preparation of amphotericin B is the first-line therapy and in neurological involvement liposomal preparation should be used. Avoid slow escalation of amphotericin B dose. Salvage therapy includes posaconazole and isavuconazole.
- Hyperbaric oxygen, deferasirox, and combination therapy may be used in desperate situation but requires randomized control trial to confirm their efficacy.

19.1 Introduction

Mucormycosis, a polymorphic disease, is caused by the fungi classified under the order *Mucorales*. The disease is considered as a "fungal emergency" as the fungus often leads to devastation by causing thrombosis, infarction, and necrosis in the vital organs. In spite of active management, the mortality due to mucormycosis remains high (>50%) [1–3].

The disease was earlier known as zygomycosis, as the order *Mucorales* was classified under so-called class *Zygomycetes* and phylum *Zygomycota*. Medically important fungi were classified under two orders (*Mucorales* and *Entomophthorales*) and class *Zygomycetes*. With the development of molecular technique, the classification of the *Zygomycota* has undergone many changes. The latest classification has put medically important fungi under phylum—*Glomeromycota* with two sub-phylum—*Mucormycotina* and *Entomophthoromycotina* [4]. The fungi under *Mucormycotina* produce rapidly progressive acute inflammatory disease (mucormycosis) in contrast to fungi under *Entomophthoromycotina*, which is responsible for slow progressive granulomatous disease (entomophthoromycosis). The causative agents, clinical course, pathology, and management of both diseases are different (Table 19.1), and the experts prefer to keep the two disease mucormycosis and entomophthoromycosis separate instead of clubbing together under the name zygomycosis.

Entomophthoromycosis is prevalent in India, China, Saudi Arabia and Thailand. The disease is restricted to subcutaneous tissues though occasionally it can lead to systemic manifestations especially gastrointestinal basidiobolomycosis. Many cases of gastrointestinal basidiobolomycosis have been reported from middle-east of Asia. Entomophthoromycosis is described in details under the chapter of "Rare fungal infection in Asia" while the present chapter is restricted to the description of the very aggressive disease, mucormycosis. The fungi in mucormycosis are aseptate/pauci-septate, thin walled, broad, ribbon-shaped hyphae, which are usually soil saprobes and ubiquitous in distribution.

Table 19.1 Difference of entomophthoromycosis and mucormycosis

	Entomophthoromycosis	Mucormycosis
Subphylum Order	*Entomophthoromycotina* *Entomophthorales*	*Mucormycotina* *Mucorales*
Clinical course	Slow progressing	Rapidly progressing
Acquisition	Traumatic implantation	Inhalation/ingestion/iatrogenic
Tissue reaction	Granulomatous, eosinophils, Splender–Hoeppli phenomenon	Acute inflammatory reaction with vascular invasion
Angio-invasion	Rare	Common
Septation in hyphae	Infrequent, when present prominent	Infrequent, less prominent
Susceptible host	Children and young adult (80%—<20 years), immunocompetent	Any age, immunocompromised
Growth	Waxy and folded	Cottony
Spores	Forcibly discharged	Passively discharged
Sequence analysis	Distinct from Mucorales	Distinct from Entomophthorales
Management	Itraconazole, potassium iodide (KI), amphotericin B, terbinafine, voriconazole	Surgery, amphotericin B & posaconazole, reversal of immunosuppression

19.2 Epidemiology

19.2.1 Incidence/Prevalence

Arnold Paltanf in 1885 first reported the disease as "mycosis mucorina" from Austria [5]. Though known for a long time, it was considered as a rare disease. In recent years, the disease is increasingly reported in patients with hematological malignancies undergoing chemotherapy, transplant recipients, uncontrolled diabetes, iron overload, prematurity, and malnutrition [1–3, 6, 7]. The paucity of information about the disease is a challenge to describe the detailed epidemiology. In an autopsy study from MD Anderson Centre, USA, documented a rise in the incidence of mucormycosis in hematological malignancy patients from 0.006 cases per 100 autopsies in 1989–1993 to 0.018 cases in 2004–2008 [8]. The prevalence of mucormycosis related hospitalizations was estimated at 0.12 per 10,000 discharges among 104 million patients in 560 hospitals of the United States from January 2005 to June 2014 [9]. Population surveillance studies from Spain and California reported mucormycosis at 0.4–1.7 cases per million population per year [10, 11]. Country wise data from France reported a rise in mucormycosis cases from 0.7 in 1997 to 1.2 cases/million populations in 2006 [12]. Hematological malignancies (22–44%) and bone marrow transplant patients (5–9%) are major risk factors for the disease in Europe and the USA [1, 2, 13, 14].

In comparison to western world, the rise in mucormycosis cases in Asian countries is much higher. A recent study from a tertiary-care center in India reported a rise of mucormycosis cases from 24.7 cases per year (1990–2007) to 89 cases per year (2013–2015) [15]. Mucormycosis has been reported at 24% of all invasive mold infections in a multi-center study on patients in intensive care unit (ICU) [16]. A rising trend of mucormycosis from 9.7% in 2008 to 23.7% in 2014 has also been reported from Iran [17]. The rise from 0.01% mucormycosis cases in 1969 to 0.16% of cases in 1989 in national medical autopsy survey of Japan is also significant [18].

Though mucormycosis is commonly known as community acquired disease, nosocomial infections have been reported in recent years. In such patients the infection is acquired from hospital environment having high load of fungal spore after construction activities or from health-care-related procedures using elastoplasts, wooden tongue depressor, osteotomy bag, or drainage catheters [19]. An outbreak of gastrointestinal mucormycosis has been reported in a hospital of China where the primary source of possible contaminating fungus was found in cornstarch used in manufacturing allopurinol tablet and ready-to-eat food [20].

Mucormycosis is classified clinically into different types depending on anatomical localization: rhino-orbito-cerebral, pulmonary, gastrointestinal, cutaneous, and disseminated types. The clinical types are often linked with specific underlying illness like rhino-orbito-cerebral types to diabetic ketoacidosis; pulmonary and disseminated varieties to acute leukemia, transplantation, and desferoxamine therapy; gastrointestinal to prematurity and malnutrition, and cutaneous lesion to trauma or burn [14].

The fungi causing mucormycosis usually thrive well on decaying organic matter, vegetation, and soil. Seasonal variation of temperature, wind, and humidity possibly play an important role in the growth of fungi, as the disease is more prevalent in autumn months in Israel and Japan and post-monsoon and autumn seasons in India [21–24]. High incidence of cutaneous mucormycosis has been reported after tsunami or hurricanes in affected areas.

19.3 Underlying Illness/Risk Factors

19.3.1 Hematological Malignancy and Hematopoietic Stem Cell Transplant (HSCT)

- Increase in incidence has been reported from many centers. At MD Anderson Centre, USA—the rise is from 8/100,000 admission in 1989–1993 to 20 cases/100,000 admission in 1994–1998 [25].
- Among hematological malignancies acute myeloid leukemia patients are more prone (1–8%) to develop the disease [25].
- HSCT—important risk factor for pulmonary mucormycosis, the incidence vary at 0.9–2% [1], but TRANSNET data showed higher rate (8%) [26]; annual incidence increased to 15% in France and Belgium [12, 27].
- Autopsy data from patients with hematological malignancy reported mucormycosis at a rate of 7% of all fungal infections [28].
- Mucormycosis is prevalent in prolonged (>3 week) and severe (<200/mm^3) neutropenia, monocytopenia (<100/mm^3), prolonged high dose of corticosteroids (prednisone >1 mg/kg/day), iron overload, high-risk stem cell transplant

(matched unrelated donor, haploidentical donor, cord blood, T-cell depleted SCT), severe GVHD and its treatment (especially corticosteroids), prolonged hyperglycemia, (fasting >200 mg/dL), colonization or heavy environmental exposure, previous exposure to *Aspergillus*-active antifungal agents (voriconazole, echinocandins), and relapsed leukemia [29].

- Comparing the risk factors of invasive aspergillosis and mucormycosis, voriconazole prophylaxis and paranasal sinus involvement significantly associated with mucormycosis in multivariate analysis; and additionally malnutrition and diabetes in univariate analysis [8].
- Clinical types: pulmonary mucormycosis is the commonest presentation followed by rhino-orbito-cerebral and cutaneous type [14].
- Mortality rates of 65% in patients with hematological malignancy and 90% in HSCT patients have been reported [30].

19.3.2 Solid Organ Transplant

- Incidence of mucormycosis at lower rate (0.2–3%) compared to HSCT but recent studies reported higher incidence (0.4–16%) [31].
- Confounding factors: Diabetes mellitus, renal failure at baseline, prior voriconazole/echinocandin use [32].
- Tacrolimus use in these patients minimizes the chance of mucormycosis, as tacrolimus possibly has anti-mucor activity [32].
- Pulmonary mucormycosis is the most common presentation followed by sinus involvement [14].

19.3.3 Diabetes

- Formidable risk factor in developing countries.
- Mucormycosis has been reported as diabetes-defining illness in 16–23% patients in Asian countries [2, 7].
- More common in ketoacidosis state [2, 6, 7].
- High risk in steroid induced diabetes in patients with hematological malignancy and transplant recipients.
- It is claimed that the incidence of mucormycosis in diabetes has come down in the USA due to use of statins and statin has anti-cancer property [33].
- Possible pathogenic mechanism in diabetes for development of mucormycosis—defective phagocytic function, impaired neutrophilic activation, impairment of iron binding, and transportation leading to more availability of iron for mucoraceous fungi. Iron helps in growth of fungi [6, 7].
- Rhino-orbito-cerebral type is the commonest presentation in these patients followed by pulmonary and cutaneous mucormycosis [6, 7, 14].
- Mortality in these patients is much less (~40%) compared to hematological malignancy and HSCT [2, 14].

19.3.4 Deferoxamine Therapy

- Disseminated mucormycosis is the most common form of presentation in these patients followed by lung involvement.
- Mortality is very high at ~80% [34].
- Iron overload in any form increases the risk of mucormycosis.
- Direct relation with deferoxamine use—78% of dialysis recipients with mucormycosis were reported to have deferoxamine [35].
- Chelated and free iron gets attached to siderophore of mucoraceous fungi and helps in growth of fungi.
- Contrasting fact—the children with hemoglobinopathies are not reported to be at higher risk for mucormycosis despite deferoxamine use.

19.3.5 Voriconazole/Echinocandins Use

- Possibly mucormycosis is a breakthrough infection in these patents [36].
- Mucoraceous fungi possibly become more virulent after voriconazole exposure, as was shown in fly and mouse models [37].
- Both sinus and pulmonary mucormycosis have been observed [14].
- More studies are required to confirm the role of antifungal agents in breakthrough infection, as echinocandins in combination with liposomal amphotericin B played the role of anti-mucor agents in animal studies.

19.3.6 Prematurity

- Gastrointestinal mucormycosis is a common presentation in these neonates or children [6, 7].
- Possibly the replacement of normal bacterial biota by ingested spore predisposes mucormycosis.
- Diagnosis of gastrointestinal mucormycosis is mostly accidental or at postmortem due to lack of clinical suspicion and difficulty in diagnosis.

19.3.7 Break in Cutaneous Barrier

- Trauma, burn, intravenous drug abuse can cause mucormycosis even in immunocompetent host [1, 2, 6, 7].
- Trauma, burn cause cutaneous mucormycosis and intravenous drug abuse lead to cerebral mucormycosis.

19.3.8 Miscellaneous

- Steroid use, alcoholic chronic liver disease, renal failure, metabolic acidosis, and prolonged stay in intensive care units are claimed to be either risk or confounding factors in development of mucormycosis [7].

19.3.9 Agents

Rhizopus oryzae is the most common agent causing mucormycosis in all studies. Other species like *Rhizopus microsporus, Lichtheimia* (previously called *Absidia*) *corymbifera, Mucor circinelloides, and Rhizomucor pusillus* are the next common agents. *Apophysomyces variabilis, Saksenaea vasiformis, Cunninghamella bertholletiae, Syncephalastrum racemosum, and Cokeromyces recurvatus* have been isolated rarely. However, the spectrum of mucoraceous fungi, causing mucormycosis vary geographically. *Apophysomyces variabilis* and *Saksenaea vasiformis* have been reported mainly from India and *Cunninghamella bertholletiae* from the USA.

19.3.10 Mucormycosis in Asia

Majority cases of mucormycosis in Asia have been reported from India. Few case series have been reported from Taiwan, Korea, Indonesia, and Japan. In Japan, nation-wide autopsy series reported mucormycosis at 0.1% of all autopsy cases and 4% of all invasive fungal infections [18]. Compared to that, in an Indian hospital, mucormycosis was seen at a six times higher rate—0.6% of all autopsy cases and 23% of all invasive fungal infections. This indicates a very high prevalence of mucormycosis in India especially associated with uncontrolled diabetes. Though the association of diabetes has been shown also in the series from Japan and Taiwan, it is overwhelming in India and overshadows all other risk factors. In a series of 22,316 consecutive diabetes cases screened in India, mucormycosis was reported at a rate of 1.6 cases/1000 diabetics [38]. A computational-based approach estimated the prevalence of mucormycosis at 140 cases per million populations in India, with prevalence ranged between 137,807 cases to 208,177 with the mean of 171,504 (SD: 12,365.6; 95% CI: 195,777–147,688) and a mean attributable mortality at 65,500 (38.2%) per year [39].

The majority people of Asian countries avoid seeking regular health checkup due to poor infrastructure and economic constraints. It is reflected in the fact that considerable (23–43%) proportion of mucormycosis patients was unaware of background diabetes before diagnosis for mucormycosis [6, 7]. In those patients, mucormycosis acted as diabetes-defining illness. The mean informed duration of diabetes was 6.7 ± 4.6 years before acquiring mucormycosis. The majority of patients with rhino-orbito-cerebral types have uncontrolled diabetes as underlying disease. However, diabetes has been associated as confounding factor in other clinical types as well, except renal mucormycosis. As the patients attend the hospital late in the course of disease, the patients with rhino-orbito-cerebral type present frequently with classical orbital (>80%) and intracranial extension (20%).

In disseminated mucormycosis, kidney is involved in ~20% of patients and isolated kidney involvement cases are rare. However, in India and China, a distinct group of population has been reported with isolated kidney involvement. The patients are young and immunocompetent. They develop acute progressive disease with loin pain, fever, hematuria, or anuria and on imaging unilateral or bilateral enlarged non-hydronephrotic kidneys with hypodensities, cortical rim sign are visualized. These cases were diagnosed only on postmortem initially but, with the increase in awareness and characteristic radiological observations, most of the cases are now diagnosed antemortem [40]. Mortality still remains high (~50%) in these cases despite active management. It is not clear, how the patients acquire renal mucormycosis. In a recent study, bladder involvement in occasional cases predicts ascending infection. However, majority experts believe the acquisition is through pulmonary route. After innocuous lesion in lung, the fungi possibly get the opportunity to invade the blood vessels and reach kidney. More studies are required to prove either hypothesis. Contrary to India, 70% of the adult renal mucormycosis patients in China have intravenous drug abuse, diabetes, steroid therapy, and kidney transplantation as risk factor or underlying disease [7, 41, 42].

Due to congenial weather condition, many mucoraceous fungi thrive well in the environment of Asian countries. The spectrum of agents causing mucormycosis is also wide. *Rhizopus arrhizus* is the most common agent isolated from these patients. *Apophysomyces variabilis* is the second frequent agent from Indian hospitals and India accounts for approximately 60% of the documented mucormycosis cases due to *Apophysomyces* species. The fungus is known to produce cutaneous and subcutaneous disease in immunocompetent patients. It is believed that contamination of wound with soil following trauma or accident is the common mode of acquisition of *Apophysomyces* species. However, this agent has been isolated from rhino-orbito-cerberal, renal, and disseminated mucormycosis as well. The mode of entry in those patients is not clear [15, 43, 44]. *R. microsporus* and *R. homothallicus* are the new emerging species in India. *R. homothallicus* has been reported from few cases of pulmonary mucormycosis with cavitary lesions [15, 45]. A detailed ecological study in India showed an abundant presence of diverse *Mucorales* species including *Apophysomyces variabilis* and *Rhizopus homothallicus* in soils [46]. Other rare mucoraceous fungi isolated from clinical samples includes *Saksenaea vasiformis, Rhizopus homothallicus, Mucor irregularis, Thamnostylum lucknowense, Syncephalastrum racemosum,* and *Cunninghamella bertholletiae. S. vasiformis* has been reported to cause necrotizing fasciitis. *T. lucknowense* has been reported to cause rhino-orbital mucormycosis [47]. *Mucor irregularis* (*Rhizomucor variabilis*) has been reported from multiple cases of cutaneous mucormycosis in China, mainly from Jiangsu, Shandong & Hebei, and Shaanxi provinces. The farmers acquire this lesion in exposed area of the body, commonly on the face, after innocuous trauma, insect bite, or surgery. The same agent has been isolated recently from a patient with sinus mucormycosis in India; hence, the agent may not be only China specific [48, 49].

19.3.11 Diagnostic Challenge

The major diagnostic challenge in mucormycosis is suspicion of the disease and collection of material from deep tissues while the patient is neutropenic and thrombocytopenic. Lack of serological and molecular diagnosis makes conventional techniques the only available method of diagnosis in mucormycosis. Conventional techniques include direct microscopy and histopathology of specimen and isolation of fungi. In patients with rhino-orbito-cereberal and cutaneous mucormycosis, the sample collection may be relatively easier, but it is difficult in other form of mucormycosis. However, after fresh plasma or platelet infusion, invasive procedure like fluoroscopy guided fine needle aspirations has improved the chance of antemortem diagnosis in pulmonary mucormycosis. A considerable number of mucormycosis cases are still diagnosed only postmortem. Direct microscopy using optical brightener and histopathology are strongly recommended for early diagnosis of mucormycosis. Demonstration of 6–25 μm, non-septate or pauci-septate, hyaline, and ribbon-like hyphae on direct microscopy helps to presumptively diagnose mucormycosis [50]. Occasionally, presence of small hyphal segments without characteristics hyphae may create problem in diagnosis. Immunohistochemistry using monoclonal antibody or extraction of DNA from specimen and sequencing may help in confirmation of such cases [51, 52].The yield of fungal DNA from fresh tissue is better than formalin-fixed paraffin-embedded tissue [53, 54]. Isolation of fungi may not be possible in all cases due to aseptate, thin, and fragile hyphae of mucoraceous fungi. While processing a sample for culture, the tissue should be minced with sterile scissor to avoid damage to hyphae. Isolation of mucoraceous fungi from non-sterile respiratory sample in an immunosuppressed patient may qualify a patient for probable mucormycosis according to EORTC-MSG guideline.

Imaging may help in suspicion of mucormycosis especially when reverse halo sign, more than 10 nodular infiltrates, and pleural effusion are present. But such characteristics findings are only occasionally visible and present in immunosuppressed patients [55, 56]. In such cases, biopsy or fine needle aspiration should be actively pursued. Pleural effusion may independently predict mucormycosis. In the absence of any known biomarker, a negative galactomannan test may increase the suspicion for mucormycosis, as patients with aspergillosis and mucormycosis have similar risk factors.

19.3.12 Treatment Challenges

The management of mucormycosis has major problems due to aggressive nature of the disease and associated serious life-threatening underlying diseases [57]. The four principles of management of mucormycosis are:

- Aggressive surgery wherever possible to minimize fungal load and to remove necrosed tissue so that antifungal drug may reach the site of fungal infection.

Antifungal drugs—Amphotericin B, posaconazole, and isavuconazole (a new water soluble azole drug, may be available soon in Asian market) have anti-mucor activity though variation of activity of these agents is reported among species and isolates; early initiation of lipid formulations of amphotericin B at high dose (3–5 mg/kg/day) is recommended to treat mucormycosis. There is no clear recommendation for the duration of antifungal therapy [29]. Conventional amphotericin B deoxycholate may be used in resource limited situation despite its nephrotoxicity; posaconazole and isavuconazole are used as salvage therapy or as maintenance therapy after containment of infection following amphotericin B therapy. Echinocandins in combination with liposomal amphotericin B have shown beneficial role in animal study, but no strong evidence has been noted in human infections as yet. The new iron chelator deferasirox has anti-mucor activity as reported in animal study, but there is no supportive evidence in human infections, rather DEFEAT study revealed contrary evidence [58, 59]. The study had many shortcomings and certain centers in India have used deferasirox with some success [60]. A control trial is required to confirm its role in either way.

Reversal of risk factors—control of diabetes, reduction of steroid dose to minimum requirement, recovery of neutropenia after granulocyte transfusion, or using growth factors (G-CSF/GM-CSF) play important supportive role during management of mucormycosis.

Improvement of immune function—γ interferon may improve immunity [61].

Due to low incidence of mucormycosis, the role of prophylaxis is not clear. However, posaconazole as prophylaxis may be used in high-risk groups like GVHD with augmented immunosuppression or in outbreak situation. The use of empiric therapy in fever-driven approach is controversial and there is no strong recommendation unless a high incidence of mucormycosis is expected. The adjunctive treatments like hyperbaric oxygen, lovastatin have been used in certain situation, but no clear recommendation is yet available.

19.4 Conclusion

The epidemiology of mucormycosis of the two worlds (Western and Asian) is different. Very high incidence, diabetes as predominant risk factor, isolated renal mucormycosis as a new clinical entity, wide spectrum of mucoraceous fungal etiology are the distinct characters of mucormycosis in Asia. Despite active intervention the mortality in mucormycosis remains high. A high index of suspicion and invasive diagnostic procedures may possibly help in early diagnosis and effective management of this disease. More studies are required to overcome the gap in knowledge of mucormycosis.

When to Suspect Mucormycosis?

- High suspicion in centers having high rate
- In patients with suspicion of invasive fungal infection
  - When galactomannan is negative
  - When beta-glucan is negative, though the issue is not clear
  - When the patient is on voriconazole/echinocandin therapy—breakthrough infection.
  - Eschar in nose, face, skin with surrounding erythema and induration, necrotic lesion on hard palate
  - Acute and aggregative vascular event
  - CT scan of paranasal sinuses showing lesions in sinuses, orbit and brain
  - Nasal—aggressive bone destruction
  - Chest CT—multiple nodule, reverse halo organ, pleural effusion
  - Abdomen—enlarged and infracted kidney
- Rhino-cerebral disease
  - Uncontrolled diabetes with diplopia, cranial nerve palsy, sinus pain, proptosis, orbital apex syndrome, palatine ulcer
- Pulmonary disease
  - Nonproductive cough, pleural pain
- Renal disease
  - Flank pain, fever, and hematuria/anuria in otherwise healthy individual.

References

1. Petrikkos G, Skiada A, Lortholary O, et al. Epidemiology and clinical manifestations of mucormycosis. Clin Infect Dis. 2012;54(Suppl 1):S23–34.
2. Roden MM, Zaoutis TE, Buchanan WL, et al. Epidemiology and outcome of zygomycosis: a review of 929 reported cases. Clin Infect Dis. 2005;41:634–53.
3. Sugar AM. Agents of mucormycosis and related species. In: Mandell G, Bennett J, Dolin R, editors. Principles and practices of infectious diseases. 4th ed. New York: Churchill Livingstone, 1995. p. 2311–21.
4. Hibbett DS, Binder M, Bischoff JF, et al. A higher-level phylogenetic classification of the Fungi. Mycol Res. 2007;111(Pt 5):509–47.
5. Paltauf A. Mycosis mucorina. Ein Beitrag zur Kenntniss der menschlichen Fadenpilzerkrankungen (sic!). Archiv für pathologische Anatomie. 1885;102:543–64.
6. Chakrabarti A, Das A, Mandal J, et al. The rising trend of invasive zygomycosis in patients with uncontrolled diabetes mellitus. Med Mycol. 2006;44:335–42.
7. Chakrabarti A, Chatterjee SS, Das A, et al. Invasive zygomycosis in India: experience in a tertiary care hospital. Postgrad Med J. 2009;85:573–81.
8. Lewis RE, Cahyame-Zuniga L, Leventakos K, et al. Epidemiology and sites of involvement of invasive fungal infections in patients with haematological malignancies: a 20-year autopsy study. Mycoses. 2013;56:638–45.

9. Kontoyiannis DP, Yang H, Song J, et al. Prevalence, clinical and economic burden of mucormycosis-related hospitalizations in the United States: a retrospective study. BMC Infect Dis. 2016;16:730.
10. Rees JR, Pinner RW, Hajjeh RA, Brandt ME, Reingold AL. The epidemiological features of invasive mycotic infections in the San Francisco Bay area, 1992–1993: results of population-based laboratory active surveillance. Clin Infect Dis. 1998;27:1138–47.
11. Torres-Narbona M, Guinea J, Martinez-Alarcon J, Pelaez T, Bouza E. In vitro activities of amphotericin B, caspofungin, itraconazole, posaconazole, and voriconazole against 45 clinical isolates of zygomycetes: comparison of CLSI M38-A, Sensititre YeastOne, and the Etest. Antimicrob Agents Chemother. 2007;51:1126–9.
12. Bitar D, Van Cauteren D, Lanternier F, Dannaoui E, Che D, Dromer F, et al. Increasing incidence of zygomycosis (mucormycosis), France, 1997–2006. Emerg Infect Dis. 2009;15:1395–401.
13. Lanternier F, Dannaoui E, Morizot G, Elie C, Garcia-Hermoso D, Huerre M, et al. A global analysis of mucormycosis in France: the RetroZygo Study (2005–2007). Clin Infect Dis. 2012;54(Suppl 1):S35–43.
14. Ribes JA, Vanover-Sams CL, Baker DJ. Zygomycetes in human disease. Clin Microbiol Rev. 2000;13:236–301.
15. Prakash H, Ghosh AK, Rudramurthy SM, et al. A prospective multicenter study on mucormycosis in India: epidemiology, diagnosis, and treatment. Med Mycol. 2019;57(4):395–402. https://doi.org/10.1093/mmy/myy060.
16. Chakrabarti A, Kaur H, Savio J, et al. Epidemiology and clinical outcomes of invasive mould infections in Indian intensive care units (FISF study). J Crit Care. 2019;5:64–70.
17. Dolatabadi S, Ahmadi B, Rezaei-Matehkolaei A, et al. Mucormycosis in Iran: a six-year retrospective experience. J Mycol Med. 2018;28:269–73.
18. Yamazaki T, Kume H, Murase S, Yamashita E, Arisawa M. Epidemiology of visceral mycoses: analysis of data in annual of the pathological autopsy cases in Japan. J Clin Microbiol. 1999;37:1732–8.
19. Rammaert B, Lanternier F, Zahar JR, et al. Healthcare-associated mucormycosis. Clin Infect Dis. 2012;54(Suppl 1):S44–54.
20. Cheng VC, Chan JF, Ngan AH, et al. Outbreak of intestinal infection due to Rhizopus microsporus. J Clin Microbiol. 2009;47:2834–43.
21. Al-Ajam MR, Bizri AR, Mokhbat J, et al. Mucormycosis in the Eastern Mediterranean: a seasonal disease. Epidemiol Infect. 2006;134:341–6.
22. Funada H, Matsuda T. Pulmonary mucormycosis in a hematology ward. Intern Med. 1996;35:540–4.
23. Shpitzer T, Keller N, Wolf M, et al. Seasonal variations in rhino-cerebral Mucor infection. Ann Otol Rhinol Laryngol. 2005;114:695–8.
24. Nithyanandam S, Jacob MS, Battu RR, et al. Rhino-orbito-cerebral mucormycosis. A retrospective analysis of clinical features and treatment outcomes. Indian J Ophthalmol. 2003;51:231–6.
25. Kontoyiannis DP, Wessel VC, Bodey GP, Rolston KV. Zygomycosis in the 1990s in a tertiary-care cancer center. Clin Infect Dis. 2000;30:851–6.
26. Pappas PG, Alexander BD, Andes DR, et al. Invasive fungal infections among organ transplant recipients: results of the Transplant-Associated Infection Surveillance Network (TRANSNET). Clin Infect Dis. 2010;50:1101–11.
27. Saegeman V, Maertens J, Meersseman W, Spriet I, Verbeken E, Lagrou K. Increasing incidence of mucormycosis in University Hospital, Belgium. Emerg Infect Dis. 2010;16:1456–8.
28. Chamilos G, Luna M, Lewis RE, Bodey GP, Chemaly R, Tarrand JJ, et al. Invasive fungal infections in patients with hematologic malignancies in a tertiary care cancer center: an autopsy study over a 15-year period (1989–2003). Haematologica. 2006;91:986–9.
29. Kontoyiannis DP, Lewis RE. How I treat mucormycosis. Blood. 2011;118:1216–24.
30. Spellberg B, Ibrahim AS. Recent advances in the treatment of mucormycosis. Curr Infect Dis Rep. 2010;12:423–9.
31. Lanternier F, Sun HY, Ribaud P, Singh N, Kontoyiannis DP, Lortholary O. Mucormycosis in organ and stem cell transplant recipients. Clin Infect Dis. 2012;54:1629–36.

32. Singh N, Aguado JM, Bonatti H, Forrest G, Gupta KL, Safdar N, et al. Zygomycosis in solid organ transplant recipients: a prospective, matched case-control study to assess risks for disease and outcome. J Infect Dis. 2009;200:1002–11.
33. Kontoyiannis DP. Decrease in the number of reported cases of zygomycosis among patients with diabetes mellitus: a hypothesis. Clin Infect Dis. 2007;44:1089–90.
34. Torres-Narbona M, Guinea J, Martínez-Alarcón J, Muñoz P, Gadea I, Bouza E, MYCOMED Zygomycosis Study Group. Impact of zygomycosis on microbiology workload: a survey study in Spain. J Clin Microbiol. 2007;45:2051–3.
35. McNab AA, McKelvie P. Iron overload is a risk factor for zygomycosis. Arch Ophthalmol. 1997;115:919–21.
36. Pongas GN, Lewis RE, Samonis G, Kontoyiannis DP. Voriconazole-associated zygomycosis: a significant consequence of evolving antifungal prophylaxis and immunosuppression practices? Clin Microbiol Infect. 2009;15(Suppl 5):93–7.
37. Lamaris GA, Ben-Ami R, Lewis RE, Chamilos G, Samonis G, Kontoyiannis DP. Increased virulence of Zygomycetes organisms following exposure to voriconazole: a study involving fly and murine models of zygomycosis. J Infect Dis. 2009;199:1399–406.
38. Bhansali A, Bhadada S, Sharma A, et al. Presentation and outcome of rhino-orbital-cerebral mucormycosis in patients with diabetes. Postgrad Med J. 2004;80:670–4.
39. Bongomin F, Gago S, Oladele R, Denning D. Global and multi-national prevalence of fungal diseases—estimate precision. J Fungi. 2017;3:57.
40. Marak RS, Misra R, Ansari MS, Dixit A, Poornima PKN, Dhole TN. Successful medical management of renal zygomycosis: a summary of two cases and a review of the Indian literature. Med Mycol. 2010;48:1088–95.
41. Jianhong L, Xianliang H, Xuewu J. Isolated renal mucormycosis in children. J Urol. 2004;171:387–8.
42. Bhadauria D, Etta P, Chelappan A, et al. Isolated bilateral renal mucormycosis in apparently immunocompetent patients—a case series from India and review of the literature. Clin Kidney J. 2018;11:769–76.
43. Chakrabarti A, Ghosh A, Prasad GS, et al. Apophysomyces elegans: an emerging zygomycete in India. J Clin Microbiol. 2003;41:783–8.
44. Bala K, Chander J, Handa U, Punia RS, Attri AK. A prospective study of mucormycosis in north India: experience from a tertiary care hospital. Med Mycol. 2015;53:248–57.
45. Pandey M, Singh G, Agarwal R, et al. Emerging Rhizopus microsporus infections in India. J Clin Microbiol. 2018;56:e00433–18.
46. Prakash H, Ghosh A, Rudramurthy S, et al. The environmental source of emerging apophysomyces variabilis infection in India. Med Mycol. 2016;54:567–75.
47. Xess I, Mohapatra S, Shivaprakash MR, et al. Evidence implicating Thamnostylum lucknowense as an etiological agent of rhino-orbital mucormycosis. J Clin Microbiol. 2012;50:1491–4.
48. Hemashettar BM, Patil RN, O'Donnell K, Chaturvedi V, Ren P, Padhye AA. Chronic rhinofacial mucormycosis caused by Mucor irregularis (Rhizomucor variabilis) in India. J Clin Microbiol. 2011;49:2372–5.
49. Lu X-L, Najafzadeh MJ, Dolatabadi S, et al. Taxonomy and epidemiology of Mucor irregularis, agent of chronic cutaneous mucormycosis. Persoonia. 2013;30:48–56.
50. García-Hermoso D, Alanio A, Lortholary O, et al. Agents of systemic and subcutaneous mucormycosis and entomophthoromycosis. In: Pfaller MA, Richter SS, Funke G, Jorgensen JH, Landry ML, Carroll KC, et al., editors. Manual of clinical microbiology. 11th ed. Washington, DC: ASM Press; 2015. p. 2087–108. https://doi.org/10.1128/9781555817381.ch121.
51. Guarner J, Brandt ME. Histopathologic diagnosis of fungal infections in the 21st century. Clin Microbiol Rev. 2011;24:247–80.
52. Spellberg B, Edwards J Jr, Ibrahim A. Novel perspectives on mucormycosis: pathophysiology, presentation, and management. Clin Microbiol Rev. 2005;18:556–69.
53. Bialek R, Konrad F, Kern J, et al. PCR based identification and discrimination of agents of mucormycosis and aspergillosis in paraffin wax embedded tissue. J Clin Pathol. 2005;58:1180–4.

54. Zaman K, Rudramurthy SM, Das A, Panda N, Honnavar P, Kaur H, Chakrabarti A. Molecular diagnosis of rhino-orbito-cerebral mucormycosis from fresh tissue samples. J Med Microbiol. 2017;66:1124–9.
55. Chamilos G, Marom EM, Lewis RE, Lionakis MS, Kontoyiannis DP. Predictors of pulmonary zygomycosis versus invasive pulmonary aspergillosis in patients with cancer. Clin Infect Dis. 2005;41:60–6.
56. Jung J, Kim MY, Lee HJ, et al. Comparison of computed tomographic findings in pulmonary mucormycosis and invasive pulmonary aspergillosis. Clin Microbiol Infect. 2015;21:684.e11–8.
57. Cornely OA, Arikan-Akdagli S, Dannaoui E, et al. ESCMID and ECMM joint clinical guidelines for the diagnosis and management of mucormycosis 2013. Clin Microbiol Infect. 2014;20(Suppl 3):5–26.
58. Chitasombat MN, Niparuck P. Deferiprone as adjunctive treatment for patients with invasive mucormycosis: a retrospective case series. Infect Dis Rep. 2018;10:7765.
59. Spellberg B, Ibrahim AS, Chin-Hong PV, et al. The Deferasirox–AmBisome Therapy for Mucormycosis (DEFEAT Mucor) study: a randomized, double-blinded, placebo-controlled trial. J Antimicrob Chemother. 2012;67:715–22.
60. Soman R, Gupta N, Shetty A, Rodrigues C. Deferasirox in mucormycosis: hopefully, not defeated. J Antimicrob Chemother. 2012;67:783–4.
61. Grimaldi D, Pradier O, Hotchkiss RS, et al. Nivolumab plus interferon-γ in the treatment of intractable mucormycosis. Lancet Infect Dis. 2017;17:18.

Rare Fungal Infections in Asia

20

Ariya Chindamporn and Navaporn Worasilchai

Key Points

Rare fungi

- Yeast: *Fereydounia khargensis, Pichia anomala, Kodamaea ohmeri, Trichosporon inkin, T. mucoides, Rhodotorula mucilaginosa, Saccharomyces cerevisiae, Blastoschizomyces capitatus*
- Septate mold: *Alternaria* spp., *A. alternata, A. malorum, Chaetomium globosum, Exserohilum* spp., *Paecilomyces formosus, Pyrenochaeta romeroi, Scedosporium apiospermum, S. prolificans*
- Non-septate mold: *Conidiobolus coronatus, Cunninghamella bertholletiae, Rhizomucor* spp., *Saksenaea erythrospora*
- Dimorphic fungi—Emergomyces
- Fungus-like microbes: *Lagenidium albertoi, Prototheca wickerhamii, Pythium insidiosum, Rhinosporidium seeberi*

Cause of Emergence

- Fungi adapting higher temperature and acquire virulence factors
- Advancement of medical devices and management
- Broad-spectrum and steroid use
- International travel and natural disasters

Challenges

- Epidemiology not well understood with regard to environmental reservoirs, modes of transmission, and ways to detect them
- Because of their relative rarity, laboratory diagnosis of these potential pathogens is challenging

A. Chindamporn (✉) · N. Worasilchai
Mycology Unit, Department of Microbiology, Faculty of Medicine, Chulalongkorn University, Bangkok, Thailand

A. Chakrabarti (ed.), *Clinical Practice of Medical Mycology in Asia*,
https://doi.org/10.1007/978-981-13-9459-1_20

- Specific identification requires expertise
- Antifungal susceptibility testing challenging because reliable methodology & antifungal breakpoints not available
- Quality-assured diagnosis requires reference laboratories
- Reference laboratory facilities are not available in majority of Asian countries

Some rare fungal infection cases caused by true fungi (yeasts and filamentous fungi), fungal-like microbes, and algae in Asian countries were summarized in this chapter. The habitat of the majority of rare fungi are in the environment like soil, plants, animals, and clean or dirty water, agriculture bound water resources. The organisms are considered non-pathogenic to human, but may accidentally enter the hosts through trauma, abrasion, or via respiratory tract. For example, cases infected by soil mold, *Saksenaea erythrospora,* which enters via contaminated intramuscular injection, resulting in the severe necrotizing fasciitis in apparently healthy hosts (Table 20.5), [1]. The early accurate diagnosis with the appropriate treatment plays the key role managing such patients. As culture and identification take long time, direct microscopy of clinical samples helps in early management. However, direct microscopy does not identify the fungi accurately as yeast cells, non-septate hyphae, hyaline or dematiaceous septate hyphae may represent many fungi. Some of the reported cases due to rare fungi are tabulated based on the morphology of fungi, yeast (Table 20.1), mold (Tables 20.3 and 20.5), and fungal-like microbes (Table 20.7) adjunct with their susceptibility profiles (Tables 20.2, 20.4, 20.6, and 20.8) to guide the clinical practices and managements.

It has been claimed that the new antifungal agents, the growing population of immunocompromised patients and also global warming have a tremendous impact on new opportunistic yeast infections [2]. Interestingly, the emergence of yeast infection changes period to period. In the last two decade, non-*albicans Candida* species account for up to 90% of candidemia cases instead of *C. albicans*. In the last decade, certain unusual opportunistic yeast species have emerged for the first time and those rare yeasts have appeared more often, for example, *Fereydounia khargensis* (multi-drug resistance yeast) [3], *Pichia anomala* [4, 5], *P. fabianii* [6], *Kodamaea ohmeri (outbreak in India)* [7], *Trichosporon asahii* (multidrug-resistant yeast) [8], etc. Fungal identification using molecular technique, which is more available in laboratories, seems to be one of the factors leading to the definite genus and species level identification. Immunocompromised hosts, ICU patients with prolong hospitalization, etc. are the common susceptible hosts (Table 20.1). In the perspective of physicians, they depend on definite identification in genus and species level and/or drug resistance characteristics leading to effective treatment. For example,

Table 20.1 Summary of rare yeast infections in Asian countries includes specimens, disease spectrum, underlying conditions/history, microbiological diagnosis, reported successful treatment, misdiagnosis, and country

Organisms	Specimens (*n*)	Disease spectrum (*n*)	Underlying conditions/history (*n*)	Microbiological laboratory diagnosis	Reported successful treatment	Misdiagnosed by common identification methods	Country; case number: year (Reference)
Fereydounia khargensis (Order Urocystidales)—Basidiomycetous yeast	Blood (1), pleural fluid (1)	Bloodstream infection (1), respiratory track (1)	Low CD4 count (1), complicated medical conditions, DM, and hepatitis B (1)	**Macro:** Dry, slightly wrinkled and fringed margins colony at 48 h on SDA then turn darker after 72-120 h **Micro:** Vegetative cells W or W/O blastospores produced by polar budding on short stalks. Pseudohyphae are occasionally observed	**ITR** 200 mg twice daily (IV) then 200 mg/day (IV) or **FLC** 400 mg/day (IV) once a day	*F. khargensis* can be misdiagnosed by **API 20C** (*Cr. neoformans*) and **VITEK 2** (*Cr. laurentii*)	**Malaysia**; 2: 2016 [3]
Pichia anomala (Order Saccharomycetales)—Ascomycetous yeast	Blood	Bloodstream infection	Very low birth weight baby. Prolong hospitalization and cross-contamination by hand staffs	**Macro:** Cream-colored colony **Micro:** Spherical, elliptical acuminate cells	**MIC** 300 mg/day (IV), **AMB**	NM	**Northern India**-outbreak; 379: Apr 1996–Feb 1998 [5] **South Korea**-outbreak; 11: Nov-Dec 2015 [4]

(continued)

Table 20.1 (continued)

Organisms	Specimens (*n*)	Disease spectrum (*n*)	Underlying conditions/history (*n*)	Microbiological laboratory diagnosis	Reported successful treatment	Misdiagnosed by common identification methods	Country; case number: year (Reference)
Kodamaea ohmeri (Order Saccharomycetales) – Ascomycetous yeast	Blood	Bloodstream infection	Immunocompromised pt, DM, hematological malignancy, patient with lines and tubes (i.e., breathing tubes, feeding tubes, and central venous catheters)	**Macro:** Cream-colored colony **Micro:** Single blastoconidia along the sides of pseudohyphae	**AMB** or **FLU** or **FLU** then **ITR** or **CAS** or **MIC**	NM	**Taiwan**; 22, 1998–2008 [7]
Trichosporon inkin and *T. mucoides* (Order Tremellales)—Basidiomycetous yeast	Skin (1), hair (2), tissue biopsy (1)	(sub) cutaneous infection (3), sinus tract (1)	Immunocompromised pt, hair dressing (3), previous or long-term antibiotic therapy (1), use of a tube, i.e., central catheter (2)	**Macro:** Soft pasty colony with cerebriform folds **Micro:** Hyaline septate hyphae with arthrospores and blastospores	**ITR** 100 mg/DIB for 15 days	NM	**South India**; 1: 2011 [23] **India**; 2: 2014 [24] **China**; 1: 2017 [25]

Rhodotorula mucilaginosa (Order Sporidiales)—Basidiomycetous yeast	Blood (2)	Bloodstream infection (2)	Immunocompromised pt (1), pt with indwelling vascular catheters, granulocytopenia, damage to the normal anatomic barriers (skin, mucosa, especially gastrointestinal), cellular immune dysfunction and parenteral nutrition (1)	**Macro:** Moist orange-colored colony **Micro:** Budding yeast cell	**AMB + Flucytosine** then **FLU**	NM	**India**; 2: 2011 [26]
Saccharomyces cerevisiae (Order Saccharomycetales)	Blood (7)	Bloodstream infection (7)	Pt with intravascular catheter and antibiotic therapy and prolong hospitalization (7)	**Macro:** Rough colonies **Micro:** Budding yeast cell with pseudohyphae	**AMB w or w/o flucytosine**	NM	**India**; 7: 2014–2015 [27]

(continued)

Table 20.1 (continued)

Organisms	Specimens (*n*)	Disease spectrum (*n*)	Underlying conditions/history (*n*)	Microbiological laboratory diagnosis	Reported successful treatment	Misdiagnosed by common identification methods	Country; case number: year (Reference)
Blastoschizomyces capitatus (Magnusiomyces capitatus, Geotrichum capitatum) (Order Saccharomycetales)—Ascomycetous yeast	Blood (2), cornea scrapings (1), sputum (4), bronchial aspirate (3), endotracheal aspirate (2), pus (1)	Bloodstream infection (2), keratomycosis (1), lower zone CAP (3)	Pt with immunosuppressive drug (1), Pt with foreign body in the eye for 5 days, no evidence of immunological suppression status (1), DM with hypertension and ischemic stroke (1), CAP (3), COPD (2), accident and injury (1), Alzheimer (1)	**KOH prep:** Branching hyphae (possible to see yeast-like cells and/or pseudohyphae). Able to grow at 45 °C and resist to cycloheximide **Macro:** Cream colored, dry, and wrinkled yeast-like colony on SDA **Micro:** Septate hyphae with branched and break up into chains of hyaline, smooth, one-celled, subglobose to cylindrical arthroconidia. (*molecular technique using ITS and D1D2 primer and 26S rDNA is recommended for definite genus species identification*)	**AMB with or without flucytosine** or **VOR** (promising agent as suggested by good in vitro susceptibility) or **FLC** 400 mg/day	NM	**Japan**; 1: 2010 [28] **China**; 1: 2015 [29], **India**; 1:2016 [30] **Western Nepal**; 1, colonization/probable 6: 2015 [31]

Note:
CAP community acquired pneumonia, *COPD* chronic obstructive pulmonary disorder, *CVA* cerebrovascular accident, *AFLP* amplified fragment length polymorphism, *ICU* intensive care unit, *IV* intravenous, *mg* milligram, *Pt* patient, *DM* diabetes mellitus, *IV* intravenous, *ANI* anidulafungin, *CAS* caspofungin, *MIC* micafungin, *ITR* itraconazole, *FLC* fluconazole, *VOR* voriconazole, *AMB* amphotericin B, *R. glutinis*: *Rhodotorula glutinis*, *Cr. neoformans*: *Cryptococcus neoformans*, *NM* No misidentification by common commercial kit has been published, *KOH prep* Potassium hydroxide preparation, *Macro* macroscopic morphology, *Micro* microscopic morphology

Table 20.2 Susceptibility profiles of rare causative yeast organisms in Asian countries published in literatures

Organisms	The MIC values (μg/mL)[a]								Reference (s)
	Azoles				Polyenes	Echinocandins			
	FLC	VOR	POS	ITR	AMB	CAS	MIC	ANI	
Fereydounia khargensis	2–8	0.03–2	ND	0.09–0.125	>32	4– >32	ND	>32	[3]
Pichia anomala	≤1–2	≤0.12	ND	ND	≤0.25–0.5	≤0.25	≤0.06	ND	[4]
Kodamaea ohmeri	4–64 (one resistant strain was reported)	0.047	0.012	0.125–0.5	0.02–0.5	0.25	0.125	0.064	[7]
Trichosporon inkin	1–32	0.03–0.5	ND	0.06–1	0.12–1	ND	ND	ND	[25]
Trichosporon mucoides	8	0.5	ND	0.125	2	ND	ND	ND	[25]
Rhodotorula mucilaginosa	>256	16– >32	ND	ND	0.5–1.5	>256	ND	ND	[26]
Saccharomyces cerevisiae	0.03–0.12	0.06–0.5	0.03–0.06	0.06–0.5	0.03–0.06	0.03–0.25	0.0075–0.5	0.03–0.5	[27]
Blastoschizomyces capitatus	8–16	0.12–0.5	ND	0.01–0.25	0.25–1	ND	1	ND	[28–31]

Note:
FLC fluconazole, *VOR* voriconazole, *POS* posaconazole, *ITR* itraconazole, *AMB* amphotericin B, *CAS* caspofungin, *MIC* micafungin, *ANI* anidulafungin, *ND* No data available

[a]The MICs (minimum inhibitory concentrations) values were determined by broth microdilution method according to Clinical and Laboratory Standards Institute document (M27-A3; 2008)

trichosporonosis, the second most common deep-seated yeast infection, is found in China, India, Japan, Taiwan, and Thailand. Invasive *Trichosporon* infections are usually misidentified as *Cryptococcus neoformans* by commercial kit due to similar antigenic determinants sharing with the capsular polysaccharide of *Cryptococcus neoformans* [9]. Variable susceptibility to Amphotericin B has been observed among *Trichosporon* species. Recent studies have documented high in vitro resistance to amphotericin B of *T. asahii, T. cutaneum*, and *T. inkii* which is one of the first line drugs for cryptococcosis treatment [10, 11]. By the reason mentioned above, species level identification in *Trichosporon* using molecular technique seems to be the necessary process. Thus, the awareness of clinicians about rare yeasts, the rapid and accurate identification by molecular technique including routine in vitro susceptibility test to guide antifungal therapy are the urgently needed (Tables 20.1 and 20.2).

Geographic condition, temperature, humidity, and natural sources bound to water and soil in Asia are the favorable conditions for fungal growth. Moreover, agriculture-related occupation and lifestyle in Asian population are accounted as parts of predisposing factors for saprophytic fungal infection. With the advent of advanced technology in medication using corticosteroid or immunosuppressants, medication to suppress the status of immune response for further treatment, i.e., transplantation, provides the advantage for fungus to play the opportunistic role in such a host, like the case infected by *Scedosporium prolificans* [12] and *Cunninghamella bertholletiae* [13, 14]. Not only the low immune status host but also the less or no immune defect host may also acquire opportunistic mold infection, especially for the latter group after exposure to the fungi intentionally or not, such as the case infected by *Conidiobolus coronatus* [15]. It is of interest that the different profile of underlying diseases, socioeconomic and living style status make one prone for fungal infection. Diabetes mellitus (DM) was common predisposing factor for mucormycosis in Asian countries, whereas haematological malignancey and solid organ transplant were risk factors in developed countries [16]. The rare cases infected by *Rhizomucor, Saksenaea erythrospora* were found in DM patients [1, 17]. Similar to rare yeast infection, the infection was first diagnosed by the awareness of the physicians, then with collaboration of laboratory. The advantage of non-cultural diagnosis/identification is shortened turnaround time, but the method is unable to perform the minimum inhibitory concentration (MIC) and/or minimum effective concentration (MEC) assay. The information of both assays is able to guide the antifungal drug of choice since the variety of MIC and MEC has been found regardless of the genus or species (Tables 20.3, 20.4, 20.5, and 20.6).

Table 20.3 Summary of rare fungal infections caused by septate mold in Asian countries

Organisms	Specimens (*n*)	Disease spectrum (*n*)	Underlying conditions/ history (*n*)	Microbiological laboratory diagnosis	Reported successful treatment	Country; case number: year (Reference)
Alternaria spp. (Order Pleosporales)	Cornea (7)	Keratitis (7)	Patient with corneal trauma (6) or associated with soft contact lenses (1) (note: This group of patients was early diagnosed within 10 d–4 mo after disease onset)	**KOH prep:** Brownish branched septate phaeoid hyphae; **GMS, PAS, H&E:** Irregular unbranched septate hyphae surrounded by the epitheloid cells and peripheral giant	**Natamycin** or **Natamycin + AMB**	**Taiwan**; 7: 2003–2012 [32]
A. alternata	Fistula swab (1) Sputum and BAL (1)	Osteomyelitis of maxilla (1) allergic bronchopulmonary mycosis (high specific IgE to *A. alternata*)	Patient with DM acquired the infection during an extraction of tooth (1) generalized, urticarial skin rash recurring periodically for the last 5 years and occasional painin the right lower chest and flank of a month	Cells outlined with neutrophils and eosinophils. **Macro:** Fast-growing, grayish-white, sued-like colony is the character definition of colony which looks like leather on the flesh side; to downy colony: short hair leather like colony. **Micro:** Dark septate hyphae with alternate direction of septa in muriform conidia	**FLC** 150 mg/d or **ITR** (treatment of choice) or **AMB** (second choice) (15 days of prednisolone 25 mg daily and thereafter on alternate days) in addition to ITR 200 mg in daily divided doses	**India**; 1: 2013 [33, 34]

(continued)

Table 20.3 (continued)

Organisms	Specimens (*n*)	Disease spectrum (*n*)	Underlying conditions/history (*n*)	Microbiological laboratory diagnosis	Reported successful treatment	Country; case number: year (Reference)
A. malorum	Biopsy tissue from necroticswollen lesions localized on the hard palate and the subcutaneous lesions (1)	Subcutaneous infection (1)	Immunocompetent host with the gradually developed the subcutaneous single well-defined localized verrucous plaques on the anterior chest, neck and face for 11 y (1)		**AMB deoxycholate** 5 mg/kg/d, 1 mo combined with **ITR** 400 mg/d, 6 mo	**Iran**; 1: 2012 [35] (Mirhendi H et al. 2013)
Chaetomium globosum (Order Sordariales)	Pus from blisters and scraping from white plaques (1)	Multiple blisters, well-defined whitish plaques with diffuse scales, surrounding erythema on right foot with cellulitis (1)	11-year-old girl with no evidence of immune status (1)	**Macro:** White to tan colony **Micro:** Flask-shaped black perithecia, covered with long hair-like setae inside contained olive brown oval-shaped ascospores in asci	**Cloxacillin** (IV) + **penicillin** (IV), 1 wk + topical **miconazole**, 4 mo	**Malaysia**; 1: 2015 [36]
Exserohilum spp. (Order Pleosporales)	Eschar	Invasive nasal infection	Patient with intractable headache at right temporal and postauricular areas in accompanying with pain at right nasal ala for 2 month. History of DM, hypertension, and dyslipidemia for 30 y, rhinoplasty with silicone implant 10 y ago	**KOH prep:** Brown septate hyphae with dichotomous branching	**POS** 400 mg/dib for 1 mo	**Thailand**; 1: 2013[a] *(poster presentation by Wannal-erdsakun S* et al. *2013)*

Paecilomyces formosus (Order Eurotiales)	Skin lesion (1)	Cutaneous: Yellowish-brown nodule on skin from back to buttocks (1)	Premature infant, required stay in incubator with high temperature and humidity (1)	**Macro:** Mold with yellowish-gray surface and black reverse colony **Micro:** Septate hyphae, branching solitary phialide with ellipsoidal conidia with long chain arrangement and chlamydospores.	**MIC** (IV) + **lanoconazole**	**Japan**; 1: 2016 [37]
Pyrenochaeta romeroi (Order Pleosporales)	Pus from finger	Subcutaneous infection	Rheumatoid arthritis and history of early morning stiffness with multiple joint pains involving hands and feet since last 10 y	**KOH prep, PAS:** Dematiaceous branched septate hyphae with irregular swellings **Macro:** Grey-black velvety colony **Micro:** Brown septatehyphae with brown-black pycnidia presents at 5-wk-old on oat meal agar (note: Based on its morphology, misdiagnosis as *Pyrenochaeta* spp. has been reported)	**ITR** 200 mg/d, 3 mo	**India**; 1: 2016 [38]

(continued)

Table 20.3 (continued)

Organisms	Specimens (*n*)	Disease spectrum (*n*)	Underlying conditions/ history (*n*)	Microbiological laboratory diagnosis	Reported successful treatment	Country; case number: year (Reference)
Scedosporium apiospermum (Order Microscales)	Aspirated fluid (1), nasal polyp biopsy (1), biopsy from lesion with clustering of rice grain size on the surface of forearm (1), corneal scraping (8)	Tenosynovitis on the dorsum of the proximal left wrist and hand (1), nasal polyp (1), sinusitis along with squamous cell carcinoma of left pterygopalatine fossa (1), fusion of two soft dome-shaped nodes on the right forearm after pulling up weeds (1) keratitis (7)	20 y with hypertension, 2 mo. DM, history of left distal radial and ulnar styloid process fracture for 2 y before and undergone L4–5 discectomy for 1 y before (1), IgA neuropathy, hypertension, and hypothyroidism without immune suppression drug treatment (2), 5 y of 100 mg/d oral cyclosporine idiopathic interstitial pneumonia (1) DM (2), with vegetable-related trauma (2), with bird wing trauma (1), without trauma (2)	**KOH prep:** Branched hyaline septate hyphae; **GMS: Hyphae H&E:** Various sizes of microabscesses covered with fibrous capsules. **Macro:** Greyish-white fluffy, sued-like to downy colony **Micro:** Septate hyphae with slender short conidiophore, bearing oval single conidium, presentation of graphium.	**FLC** 200 mg or **Natamycin + VOR** (eyedrops) or **VOR** 250 mg/day or **ITR** 40 mg/d for 7 d/mo or **AMP** or **ITR + FLC** or **VOR** and **Natamycin** (eyedrop)	**Korea**; 1: 2017 [39] **India;** 2: 2013–2015 [40], **Japan**; 1: 2015 [41], **India** (5:2007–2015) **Malaysia**; 1: 2013 [42] **Korea;** 1: 2008 [43]
S. prolificans (*Lomentospora prolificans*)	Bronchial aspirate (1)	Pulmonary chromomycosis (1)	8 y after lung transplantation and received routine immunosuppressants (1)		Endobronchial topical **AMB**	**Japan**; 1: 2017 [12]

Note:
Pt patient, *IV* intravenous, *DM* diabetes mellitus, *d* day(s), *mo* month(s), *y* year(s), *MIC* micafungin, *ITR* itraconazole, *FLC* fluconazole, *VOR* voriconazole, *AMB* amphotericin B, *IV* intravenous, *mg* milligram, *KOH prep* Potassium hydroxide preparation, *Macro* macroscopic examination, *Micro* microscopic examination, *GMS* Gomori methenamine silver stain, *PAS* periodic acid–Schiff, *H&E* hematoxylin and eosin

[a]*Poster presentation: Exserohilum rostratum* invasive nasal infection in a renal transplant recipient: the first case report *(poster number P1318) by Wannalerdsakun S* et al. *on Monday 12th May 2014 at the 24th* European Congress of Clinical Microbiology and Infectious Diseases. Barcelona, Spain

Table 20.4 Susceptibility profiles of rare causative septate mold in Asian countries published in literatures

Organisms	The MIC values (μg/mL)[a]								Reference (s)
	Azoles				Polyene	Echinocandins			
	FLC	VOR	POS	ITR	AMB	CAS	MIC	ANI	
Alternaria spp.	16– >64	0.25– >8	0.03–0.25[b]	0.03–2[b]	0.12–1[c]	0125– >32	ND	ND	[35, 44, 45]
Chaetomium globosum	ND	0.5	ND	ND	2–8	ND	64	ND	[46]
Exserohilum spp.	ND	1–2	0.1	0.02–10	<0.125–1	ND	<0.5	ND	[47]
Paecilomyces spp.	0.125– >64	ND	ND	0.03– >16	0.03– >16	ND	ND	ND	[48]
Pyrenochaeta romeroi	>64	4	0.5	0.5	4	8	ND	1[d]	[49]
Scedosporium apiospermum	ND	0.03–8	0.03–16	0.03–16	0.06–16	ND	ND	ND	[41, 45]
Scedosporium prolificans	ND	4– >16	ND	>16	8– >16	2– >8	0.125– >8	0.5– >8	[50]

Note:
FLC fluconazole, *VOR* voriconazole, *POS* posaconazole, *ITR* itraconazole, *AMB* amphotericin B, *CAS* caspofungin, *MIC* micafungin, *ANI* anidulafungin, *ND* no data available

[a]The MICs (minimum inhibitory concentrations) values were determined by broth microdilution method according to Clinical and Laboratory Standards Institute document (M38-A2; 2008)

[b]Some isolate of *A. alternata* showed MICs >8 mg/mL

[c]Some isolate of *A. alternata* showed MICs 16 mg/mL

[d]*MEC* minimum effective concentration

Table 20.5 Summary of rare fungal infections caused by non-septate mold in Asian countries

Organisms	Specimens (*n*)	Disease spectrum (*n*)	Underlying conditions/ history (*n*)	Microbiological laboratory diagnosis	Reported successful treatment	Country; case number: year (Reference)
Conidiobolus coronatus (Subphylum Entomophthoro-mycotina)	Tissue from nasopharyngeal mass (2)	Nasal cavity (2)	No underlying dis. Indicated/ unilateral nasal mass/surface antigen of hepatitis and HIV: −ve (2)	**PAS, GMS:** Chronic granulomatous inflammation with branching and broad hyphae, positive for Splendore-Hoeppli reaction **Macro:** Rapid growing tan to brown colony which are glabrous and waxy, then it becomes powdery after aerial hyphae development. Its spore can be discharged by sporangiophores. **Micro:** Sparsely septate hyphae with unbranched sporangiophores, spores, zygospores, and chlamydoconidia	**AMB**	**India**; 2: 2015 [15, 51]
Cunninghamella bertholletiae (Subphylum Mucoromycotina)	Lung biopsy (2), BAL (1) BAL and pus from L5-S1-laminectomy (1)	Lung infarction (2), fever, dry cough, radicular pain (1), disseminated mucormycosis (1)	Patient with hyperleukocytosis (Ph + ALL) and on prophylaxis: Fluconazole and cotrimazole with acute myeloid leukemia (AML) and on GVHD prophylaxis (2), with pulmonary eosinophilia and emergency surgery due to the ruptured of abdominal aortic aneurysm of well-controlled asthma-COPD overlap with inhaled steroid (1), with kidney transplant (1)	**KOH prep, Papanicalaou, GMS:** Right angles branching of broad, thin-wall aseptate hyphae **Macro:** Rapid growing of white to grey colony **Micro:** Hyaline broad non-septate hyphae, sporangiophores branched, terminating in a swollen vesicle with 1 sporangiola (each becoming a sporangiospore) covering the entire surface, sporangiospores spherical to ovoidal	**AMB** 5–10 mg/kg/d	**Taiwan**; 1: 2013 [14] **Japan**; 2: 2017 [52] **Thailand**; 1: 2014 [13]

Rhizomucor spp. (Subphylum Mucoromycotina) + *Candida albicans* + *Klebsiella pneumoniae*	Biopsy tissue from nasal cavity (1)	Rhono-facial-cranial infection (1)	DM with right check swelling after tooth extraction (1)	**KOH prep:** Mix of sterile non-septate hyphae and yeast cells **Macro:** Mix of rapid growing of white aerial mold, yeast cells, and bacterial cells **Micro:** Sparsely broad non-septate hyphae with rudimentary rhizoids (few in number and are located on stolons between the sporangiophores), sporangia, and sporangiospores (irregularly branched and end in sporangia at their apices). **Gram stain of bacterial colony:** Gram-negative cells with rod shape	Patient dies of sepsis and cardiac arrest during 5 mg/kg intravenous liposomal AMB and other supportive medications, including diabetic control	**Bahrain**; 1: 2018 [17]
Saksenaea erythrospora (Subphylum Mucoromycotina)	Tissue biopsy	Large ulcerative lesion on gluteal area, large necrotic area related to the history of each patient	No underlying disease, with DM, with I/M injection 7–15 d prior on left gluteal area, medication using bandage	**KOH/KOH-calcofluor prep, H&E, PAS, GMS:** Right angle branching of sparsely septate ribbon-like hyphae. **Macro:** Fast growing of white aerial mycelia colony **Micro:** Sterile broad non-septate hyphae with sporadic hemispherical columella	**Liposomal AMB**	**North India**; 5: Nov.2013-Oct.2014 [1]

Note:
Pt patient, *DM* diabetes mellitus, *GVHD* graft versus host disease, *d* day(s), *mo* month(s), *y* year(s), *MIC* micafungin, *ITR* itraconazole, *FLC* fluconazole, *VOR* voriconazole, *AMB* amphotericin B, *IV* intravenous, *mg* milligram, *I/M* intramuscular, *KOH prep* potassium hydroxide preparation, *Macro* macroscopic examination, *Micro* microscopic examination, *GMS* Gomori methenamine silver stain, *PAS* periodic acid–Schiff, *H&E* hematoxylin and eosin

Table 20.6 Susceptibility profiles of rare causative non-septate mold in Asian countries published in literatures

Organisms	The MIC values (μg/mL)[a]								Reference (s)
	Azoles				Polyene	Echinocandins			
	FLC	VOR	POS	ITR	AMB	CAS	MIC	ANI	
Conidiobolus coronatus	128	ND	ND	0.25–32	2–4	ND	ND	ND	[53]
Cunninghamella bertholletiae	>64	>8[b]	ND	>8[b]	4[b]	ND	>64[b]	ND	[54]
Rhizomucor spp.	>64	>16	ND	2–4	2–4	ND	>16	ND	[55]
Saksenaea spp.	ND	ND	ND	0.01	ND	ND	ND	ND	[56]

Note:
FLC fluconazole, *VOR* voriconazole, *POS* posaconazole, *ITR* itraconazole, *AMB* amphotericin B, *CAS* caspofungin, *MIC* micafungin, *ANI* anidulafungin, *ND* no data available

[a]The MICs (minimum inhibitory concentrations) values were determined by broth microdilution method according to Clinical and Laboratory Standards Institute document (M38-A2; 2008)

[b]*MEC* minimum effective concentration

Another life-threatening disease that should be addressed in Asia is pythiosis, caused by the fungal-like microbes with the similar morphology to mold, called *Pythium insidiosum* (Tables 20.7 and 20.8). This was found as the highest incidence in the world. Underlying disease and/or history play the key role to aid the diagnosis. More than 95% of these patients in Thailand have the hematological abnormality with history of exposure to water related to agricultural field. In contrast to the risk factors in majority of keratitis patients, they are healthy persons with water spilled into corneas [18]. The favorable habitat of this parafungus is in water or soil near the water related to the agricultural area. This is the strong evidence to say that more cases might be present in Asia countries. Due to the presence of non-septate hyphal morphology in artery or corneal samples the patient may be misdiagnosed as mucormycosis or entomophthoromycosis, resulting in unsuccessful treatment. Thus, early and accurate diagnosis is required. Since *P. insidiosum* is not fungus, majority of antifungal drug treatment is not effective. Amputation with antifungal agent, combined with immunotherapy, to balance the immune system is the practical treatment. With better recognition and diagnosis, the sporadic cases were published in Asian countries, such as South China, and India [19–21]. In addition, another similar parafungus, *Lagenidium albertoi,* which has a very similar phenotype that caused keratitis was published. This organism mostly infected dogs. In addition, the unculturable fungus, *Rhinosporidium seeberi* is commonly found in Sri Lanka, and India. The diagnosis needs the direct examination, histopathology, or molecular approach. Moreover, there is one more yeast-like organism that should be mentioned even though the case is rare. The algae, *Prototheca* spp., has the yeast-like colony but without budding cells under microscope (Tables 20.7 and 20.8).

Thus, the suspicious index of fungal or fungal-like infection by physicians and the awareness of the laboratory staff are the important keys to start early treatment and to save the patients' life. The online survey of laboratory situations for fungal diagnosis at 241 laboratories of 7 Asian countries reported that majority of them perform only the direct examination and culture. The incorporation of molecular and serological techniques is essential to improve diagnosis of rare fungal infections [22]. The training of laboratory personnel in this field is also essential to improve diagnosis.

Table 20.7 Summary of rare fungal infections caused by fungus-like microbes in Asian countries

Organisms	Specimens (*n*)	Disease spectrum (*n*)	Underlying conditions/ history (*n*)	Microbiological laboratory diagnosis	Reported successful treatment	Country; case number: year (Reference)
Lagenidium albertoi (Kingdom Chromalveolata, Order Lagenidiales)	Cornea scrapings	Keratitis	Immunocompetent host/ flushed eye with tap water	**KOH prep, H&E, GMS:** Longitudinal and transverse non-septate hyphae. **Macro:** Very rapid growth, submerged glabrous white/yellowish colony. **Micro:** Broad rarely septate hyaline hyphae	**Terbinafine + ITR + topical natamycin**	**Thailand**; 1, 2013 [57]
Prototheca wickerhamii or P. zopffii (Order Chlorellales)	CSF (1), skin biopsy (19)	Meningoencephalitis (1), cutaneous infection (19)	Immunocompetent host (9), Pt, farmer by professional, with itchy rashes on hisarm since 1 year (1) Pt with DM (9), with hypoalbuminemia (1)	**Giemsa and Wright stain, PAS:** Eosinophilic pleocytosis and clusters of *Prototheca* with purple spherical sporangia (symmetrical morula-like sporangia and endospores) **KOH prep:** Hyaline yeast-like cells with various sizes **Macro:** Smooth creamy white, yeast-like colonies **Micro:** 2–8 tightly packed endospores within a sporangium (the hallmark morula form or a daisy)	**AMB** (IV) 10 mg/d then increased to 40 mg/d for 3 mo + **hydrocortisone** 100 mg/d or **FLC** (IV) 400 mg/d for 7 d then **FLC** 100 mg/ DIB for 3 wk or **ITR** or **VOR**	**Korea**; 1, 2017 [58] **China and Taiwan**; 19, 1964–2018 [59]

Pythium insidiosum (Kingdom Stramenopila, Order Pythiales)	Tissue, corneal scraping, artery, cerebral emboli	(Sub)cutaneous, vascular, ocular and systemic infection	*Vascular type*: Pt with abnormal red blood cells (mostly in Thailand); most of them are agriculturist, farmers, or presence the history of water exposure in rice field or irritation area. Recently, hypertension, smoking, and heavy alcohol drinker has been claimed as risk factors. *Ocular type*: Immunocompetent host and exposed to water/or injured by leaves	**KOH prep, PAS, GMS:** Irregular sparsely septate hyaline filaments (2.5–6.5 μm in diameter) **Macro:** Fast growing submerge mycelium **Micro:** Board rare septate hyphae	*Vascular type*: Amputation + **terbinafine + ITR** or **VOR** + immunotherapy *(Sub) cutaneous type*: **SSKI**	**Thailand**; 132, 1985–2013 [18, 60]
Rhinosporidium seeberi (Class Mesomycetozoea, Order Dermocystida)	Polypoidal mass protruding from the left nasal cavity (4) pedunculated mass with stalk arising from palpebral conjunctiva of lower lid (1), discharging sinus from heel	Nasal cavity (4) Keratitis (1) subcutaneous (1)	History of two conventional nasal surgeries for excision of rhinosporidiosis (1), history of animal handling and contactwith contaminated water (pond) (2), no underlying dis (3)	**KOH prep:** Sporangia filled with endospores **H&E**: Thick-walled sporangial sac filled with numerous endospores surrounded by inflammatory cells. **Macro and Micro:** Unable to be cultured	**Dapsone** or **Dapsone + KET + trimethoprime-sulphadiazine**	**India**; 3: 2011 [61] **India**; 3: 2017 [62–64]

Note:
Pt patient, *DM* diabetes mellitus, *d* day(s), *mo* month(s), *y* year(s), *ITR* itraconazole, *FLC* fluconazole, *VOR* voriconazole, *AMB* amphotericin B, *IV* intravenous, *mg* milligram, *KOH prep* potassium hydroxide preparation, *Macro* macroscopic examination, *Micro* microscopic examination, *GMS* Gomori methenamine silver stain, *PAS* periodic acid–Schiff, *H&E* hematoxylin and eosin

Table 20.8 Susceptibility profiles of rare causative fungus-like microbes in Asian countries published in literatures

Organisms	The MIC values (μg/mL)[a]								Reference (s)
	Azoles				Polyene	Echinocandins			
	FLC	VOR	POS	ITR	AMB	CAS	MIC	ANI	
Prototheca wickerhamii or *P. zopffii*	128/NI[b]	1/NI[b]	ND	1	0.5–0.25[c]	>32[c]	ND	ND	[59, 65]
Pythium insidiosum	1–8	1–8	ND	1–4	4–8	2–4	ND	2–8	[18, 60]

Note:
FLC fluconazole, *VOR* voriconazole, *POS* posaconazole, *ITR* itraconazole, *AMB* amphotericin B, *CAS* caspofungin, *MIC* micafungin, *ANI* anidulafungin, *ND* no data available

[a]The MICs (minimum inhibitory concentrations) values were determined by broth microdilution method according to Clinical and Laboratory Standards Institute document (M38-A2; 2008)

[b]NI: No zone of inhibition for either fluconazole (25 μg) (Becton Dickinson, Sparks, MD) or voriconazole (1 μg) (Becton Dickinson, Sparks, MD) on the disk diffusion test

[c]Determined by *E*-test method (BioMerieux, Marcy l'Etoile, France)

References

1. Chander J, Singla N, Kaur M, Punia RS, Attri A, Alastruey-Izquierdo A, et al. Saksenaea erythrospora, an emerging mucoralean fungus causing severe necrotizing skin and soft tissue infections—a study from a tertiary care hospital in north India. Infect Dis (Lond). 2017;49(3):170–7.
2. Skiada A, Pavleas I, Drogari-Apiranthitou M. Rare fungal infectious agents: a lurking enemy. F1000Res. 2017;6:1917.
3. Tap RM, Ramli NY, Sabaratnam P, Hashim R, Bakri AR, Bee LB, et al. First two cases of fungal infections associated with multi-drug resistant yeast, Fereydounia khargensis. Mycopathologia. 2016;181(7–8):531–7.
4. Jung J, Moon YS, Yoo JA, Lim JH, Jeong J, Jun JB. Investigation of a nosocomial outbreak of fungemia caused by Candida pelliculosa (Pichia anomala) in a Korean tertiary care center. J Microbiol Immunol Infect. 2018;51(6):794–801.
5. Chakrabarti A, Singh K, Narang A, Singhi S, Batra R, Rao KL, et al. Outbreak of Pichia anomala infection in the pediatric service of a tertiary-care center in Northern India. J Clin Microbiol. 2001;39(5):1702–6.
6. Wu Y, Wang J, Li W, Jia H, Che J, Lu J, et al. Pichia fabianii blood infection in a premature infant in China: case report. BMC Res Notes. 2013;6:77.
7. Shang ST, Lin JC, Ho SJ, Yang YS, Chang FY, Wang NC. The emerging life-threatening opportunistic fungal pathogen Kodamaea ohmeri: optimal treatment and literature review. J Microbiol Immunol Infect. 2010;43(3):200–6.
8. de Almeida Junior JN, Hennequin C. Invasive Trichosporon infection: a systematic review on a re-emerging fungal pathogen. Front Microbiol. 2016;7:1629.
9. Davies GE, Thornton CR. Differentiation of the emerging human pathogens Trichosporon asahii and Trichosporon asteroides from other pathogenic yeasts and moulds by using species-specific monoclonal antibodies. PLoS One. 2014;9(1):e84789.
10. Al-Mahmeed M, Khan ZU, Ahmad S, Chehadeh W. Antifungal susceptibility profile of clinical Trichosporon asahii and Trichosporon asteroides isolates identified by molecular methods. J Chemother. 2009;21(3):360–2.
11. Lemes RM, Lyon JP, Moreira LM, de Resende MA. Antifungal susceptibility profile of Trichosporon isolates: correlation between CLSI and etest methodologies. Braz J Microbiol. 2010;41(2):310–5.
12. Mitomo H, Sakurada A, Matsuda Y, Notsuda H, Watanabe T, Oishi H, et al. Endobronchial topical amphotericin B instillation for pulmonary chromomycosis after lung transplantation: a case report. Transplant Proc. 2018;50(3):939–42.
13. Navanukroh O, Jitmuang A, Chayakulkeeree M, Ngamskulrungroj P. Disseminated Cunninghamella bertholletiae infection with spinal epidural abscess in a kidney transplant patient: case report and literature review. Transpl Infect Dis. 2014;16(4):658–65.
14. Su YY, Chang TY, Wang CJ, Jaing TH, Hsueh C, Chiu CH, et al. Disseminated Cunninghamella bertholletiae infection during induction chemotherapy in a girl with high-risk acute lymphoblastic leukemia. Pediatr Neonatol. 2016;57(6):531–4.
15. Varshney S, Gupta P, Bist SS, Bhagat S. Conidiobolus coronatus granuloma of the right inferior turbinate: a rare presentation. Ear Nose Throat J. 2015;94(4–5):E32–5.
16. Petrikkos G, Skiada A, Lortholary O, Roilides E, Walsh TJ, Kontoyiannis DP. Epidemiology and clinical manifestations of mucormycosis. Clin Infect Dis. 2012;54(Suppl 1):S23–34.
17. Gupta E, Verma U, Lal P, Gupta PC, Prakash P. Post tooth extraction necrotising fasciitis and rhinocerebral mucormycosis in a diabetic patient. Int J Curr Microbiol Appl Sci. 2018;7(7).
18. Worasilchai N, Permpalung N, Chongsathidkiet P, Leelahavanichkul A, Mendoza AL, Palaga T, et al. Monitoring anti-pythium insidiosum IgG antibodies and (1-->3)-beta-d-glucan in vascular pythiosis. J Clin Microbiol. 2018;56(8).
19. Agarwal S, Iyer G, Srinivasan B, Agarwal M, Panchalam Sampath Kumar S, Therese LK. Clinical profile of pythium keratitis: perioperative measures to reduce risk of recurrence. Br J Ophthalmol. 2018;102(2):153–7.

20. He H, Liu H, Chen X, Wu J, He M, Zhong X. Diagnosis and treatment of pythium insidiosum corneal ulcer in a chinese child: a case report and literature review. Am J Case Rep. 2016;17:982–8.
21. Rathi A, Chakrabarti A, Agarwal T, Pushker N, Patil M, Kamble H, et al. Pythium keratitis leading to fatal cavernous sinus thrombophlebitis. Cornea. 2018;37(4):519–22.
22. Chindamporn A, Chakrabarti A, Li R, Sun PL, Tan BH, Chua M, et al. Survey of laboratory practices for diagnosis of fungal infection in seven Asian countries: an Asia Fungal Working Group (AFWG) initiative. Med Mycol. 2018;56(4):416–25.
23. Janagond A, Krishnan KM, Kindo AJ, Sumathi G. Trichosporon inkin, an unusual agent of fungal sinusitis: a report from south India. Indian J Med Microbiol. 2012;30(2):229–32.
24. Tendolkar U, Shinde A, Baveja S, Dhurat R, Phiske M. Trichosporon inkin and Trichosporon mucoides as unusual causes of white piedra of scalp hair. Indian J Dermatol Venereol Leprol. 2014;80(4):324–7.
25. Xiaoxi X, Yaling D, Kaiwen Z, Xin R, Pradhan S, Yuping R. Trichosporon inkin causing subcutaneous sinus tract: Successfully treated by oral and ultrasound-guided intralesional itraconazole therapy. Indian J Dermatol Venereol Leprol. 2017;83(4):506–9.
26. Duggal S, Jain H, Tyagi A, Sharma A, Chugh TD. Rhodotorula fungemia: two cases and a brief review. Med Mycol. 2011;49(8):879–82.
27. Roy U, Jessani LG, Rudramurthy SM, Gopalakrishnan R, Dutta S, Chakravarty C, et al. Seven cases of Saccharomyces fungaemia related to use of probiotics. Mycoses. 2017;60(6):375–80.
28. Sipsas N, Kontoyiannis DP. Trichosporon species and Blastoschizomyces capitatus. 2010.
29. Gao GX, Tang HL, Zhang X, Xin XL, Feng J, Chen XQ. Invasive fungal infection caused by geotrichum capitatum in patients with acute lymphoblastic leukemia: a case study and literature review. Int J Clin Exp Med. 2015;8(8):14228–35.
30. Brunetti G, Visconti V, Ghezzi MC, Mantovani S, Ferretti G, Raponi G. Management and treatment of Magnusiomyces capitatus (Geotrichum capitatum) pleural infection in a non-neutropenic patient with posaconazole. A new therapeutic opportunity? New Microbiol. 2016;39(4):307–9.
31. Subramanya Supram H, Gokhale S, Chakrabarti A, Rudramurthy SM, Gupta S, Honnavar P. Emergence of Magnusiomyces capitatus infections in Western Nepal. Med Mycol. 2016;54(2):103–10.
32. Hsiao CH, Yeh LK, Chen HC, Lin HC, Chen PY, Ma DH, et al. Clinical characteristics of alternaria keratitis. J Ophthalmol. 2014;2014:536985.
33. Chhabra V, Rastogi S, Barua M, Kumar S. Alternaria alternata infection associated osteomyelitis of maxilla: a rare disease entity. Indian J Dent Res. 2013;24(5):639–41.
34. Chowdhary A, Agarwal K, Randhawa HS, Kathuria S, Gaur SN, Najafzadeh MJ, et al. A rare case of allergic bronchopulmonary mycosis caused by Alternaria alternata. Med Mycol. 2012;50(8):890–6.
35. Mirhendi H, Fatemi MJ, Bateni H, Hajabdolbaghi M, Geramishoar M, Ahmadi B, et al. First case of disseminated phaeohyphomycosis in an immunocompetent individual due to Alternaria malorum. Med Mycol. 2013;51(2):196–202.
36. Mohd Tap R, Sabaratnam P, Ahmad NA, Abd Razak MF, Hashim R, Ahmad N. Chaetomium globosum cutaneous fungal infection confirmed by molecular identification: a case report from Malaysia. Mycopathologia. 2015;180(1–2):137–41.
37. Kuboi T, Okazaki K, Inotani M, Sugino M, Sadamura T, Nakano A, et al. A case of cutaneous Paecilomyces formosus infection in an extremely premature infant. J Infect Chemother. 2016;22(5):339–41.
38. Sharma S, Capoor MR, Singh M, Kiran D, Mandal AK. Subcutaneous phaeohyphomycosis caused by pyrenochaeta romeroi in a rheumatoid arthritis patient: a case report with review of the literature. Mycopathologia. 2016;181(9–10):735–43.
39. Kim CM, Lim SC, Kim J, Jang HS, Chung JH, Yun NR, et al. Tenosynovitis caused by Scedosporium apiospermum infection misdiagnosed as an Alternaria species: a case report. BMC Infect Dis. 2017;17(1):72.

40. Rynga D, Capoor MR, Varshney S, Naik M, Gupta V. Scedosporium apiospermum, an emerging pathogen in India: case series and review of literature. Indian J Pathol Microbiol. 2017;60(4):550–5.
41. Ishii S, Hiruma M, Hayakawa Y, Sugita T, Makimura K, Hiruma M, et al. Cutaneous Pseudallescheria boydii/Scedosporium apiospermum complex (molecular type: Scedosporium apiospermum [Clade 4]) infection: a case report and literature review of cases from Japan. Med Mycol J. 2015;56(4):E25–30.
42. Fadzillah MT, Ishak SR, Ibrahim M. Refractory Scedosporium apiospermum keratitis successfully treated with combination of amphotericin B and voriconazole. Case Rep Ophthalmol Med. 2013;2013:413953.
43. Yoon S, Kim S, Lee KA, Kim H. [A case of Scedosporium apiospermum keratitis confirmed by a molecular genetic method]. Korean J Lab Med. 2008;28(4):307–11.
44. Pastor FJ, Guarro J. Alternaria infections: laboratory diagnosis and relevant clinical features. Clin Microbiol Infect. 2008;14(8):734–46.
45. Borman AM, Fraser M, Palmer MD, Szekely A, Houldsworth M, Patterson Z, et al. MIC distributions and evaluation of fungicidal activity for amphotericin B, itraconazole, voriconazole, posaconazole and caspofungin and 20 species of pathogenic filamentous fungi determined using the CLSI broth microdilution method. J Fungi (Basel). 2017;3(2).
46. Serena C, Ortoneda M, Capilla J, Pastor FJ, Sutton DA, Rinaldi MG, et al. In vitro activities of new antifungal agents against Chaetomium spp. and inoculum standardization. Antimicrob Agents Chemother. 2003;47(10):3161–4.
47. Katragkou A, Pana ZD, Perlin DS, Kontoyiannis DP, Walsh TJ, Roilides E. Exserohilum infections: review of 48 cases before the 2012 United States outbreak. Med Mycol. 2014;52(4):376–86.
48. Castelli MV, Alastruey-Izquierdo A, Cuesta I, Monzon A, Mellado E, Rodriguez-Tudela JL, et al. Susceptibility testing and molecular classification of Paecilomyces spp. Antimicrob Agents Chemother. 2008;52(8):2926–8.
49. Badali H, Chander J, Gulati N, Attri A, Chopra R, Najafzadeh MJ, et al. Subcutaneous phaeohyphomycotic cyst caused by Pyrenochaeta romeroi. Med Mycol. 2010;48(5):763–8.
50. Lackner M, de Hoog GS, Verweij PE, Najafzadeh MJ, Curfs-Breuker I, Klaassen CH, et al. Species-specific antifungal susceptibility patterns of Scedosporium and Pseudallescheria species. Antimicrob Agents Chemother. 2012;56(5):2635–42.
51. Bhalla S, Srivastava VK, Gupta RK. Rhinofacial entomophthoramycosis: a rare fungal infection in an adolescent boy. Indian J Pathol Microbiol. 2015;58(3):402–3.
52. Hirano T, Yamada M, Sato K, Murakami K, Tamai T, Mitsuhashi Y, et al. Invasive pulmonary mucormycosis: rare presentation with pulmonary eosinophilia. BMC Pulm Med. 2017;17(1):76.
53. Kimura M, Yaguchi T, Sutton DA, Fothergill AW, Thompson EH, Wickes BL. Disseminated human conidiobolomycosis due to Conidiobolus lamprauges. J Clin Microbiol. 2011;49(2):752–6.
54. Ota H, Yamamoto H, Kimura M, Araoka H, Fujii T, Umeyama T, et al. Successful treatment of pulmonary mucormycosis caused by Cunninghamella bertholletiae with high dose liposomal amphotericin B (10 mg/kg/day) followed by a lobectomy in cord blood transplant recipients. Mycopathologia. 2017;182(9–10):847–53.
55. Wang SB, Li RY, Yu J. Identification and susceptibility of Rhizomucor spp. isolated from patients with cutaneous zygomycosis in China. Med Mycol. 2011;49(8):799–805.
56. Gomez-Lopez A, Cuenca-Estrella M, Monzon A, Rodriguez-Tudela JL. In vitro susceptibility of clinical isolates of Zygomycota to amphotericin B, flucytosine, itraconazole and voriconazole. J Antimicrob Chemother. 2001;48(6):919–21.
57. Reinprayoon U, Permpalung N, Kasetsuwan N, Plongla R, Mendoza L, Chindamporn A. Lagenidium sp. ocular infection mimicking ocular pythiosis. J Clin Microbiol. 2013;51(8):2778–80.

58. Kim JE, Oh TH, Lee KH, Shin JH, Jung SI. Successful treatment of protothecal tenosynovitis in an immunocompetent patient using amphotericin B deoxycholate. Infect Chemother. 2017;49(4):293–6.
59. Wang F, Feng P, Lin Y, Chen X, Xu D, Wang Z, et al. Human cutaneous protothecosis: a case report and review of cases from Mainland China, Hong Kong, and Taiwan. Mycopathologia. 2018;183(5):821–8.
60. Permpalung N, Worasilchai N, Plongla R, Upala S, Sanguankeo A, Paitoonpong L, et al. Treatment outcomes of surgery, antifungal therapy and immunotherapy in ocular and vascular human pythiosis: a retrospective study of 18 patients. J Antimicrob Chemother. 2015;70(6):1885–92.
61. Das S, Kashyap B, Barua M, Gupta N, Saha R, Vaid L, et al. Nasal rhinosporidiosis in humans: new interpretations and a review of the literature of this enigmatic disease. Med Mycol. 2011;49(3):311–5.
62. Narayana Kurup JK, Singasani R, Mohanty SP. Rare case of disseminated rhinosporidiosis with chronic osteomyelitis of the calcaneum treated by a simple technique of negative pressure wound therapy. BMJ Case Rep. 2017;2017.
63. Kaushal S, Mathur SR, Mallick SR, Ramam M. Disseminated cutaneous, laryngeal, nasopharyngeal, and recurrent obstructive nasal rhinosporidiosis in an immunocompetent adult: a case report and review of literature. Int J Dermatol. 2011;50(3):340–2.
64. Kalamkar C, Mukherjee A. Bilateral conjunctival rhinosporidiosis in a paediatric patient. J Clin Diagn Res. 2017;11(9):NL01–NL2.
65. Ahn A, Choe YJ, Chang J, Kim D, Sung H, Kim MN, et al. Chronic eosinophilic meningoencephalitis by Prototheca wickerhamii in an immunocompetent boy. Pediatr Infect Dis J. 2017;36(7):687–9.

Challenges, Pitfalls, and Possible Solution for Asian Countries

21

Rajeev Soman and Ayesha Sunavala

Key Points
- The burden of invasive fungal infections in Asia is considerable.
- However, there is limited awareness among clinicians, paucity of diagnostic mycology laboratories and of large systematic epidemiological studies.
- Limited data show significant uniqueness of fungal infections in the Indian scenario, which is important in planning intervention strategies.
- Therefore, the western guideline and treatment recommendations may not be fully applicable in India, and a careful modification is necessary.

21.1 Introduction

The unique geo-ecological characteristics and the increasing number of at-risk populations in Asian countries are responsible for the high fungal disease burden in this part of the world. However, data on the prevalence of invasive fungal infections (IFIs) in Asia remains sparse. This lack of knowledge stems from several factors such as poor clinical awareness outside specialized units, inadequate diagnostic facilities, lack of regulated national surveillance systems, and no obligatory reporting of IFIs. Factors which contribute to suboptimal outcomes include comorbidities that reduce the potential for cure and the lack of expertise in the management of IFIs. Additionally, the high cost of treatment as well as the unregulated access to

R. Soman (✉)
Department of Medicine and Division of Infectious Diseases, P.D. Hinduja Hospital and Medical Research Centre, Mumbai, India

Jupiter Hospital, Pune, India

A. Sunavala
Department of Medicine, Division of Infectious Diseases, PD Hinduja Hospital, Mumbai, India

A. Chakrabarti (ed.), *Clinical Practice of Medical Mycology in Asia*,
https://doi.org/10.1007/978-981-13-9459-1_21

drugs leads to both under-treatment on the one hand and the misuse of antifungal agents on the other. National surveillance programs, capacity buildup in response to the increasing burden of IFIs, education of all the stake-holders and exploring low cost alternative diagnostic and therapeutic strategies is the need of the hour. In addition, there are particular challenges, pitfalls, and possible solutions that pertain to individual fungal infections.

21.2 Invasive Candidiasis

Recent data shows that 50% of the global cases of candidemia were reported from Asia. In India, the incidence is reported to be 1–12/1000 admissions which is 20–30 times higher as compared to the developed world [1, 2].

A study on ICU acquired candidemia in India found that candidemia was acquired significantly earlier after ICU admission, in patients who were considerably younger, predominantly non-neutropenic and with lower APACHE scores than in other studies. Prior exposure to broad- spectrum antibiotics, use of steroids in a large number of patients and poor infection control practices were thought to be attributable factors [3].

Specific risk factors have been described for invasive candidiasis, which are common to majority of critically ill patients in Asian countries and thus non-discriminatory. A unique subset of high risk patients with gastrointestinal factors such as recurrent bowel perforation, anastomotic leaks, and necrotizing pancreatitis has been identified. However, the most important combination of factors in an individual has not been clearly established. The multiple *Candida* prediction models developed to identify patients at risk have a high specificity but low sensitivity, thus missing many cases of invasive candidiasis.

On the other hand, the lack of clear understanding about colonization versus invasion from respiratory and urinary tracts leads to over-diagnosis and treatment with antifungal agents, e.g., renal transplant recipients were previously considered to have a higher risk for ascending infection and candidemia following asymptomatic candiduria. However, recent studies reveal that although mortality is higher in these patients, it is not reduced with antifungal therapy and hence treatment of asymptomatic candiduria in these patients may no longer be warranted. There is still considerable ambiguity regarding risk factors for invasion and further studies are needed on different risk groups [4].

The management of invasive candidiasis is also plagued by several diagnostic hurdles of which inadequate laboratory facilities for diagnosis is the most important in the developing world. Where facilities do exist, accurate identification of species with drug susceptibility may be lacking. Significant pathogens such as *C. auris* have been misidentified even by automated blood culture systems leading to mismanagement and grave infection control implications. Because *Candida* often colonizes body surfaces, the laboratory may dismiss the sample as a colonizer and not proceed further to identify it to a species level in order to save laboratory work and cost. However, Centre for Disease Control and Prevention (CDC), Atlanta in its guideline of infection control has recommended that *Candida auris* should be identified to the species level even when isolated from non-sterile body sites like urine, wounds, sputum, and bile. This is important as infection control precautions are required while handling colonized patients. Otherwise, intense local transmission may lead to nosocomial outbreaks.

Due to the poor sensitivity of blood cultures for *Candida*, fungal biomarkers like β-D-Glucan (BDG) are a promising option for prompt diagnosis. However, these assays are not widely available, expensive and technically demanding to perform. Although attractive, the pre-emptive approach in treating invasive candidiasis is difficult to follow because such an approach needs repeated BDG testing which would be presently limited by both availability and cost.

The traditional empiric approach leads to delay in treatment initiation as well as, paradoxically, overuse of antifungal agents. Terminating empiric therapy in patients with clinical improvement but negative cultures is especially challenging and a negative BDG in these situations would be invaluable to antifungal stewardship.

Echinocandins are now recommended as first-line agents for candidemia in all patients and Fluconazole is considered as an acceptable alternative in some patients [4]. However, in resource limited settings this recommendation is often impractical. Besides early de-escalation to an azole, especially if *C. parapsilosis* is identified, may be both optimization and a cost-saving strategy.

Apart from appropriate antifungals in candidemic patients, the removal of central venous catheters when necessary, fundoscopy to rule out ophthalmic involvement, echocardiography to rule out endocarditis and follow up blood cultures to document fungal clearance are of immense significance but have not been fully appreciated by the treating clinicians in developing countries.

21.3 Aspergillosis

Although the incidence of invasive aspergillosis (IA) remains largely unknown, autopsy data suggests that 42% of IFIs are due to IA [5]. The hot and humid climatic conditions in most Asian countries as well construction activities especially in the vicinity of hospitals, leads to very high environmental fungal colony counts.

Invasive pulmonary aspergillosis (IPA) poses unique diagnostic challenges in this part of the world. Suspicion of IPA maybe low as the novel, emerging risk factors such as H1N1 infection, chronic obstructive airway disease, steroids, malnutrition, AIDS, polytrauma, infection control breaches during surgery and poor storage facilities for medical equipment and drugs are not well known to treating physicians [6].

The clinical and radiological manifestations of IPA overlap with tuberculosis and other common tropical respiratory infections. The latter are often treated empirically leading to a delay in the diagnosis of IPA.

The unavailability of CT scans and fungal biomarkers and the cost of repeated testing in high risk patients make the pre-emptive approach to IA, especially difficult. Additionally, the use of generic piperacillin tazobactam and the prevalence of other cross-reacting molds such as *Talaromyces marneffei* in Northeast India and *Histoplasma capsulatum* in different parts of the country reduce the specificity of the galactomannan assay.

These diagnostic limitations coupled with the uncontrolled access to antifungal agents leads to the widespread empiric treatment of IA. Limited knowledge of the drugs, especially interactions with rifampin, anti-epileptic drugs, agents which prolong QTc interval, immunosuppressants, and acid suppressive agents may lead to inadequate antifungal drug exposures as well as serious toxicity. Additionally, a wide range of generic antifungal agents are freely available with questionable quality and bioavailability.

Therapeutic drug monitoring (TDM) of the azoles has been strongly recommended to overcome the issues of suboptimal drug exposure as well as to minimize toxicity [7]. However, the limited availability of the test precludes its use in most resource-limited settings. Polymorphisms in azole metabolizing enzymes need to be studied in developing countries to further refine the use of these drugs. Prolonged use of voriconazole both for prophylaxis and treatment of conditions like osteomyelitis or chronic granulomatous aspergillosis has been associated with late complications like periostitis and skin cancer. Awareness among physicians in developing countries about these toxicities is essential [7].

In different studies of developing countries, development of chronic pulmonary aspergillosis in post-tuberculosis managed lung has been highlighted. Simple *Aspergillus* antibody test or imaging can diagnose the condition and avoid unnecessary second-line anti-tubercular treatment due to misdiagnosis.

21.4 Cryptococcosis

The incidence of cryptococcal meningitis in the HIV population has reduced with the advent of HAART; however, there has been a steady rise in incidence in the apparently immune-competent host. Newer risk factors include diabetes mellitus, tuberculosis (TB), end-stage renal disease, liver cirrhosis, systemic lupus erythematosus (SLE), malignancy, idiopathic CD4 lymphocytopenia, and steroid therapy. Several studies have also revealed an association of cryptococcal infection with underlying TB [8, 9].

The overwhelming prevalence of TB in our country, the strong association between the two infections and the clinical resemblance to TB meningitis (TBM), leads to a very low suspicion of cryptococcal meningitis especially in the non-HIV population.

The poor diagnostic yield in TBM often compels the physician to start empiric anti-tubercular treatment (ATT) without searching for an alternative diagnosis of cryptococcal meningitis. This may change with better TB diagnostics even in resource-limited settings. In some instances, empiric ATT is continued even after cryptococcal meningitis has been diagnosed and as a result, rifampin may reduce the levels of fluconazole leading to cryptococcal relapse and resistance.

Once the diagnosis of cryptococcal meningitis is established, the cost and practical difficulties of providing treatment with amphotericin B preparations and 5FC are considerable. The need for repeated CSF drainage to reduce intracranial pressure (ICP) and to document fungal clearance and the longer induction phase of treatment for non-HIV patients is commonly missed, thus compromising the outcome of treatment.

21.5 Mucormycosis

Although uncontrolled type 2 DM is one of the strongest risk factors for invasive mucormycosis (IM); the disease remains unsuspected and underdiagnosed as 16–23% of patients who present with IM in India are unaware of their underlying diabetes [10].

The lack of suspicion of IM also poses challenges in other apparently normal hosts, especially when it presents atypically and in unusual locations. A distinct entity of isolated renal mucormycosis in young, immunocompetent adults has been reported from India and China. Due to the initial lack of awareness, these cases were first diagnosed only from autopsy specimens [11, 12]. This situation may change with better awareness, early imaging, and histopathologic diagnosis.

Mucormycosis can also occur following insect bites in developing countries [13] and following traumatic wounds grossly contaminated with soil. Lack of awareness of these risk factors hampers diagnostic suspicion and appropriate management. While biopsy is the mainstay of diagnosis, IM is not suspected unless the physician has seen a "critical number" of such patients and recognizes the necrotic lesion or black colored discharge as a hallmark of the disease. This often leads to the use of inappropriate antibiotics and even steroids which aggravate the disease. In patients with conventional risk factors like profound neutropenia, hemodynamic instability and thrombocytopenia often preclude invasive procedures and a biopsy thus leading to a delay in diagnosis. Additionally, immediate and extensive surgical debridement may not be undertaken in these patients even after the diagnosis is established.

Mucormycosis is a medical emergency and the urgency to begin appropriate treatment cannot be overemphasized. A delay in treatment of more than 6 days has been shown to double the mortality rate of this infection [14].

Distinguishing between mucormycosis and aspergillosis on biopsy requires expertise, especially when only scanty and disrupted hyphae are seen, but it is needed in a timely fashion as treatment choices differ. Treatment or prophylaxis with voriconazole increases the virulence and angio-invasiveness of *Mucorales* by up-regulation of efflux pumps, secretion of virulence factors, accumulation of alternative non-ergosterol sterols and increased adherence to endothelial surfaces or the extracellular matrix [15].

The unavailability of all preparations of antifungals, the toxicity and the cost in resource-limited settings often result in major treatment limitations. Lack of awareness, uncertain efficacy, expense, and potential for inadvertent harm often precludes the use of adjuvant therapy like echinocandins, deferasirox, statins, and G CSF.

Duration of treatment for IM is based on clinical and radiological resolution, adequate surgical debridement, and reversal of underlying risk factors. However, in reality it is practically impossible to fulfill all these criteria in every patient, thus leading to prolonged, sometimes indefinite need of antifungals.

Finally, the successful outcome of IM requires a team approach involving the microbiologist, histopathologist, surgeon, ophthalmologist, and infectious disease physician. Apart from the multispecialty, tertiary care centers in large cities—the combined efforts of skilled specialists and laboratory expertise may be difficult to come by.

21.6 Conclusion

While it is relatively easy to outline challenges and pitfalls from experience, solutions to these problems are difficult and elusive. Continuing education of clinicians across all specialties is necessary to optimize outcomes for invasive fungal infections. Awareness and implementation of fungal stewardship practices is the need of the hour in our country to prevent the emergence of new fungal superbugs. Clinical research to find acceptable, alternative/innovative diagnostic and therapeutic strategies for resource-limited countries is essential. The alternative strategies may further be validated and implemented to improve the prognosis for the difficult to manage invasive fungal infections.

References

1. Kaur H, Chakrabarti A. Strategies to reduce mortality in adult and neonatal candidemia in developing countries. J Fungi. 2017;3:41.
2. Bongomin F, Gago S, Oladele R, Denning D, et al. Global and multi-national prevalence of fungal diseases—estimate precision. J Fungi. 2017;3:57.
3. Chakrabarti A, Sood P, Rudramurthy SM, et al. Incidence, characteristics and outcome of ICU acquired candidemia in India. Intensive Care Med. 2015;41:285.
4. Pappas PG, Kauffman CA, Andes DR, et al. Clinical practice guideline for the management of candidiasis: 2016 update by the Infectious Diseases Society of America. Clin Infect Dis. 2016;62(4):e1–50.
5. Chakrabarti A. Opportunistic fungal infections in Asia. In: Fungal infections in Asia. The Eastern Frontier of Mycology. 2013; Elsevier. p. 11–21.
6. Bassetti M, Bouza E. Invasive mould infections in the ICU setting: complexities and solutions. J Antimicrob Chemother. 2017;72(1):i39–47.
7. Patterson TF, Thompson GR III, Denning DW, et al. Practice guidelines for the diagnosis and management of aspergillosis: 2016 update by the Infectious Diseases Society of America. Clin Infect Dis. 2016;63:e1–e60. https://doi.org/10.1093/cid/ciw326.
8. Chakrabarti A, Chatterjee SS, Shivaprakash MR. Overview of opportunistic fungal infections in India. Nippon Ishinkin Gakkai Zasshi. 2008;49:165–72.
9. Yuchong C, Fubin C, Jianghan C, et al. Cryptococcosis in China (1985-2010): review of cases from Chinese database. Mycopathologica. 2012;173:329–35.
10. Bhansali A, Bhadada S, Sharma A, et al. Presentation and outcome rhino-orbital-cerebral mucormycosis in patients with diabetes. Postgrad Med J. 2004;80:670–4.

11. Marak RS, Misra R, Ansari MS, et al. Successful medical management of renal zygomycosis: a summary of two cases and a review of the Indian literature. Med Mycol. 2010;48:1088–95.
12. Yu J, Li RY. Primary renal zygomycosis due to *Rhizopus oryzae*. Med Mycol. 2006;44:461–6.
13. Soman R, Gupta N, Sohanlal T, Shetty A, Hegde A, Sankhe M, Rodrigues C. Insect bite causing mucormycosis: report of two cases. JIMSA. 2010;23(1):57.
14. Chamilos G, Lewis R, Kontoyiannis D. Delaying amphotericin B–based frontline therapy significantly increases mortality among patients with hematologic malignancy who have zygomycosis. CID. 2018;47(4):503–9.
15. Lamaris GA, Ben-Ami R, Lewis RE, et al. Increased virulence of Zygomycetes organisms following exposure to voriconazole: a study involving fly and murine models of zygomycosis. J Infect Dis. 2009;199:1399–406.

An Appraisal of the Current Guidelines for the Use of Antifungals in the Treatment of Invasive Candidiasis, Aspergillosis, and Mucormycosis

22

Suganthini Krishnan Natesan
and Pranatharthi H. Chandrasekar

Key Points

A suspicion for an invasive fungal infection should be based on host risk factors, a thorough history, and good clinical examination combined with radiologic imaging. It is reasonable to initiate empiric antifungal therapy pending appropriate laboratory investigations if urgent intervention is warranted. Attempts to establish an etiologic diagnosis is crucial, but not always feasible. IDSA guidelines and other guidelines serve as reliable guides but not the final say-so for any patient. Asian setting and in particular, the Indian setting for invasive fungal infection is substantially different from that seen in the Western hemisphere. Local epidemiological data, individual host risk factors and availability of resources should be carefully considered and the guidelines may be appropriately modified for the best outcome.

22.1 Introduction

Invasive fungal infections (IFI) contribute to substantial morbidity and mortality in immunocompromised patients. Although bacterial and viral infections are more frequently encountered relative to fungal infections, the incidence of IFI has steadily

S. K. Natesan (✉)
John D. Dingell VA Medical Center, Detroit, MI, USA

Division of Infectious Diseases, Department of Medicine, Wayne State University, School of Medicine, Detroit, MI, USA
e-mail: skrishn@med.wayne.edu

P. H. Chandrasekar

Division of Infectious Diseases, Department of Medicine, Wayne State University, School of Medicine, Detroit, MI, USA

Karmanos Cancer Center, Detroit, MI, USA

A. Chakrabarti (ed.), *Clinical Practice of Medical Mycology in Asia*,
https://doi.org/10.1007/978-981-13-9459-1_22

risen over the last decade. The occurrence of IFIs parallels the extent of immunosuppression; the risk factors associated with IFIs include the type of malignancy, use of vascular catheters, gastrointestinal surgery, solid organ or hematopoietic stem cell transplantation, neutropenia, graft versus host disease, use of steroids and/or other immunosuppressants including the novel biologics. Although a vast majority (>80%) of these infections are caused by *Candida* and *Aspergillus*, emergence of mucormycosis, particularly in countries such as India, has been noted in recent years.

Several reports on the epidemiology and management guidelines of IFI have been published from various countries, mostly from Europe, Australia/New Zealand, and the USA, in the past two decades [1–23], most of them within the last 5 years. Since the publication of our last appraisal in 2013, the field of mycology has witnessed the introduction of yet another second-generation triazole in 2015, isavuconazole which has demonstrated excellent efficacy against aspergillosis and mucormycosis, favorable safety profile with minimal drug interactions [24–30]. Introduction of novel chemotherapeutic regimens, use of antifungal prophylaxis and institution-dependent transplant strategies have resulted in a changing epidemiology of IFI. Most importantly, recent epidemiological studies have reported the emergence of non-*C. albicans* and azole-resistant pathogenic fungi in several cancer centers around the world [31–34]. Epidemiological differences contribute to varied frequency of IFI in different countries. Hence, management guidelines are not universally applicable. Our current appraisal has attempted to accommodate recommendations from most recent guidelines published and includes the ESCMID-ECMM-ERS (European Society of Clinical Microbiology and Infectious Diseases-European Council on Medical Mycology-European Respiratory Society) guidelines from 2018 [7], the ECIL-6 (European Conference on Infection in Leukemia) guidelines from 2017 [3], and the Australian/New Zealand consensus guidelines for management of yeast and mold infections in hematology/oncology setting, 2014 [9–12], with a special focus on the 2016 guidelines for the diagnosis and management of Candidiasis and Aspergillosis published by the Infectious Disease Society of America [1, 2].

We have summarized the clinical practice guidelines for the management of invasive candidiasis and aspergillosis published by the Infectious Disease Society of America (IDSA) [1, 2] and examined their applicability to the Asian setting. We have also included a special section on *Candida auris*, the emerging multi-drug-resistant yeast in various centers around the world. These guidelines serve as valuable tools for the management of patients with IFIs. Although the emphasis of this chapter is on IFIs in India, the epidemiology, clinical presentation, and treatment approaches of IFI in most Asian countries are overlapping; hence, the discussion presented here is largely applicable to IFIs throughout the Asian continent.

Given the wide variation in the risk factors, epidemiology and differential microbial susceptibility, treatment practices and financial constraints in the health care setting, we have attempted to delineate the critical factors that need to be considered for therapy and the modifications needed in the guidelines for the Asian setting.

22.2 Treatment of Candidiasis

We reviewed Indian data on invasive candidiasis from several tertiary care hospitals. The exact incidence and prevalence of invasive candidiasis in different regions within India remain unclear as multicentric studies are scant. From available data, incidence of candidiasis appears to range from 5 to 16%. Importantly, there has been an emergence of azole-resistant, non-albicans *Candida species* over the last decade, particularly *C. tropicalis* [31–34]. Data including a large study from Post Graduate Institute of Medical Education & Research, Chandigarh, indicate that *C. tropicalis* accounted for 35% cases of candidemia while *C. albicans* accounted for only 15% cases [34]. Two studies that evaluated the epidemiology of invasive candidiasis in the critical care setting reported *C. tropicalis* as the predominant pathogen in 85% of cases. The risk factors reported included urinary catheters, central line catheters, mechanical ventilation, peritoneal dialysis, and corticosteroid use [35, 36]. The first largest prospective, nationwide multicentric observational study (2011–2012) of candidemia evaluated the incidence in 27 intensive care units in India, from which 1400 ICU acquired candidemia cases were reported. Overall incidence was 6.51 cases/1000 ICU admissions, 65.2% were adult patients, average time in ICU was 8 days, and predominant species was *C. tropicalis* (41.6%). Azole and multi-drug resistance were seen in 11.8% and 1.9% of isolates, respectively. *Candida auris* was mostly seen in public sector hospitals compared to private institutions (8.2% vs 3.9%). Given that blood cultures detect only 40% of the cases of candidemia, the authors estimated the incidence of candidemia to be ~675–710/year, with an estimated mortality of 50% [37]. Table 22.1 shows the high prevalence of *C. tropicalis* and relatively minor role played by *C. albicans* in India, as compared to other regions [33, 34].

Importantly, in sharp contrast to Western data, frequent fluconazole resistance was noted in *C. albicans* (10–13%) and in non-albicans Candida including *C. tropicalis* (5–19%) and *C. glabrata* (~36%). Incidence of azole resistance in *C. tropicalis* has ranged from 3.9 to 37.5%. A teaching hospital from Vellore, reported that 112 isolates of *Candida species* were isolated from various clinical specimens during the year 2012. Among them 61 (54.3%) were identified as *C. tropicalis*. All *C. tropicalis* isolates were sensitive to amphotericin B (100%) but 23 isolates (37.7%) were

Table 22.1 Percent Candida species causing bloodstream infection, worldwide and in India

Species	USA ($n = 4570$)	Europe ($n = 7659$)	L. America ($n = 1710$)	Asia ($n = 5803$)	India ($n = 2592$)
C. albicans	52	61	42	32	16
C. glabrata	20	15	5	8	5
C. parapsilosis	12	12	22	13	4
C. tropicalis	12	7	18	25	37
C. krusei	2	2	3	3	5
C. guilliermondii	0	1	3	5	11
Other Candida species	3	3	7	13	23

References: [33, 34]

resistant to fluconazole [38]. A recent study from Kolkata reported 100% susceptibility of *C. albicans* to fluconazole, but resistance to amphotericin B, 5-flucytosine, voriconazole, and itraconazole was seen in 53.6%, 64.3%, 10.7%, and 21.4% of cases, respectively. For non-*C. albicans*, resistance to amphotericin B, fluconazole, 5FC, voriconazole, and itraconazole was 30.5%, 61.1%, 33.3%, 19.4%, and 38.9%, respectively. All Candida species were susceptible to caspofungin [39]. More recently, Rajalakshmi et al. from South India reported data on candidemia in a tertiary care hospital, from 2010 to 2015. Of 206 isolates, 84% was non-albicans *Candida* (*C. tropicalis, C. parapsilosis, C. haemulonii* sensu *lato* (complex), and *C. glabrata*). Most C. *glabrata* isolates were resistant to fluconazole; among 38 *C. haemulonii* isolates, all were resistant to fluconazole and 37 of 38 were resistant to amphotericin B [40]. Overall, a great variation in both incidence and prevalence of invasive candidiasis has been reported from various centers in India. Exact reasons for the unique epidemiology and high prevalence of azole resistance are unclear although extensive use of fluconazole, improved diagnosis and susceptibility testing may contribute to this finding. Hence, it is essential that hospitals closely monitor their epidemiological shifts in *Candida species* and provide appropriate therapy based on susceptibility, as it impacts clinical outcome.

22.2.1 Candidemia in the Non-neutropenic Patient

Table 22.2 summarizes the recommendations from the IDSA for the management of invasive candidal infections [2]. The table includes suggested options for the Indian/Asian setting.

Table 22.2 Management of candidiasis based on IDSA guidelines and suggested options for the Indian setting

Clinical situation	IDSA guidelines	Suggested options for the Indian setting
Candidemia in non-neutropenic patients	1. Echinocandin 2. Fluconazole (800–400 mg/day)	1. Fluconazole (800 mg/day) 2. AMB-d (0.5–1 mg/kg/day)/ Fungisome (1–3 mg/kg/day)
Candidemia in neutropenic patients	1. Echinocandin 2. Lipid form AMB (3–5 mg/kg/day)	1. AMB-d (0.5 mg/kg/day)/ Fungisome (1–3 mg/kg/day) 2. Step down to fluconazole (800 mg/day)
Empiric therapy for invasive candidiasis in non-neutropenic patients (in ICU)	1. Echinocandin 2. Fluconazole 800 mg/day	1. Fluconazole 800 mg/day → 400 mg/day 2. AMB-d (0.5–1 mg/kg/day)/ Fungisome (1–3 mg/kg/day)
Empiric therapy for invasive candidiasis in neutropenic patients	1. Echinocandin 2. Lipid form AMB (3–5 mg/kg/day) 3. Voriconazole (6 mg/kg/day followed by 4 mg/kg/day)	1. AMB-d (0.5–1 mg/kg/day)/ Fungisome (1–3 mg/kg/day) 2. Step down to fluconazole (800 mg/day)
Asymptomatic cystitis	No treatment, remove, or change urinary catheters	No treatment, remove, or change urinary catheters

Table 22.2 (continued)

Clinical situation	IDSA guidelines	Suggested options for the Indian setting
Symptomatic cystitis	Fluconazole (200 mg/day for 2 weeks)	Fluconazole (200 mg/day for 2 weeks) or for fluconazole-R isolates, AMB-d 0.5–1 mg/day for 1–7 days
Acute pyelonephritis	Fluconazole (200–400 mg/day for 2 weeks)	Fluconazole (200–400 mg/day for 2 weeks) or for fluconazole-R isolates, AMB-d 0.3–0.6 mg/kg/day for 1–7 days with or without oral flucytosine
Fungal balls in bladder	1. Surgical removal 2. Same for cystitis/pyelonephritis	1. Surgical removal 2. Same for cystitis/pyelonephritis
Osteomyelitis	1. Surgical debridement in selected cases 2. Fluconazole 400 mg/day for 6–12 months OR an echinocandin for 2 weeks followed by fluconazole 3. Lipid form AMB for 2 weeks switch to oral fluconazole (400–800 mg/day) for 6–12 months (depending on susceptibility)	1. Surgical debridement 2. Fluconazole 400 mg/day for 6–12 months 3. AMB-d (0.5–1 mg/kg/day)/ Fungisome (1–3 mg/kg/day) for 2 weeks switch to oral fluconazole (400–800 mg/day) for 6–12 months (depending on susceptibility)
Septic arthritis	1. Joint washouts/removal of prosthesis 2. Fluconazole 400 mg/day for 6 weeks OR an echinocandin × 2 weeks, followed by fluconazole × 4 weeks 3. Lipid form AMB for 2 weeks switch to oral fluconazole (400–800 mg/day) for 4 weeks (depending on susceptibility)	1. Joint washouts/removal of prosthesis 2. Fluconazole 400 mg/day for 6 weeks 3. Lipid form AMB for several weeks switch to oral fluconazole (400–800 mg/day) for total 6 weeks (depending on susceptibility)
Central nervous system involvement	1. Removal of shunts/catheters/ prosthetic devices 2. Liposomal AMB ± 5FC for 2 weeks, switch to fluconazole 400–800 mg/day until clinical, CSF, and radiological improvement	1. Removal of shunts/catheters/ prosthetic devices 2. AMB-d (1 mg/kg/day)/ Fungisome (1–3 mg/kg/day) for 2 weeks switch to fluconazole 400–800 mg/day until clinical, CSF, and radiological improvement
Cardiovascular involvement	1. Removal of shunts/catheters/ prosthetic devices 2. Lipid form AMB ± 5FC, OR high dose echinocandin for several weeks switch to fluconazole 400–800 mg/day until clearance of candidemia plus clinical, CSF, and radiological improvement (lifelong suppression, if device cannot be removed)	1. Removal of shunts/catheters/ prosthetic devices 2. AMB-d (1 mg/kg/day)/ Fungisome (1–3 mg/kg/day) for 2 weeks switch to fluconazole 400–800 mg/day until clearance of candidemia plus clinical, CSF, and radiological improvement (lifelong suppression if device cannot be removed)

The three major classes of agents used in the treatment of candidiasis include polyenes, azoles, and echinocandins. The choice of appropriate antifungal agent should be based on the epidemiology, recent history of antifungal exposure, antifungal susceptibility pattern, severity of illness, comorbidities, and tolerability. In general, severe infections (meningeal or endocardial) and hemodynamically unstable patients requiring ICU admission benefit from the use of fungicidal agents such as polyenes and echinocandins. In the USA, *C. albicans* (52%) remains the most common *Candida* species associated with candidemia although there has been an increase in the incidence of non-*C. albicans* reported over the last decade. *C. glabrata*, *C. parapsilosis,* and *C. tropicalis* are the most frequently encountered non-albicans species causing candidemia. Other rare non-albicans pathogenic species include *C. krusei*, *C. guilliermondii* and *C. lusitaniae*.

Based on data from several clinical trials, fluconazole is recommended as first-line therapy for selected patients with candidemia. Such patients are those with mild-to-moderate illness, likely infected with *C. albicans*, have not received azoles in the recent past, have no meningeal or endocardial involvement, and are hemodynamically stable. However, in patients who are severely ill and/or hemodynamically unstable or infected with non-albicans *Candida* species or have had recent azole exposure, or with involvement of meninges or endocardium, the IDSA panel recommends echinocandins (effective against most common species) as first-line agents, and not to rely on fluconazole in view of the possibility of azole-resistant *Candida*. Polyenes, in general, have been replaced by azoles and echinocandins due to severe adverse reactions associated with amphotericin B.

The duration of therapy recommended is 2 weeks from the time of clearance of candidemia, provided there are no metastatic complications. This recommendation is based on several randomized controlled trials that have shown reduced metastatic complications and relapses with 2 weeks of therapy. However, the exact duration of therapy and the time of switch to an oral azole from intravenous therapy remain somewhat ill defined and must be based on clinical improvement, epidemiological factors, and feasibility. As most cases of Candidemia are central line- or vascular catheter-related, removal of the intravenous catheter is strongly recommended for all non-neutropenic patients with candidemia. In the presence of azole-susceptible *Candida* causing candidemia without any metastatic complication, switching to oral fluconazole (400–800 mg po once daily) after the first several days of parenteral therapy with amphotericin B deoxycholate (AMB-d) (1 mg/kg/day) or Fungisome (1–3 mg/kg/day) is acceptable, provided absorption of fluconazole in the gastrointestinal tract is not impaired. In azole-resistant candidemia, a polyene or an echinocandin would be the optimal choice. Examination of the fundus must be performed in all cases of candidemia; if retinal or vitreal involvement is seen, therapy is prolonged and surgery may be indicated.

22.2.2 Candidemia in the Neutropenic Patient

Candidemia is a serious, life-threatening infection in the neutropenic population. It is associated with an increased risk for dissemination and high mortality. There are several critical factors that need to be considered during treatment of neutropenic patients with candidemia: (1) wide use of fluconazole for prophylaxis in hematopoietic stem cell transplant patients and patients on chemotherapy, and, as a result, possible selection of azole-resistant Candida, (2) rapid dissemination of infection during neutropenia and (3) adverse drug reactions.

In the setting of neutropenia, echinocandins are recommended as first-line therapy. Echinocandins, like polyenes, are rapidly fungicidal in contrast to azoles that are fungistatic. Echinocandins have excellent anti-candidal activity against *C. glabrata* and *C. krusei*. However, for infections due to *C. parapsilosis*, since echinocandins generally have suboptimal activity in vitro, fluconazole or AMB-d (1 mg/kg/day)/ or Fungisome (1–3 mg/kg/day) may be preferred as initial therapy. Duration of therapy is 2 weeks from the time of clearance of candidemia. The potential source, i.e., intravenous device, must ideally be removed; however in the profoundly neutropenic setting, removal of the device may lead to more complications, and so the guidelines recommend use of clinical judgment regarding device removal.

22.2.3 Empiric Therapy of Candidemia in the Non-neutropenic Patient

Given the relatively common prevalence of azole resistance in Candida, fluconazole may not be a reasonable option for empiric therapy of invasive candidiasis in India (Table 22.2). In a critically ill patient, a polyene or an echinocandin may be more reliable, and both classes appear equally effective, though the former is more toxic. Lipid formulations of amphotericin B (LFAmB) as well as echinocandins are in general, expensive and so, may not be a viable option for prolonged use in resource-limited settings. Although associated with major disadvantages including infusion reactions, electrolyte abnormalities and nephrotoxicity, closely monitored use of conventional amphotericin B deoxycholate (AmB-d) remains a viable potent therapeutic option. The advantages of the lipid forms of amphotericin over conventional amphotericin B deoxycholate are easy tolerability and significantly reduced nephrotoxicity; efficacy wise, the two appear similar and there are no good data to suggest superiority of one over the other.

Amphotericin B deoxycholate (at a dosage of 0.5–1 mg/kg daily) or Fungisome (1–3 mg/kg/day) daily are reasonable options. Once the organism is identified to be fluconazole-susceptible, a switch to therapy with fluconazole is acceptable. With the prevalence of azole resistance, routine susceptibility testing is prudent when managing infections due to *C albicans, C. tropicalis* and other potentially resistant species. Unfortunately, susceptibility testing of *Candida* isolates is not readily available in most hospital laboratories.

22.2.4 Empiric Therapy of Candidemia in the Neutropenic Patient

Neutropenic patients who remain febrile despite broad spectrum antibacterial agents may be suspected to have invasive candidal infections and empirically treated with antifungal drugs. Serum beta-D-glucan test, commonly used biomarker in the USA, may not be readily available in the Asian setting for an early diagnosis of invasive candidiasis. Since diagnosis of candidiasis is not always easily established, empiric anti-candidal therapy in this setting is acceptable and has been associated with improved outcome.

The IDSA guidelines recommend lipid formulation of AMB, caspofungin, or voriconazole intravenously as primary empiric therapy, and high dose fluconazole or itraconazole as alternative agents. Following options may be suitable for the resource-limited setting: an echinocandin or amphotericin B deoxycholate or Fungisome (1–3 mg/kg/day) or a lipid formulation of AmB. Once the susceptibility is known, transition to fluconazole is acceptable if the isolate is fluconazole-susceptible. Until susceptibility data are known, azoles should not be used for empiric therapy in patients who had received an azole for prophylaxis.

22.2.4.1 Candidal Urinary Tract Infection

IDSA guidelines focus on fluconazole-susceptible *C. albicans* and fluconazole-resistant *C. glabrata* candiduria (Table 22.2). The recommendation is to defer antifungal treatment and eliminate the predisposing factors such as change or removal of indwelling urinary catheters for asymptomatic candiduria. Treatment is indicated in situations where there is a high risk of dissemination such as in neonates and infants with low birth weights, neutropenic patients, and patients prior to urological procedures. Fluconazole at 200 mg daily for 7 days for fluconazole-susceptible *Candida* and AmB-d 0.3–0.6 mg/kg IV daily for 1–7 days for fluconazole-resistant *Candida* are recommended.

Data on the exact incidence of asymptomatic and symptomatic candiduria are not available from India. Few institutions have reported that *C. tropicalis* has replaced *C. albicans* as the most frequently isolated yeast from urine specimens [35, 36]. As fluconazole is highly water soluble, primarily excreted in the urine, and achieves urine concentrations that are 10–20 times higher than serum concentrations, most Candida infections may be treated with fluconazole at 400–800 mg once daily for 2 weeks. This regimen may be effective against selected cases of *C. tropicalis* and *C. glabrata* infections as well. If the isolate is fluconazole-resistant (commonly with *C. glabrata* or *C. krusei*), IV AMB-d at 0.3–0.5 mg/kg daily for 1–7 days may be appropriate. In severely ill patients, continued treatment with IV AMB-d is appropriate until susceptibility data are available. Lipid formulations of AMB and echinocandins achieve low urinary concentrations and are not recommended. Fluconazole may be given orally, thus eliminating the need for IV access. *Candida* prostatitis and epididymo-orchitis are infrequently reported and involve surgical drainage/debridement of the infected site plus antifungal therapy based on the specific pathogen isolated and its antifungal susceptibility.

22.2.4.2 Candidal Osteoarticular Infection

The mainstay of therapy involves surgical debridement in conjunction with antifungal therapy. Fluconazole, caspofungin, and AmB-d have been used with success. IDSA recommends the use of AmB-d at 0.5–1 mg/kg daily for 6–10 weeks. Surgical debridement along with AMB-d or Fungisome (1–3 mg/kg/day) for 1–2 weeks followed by oral fluconazole (400–800 mg daily) for 6–12 months, based on the specific pathogen isolated, is a reasonable strategy. *Candida* prosthetic joint infections necessitate resection arthroplasty in most situations, and if the device cannot be removed, chronic or lifelong suppression with fluconazole is recommended. The data are scarce on fungal osteoarticular infections in India. Few case reports suggest the incidence of primary septic arthritis and osteomyelitis in neonates caused by *Candida* species to be about 7%.

22.2.4.3 Candidal Central Nervous System (CNS) Infection

Data on CNS candidiasis are sparse. Sundaram et al. reported six patients with multiple intracerebral abscesses, none had any identifiable immunocompromise [41]. A study from Indore, examining the causes of fungal meningitis in HIV-positive and negative subjects, found *Candida* to be the most common cause of fungal meningitis in both patient groups, after cryptococcal meningitis. In the HIV-negative group, diabetes, renal transplantation, and prematurity were recognized as risk factors. CNS candidiasis has been seen as a co-infection with *A. fumigatus* and *Mucorales*. *C. albicans* and *C. tropicalis* were the common *Candida* species involved [42].

Fluconazole achieves excellent levels in the CSF and brain parenchyma. Guidelines recommend the combination of liposomal AmB at 3–5 mg/kg daily with or without flucytosine at 25 mg/kg four times daily for several weeks, followed by maintenance therapy with oral fluconazole at 400–800 mg daily until there is complete resolution of clinical, CSF, and radiological abnormalities. Removal of all prosthetic devices related to CNS infection is strongly recommended.

Most of these recommendations were not based on randomized controlled trials, but were based on case series, case reports, and clinical expertise. Surgical debridement in selected cases of brain abscess, especially if solitary, and removal of all CNS devices appear prudent. Initial therapy with intravenous AMB-d (1 mg/kg/day) or Fungisome (1–3 mg/kg/day) until clinical stability, and then therapy with fluconazole 800 mg daily for long-term maintenance is a reasonable alternative. Obviously, susceptibility data play an important role. It needs to be remembered that echinocandins do not achieve high concentrations across the blood–brain barrier and are not recommended in the treatment of CNS candidiasis.

22.2.5 Candidal Endophthalmitis

IDSA recommendations are based on published case reports and suggest a combination of conventional AmB-d at a dose of 0.7–1 mg/kg daily with flucytosine at 25 mg/kg four times daily as first-line therapy for candidal endophthalmitis. High dose fluconazole (400–800 mg daily) may be used as monotherapy for less severe cases. Lipid form of AmB and voriconazole are useful alternative agents in case of intolerance to conventional amphotericin B deoxycholate. Endophthalmitis may be due to an endogenous source (such as during candidemia) or due to an exogenous cause (such as following surgery or trauma); the latter is common in non-neutropenic patients. In a single center study (14-year case series) from Chandigarh, fungal endophthalmitis was reported in 113 patients and the distribution of cases was: post-cataract surgery (53 patients), post-trauma (48 patients), and acquisition via endogenous route (12 patients). *Aspergillus* species was the most common (54.4%) mold isolated, followed by yeasts (24.6%), and melanized fungi (10.5%). Among aspergilli, *Aspergillus flavus* was the most common (24.6%) species, whereas *Candida tropicalis* (8.8%) was the most common yeast isolated [43].

A diagnostic and therapeutic vitreal aspirate with vitrectomy and intravitreal antifungal therapy with conventional IV AmB deoxycholate (AMB-d) is recommended in all patients with severe endophthalmitis and vitritis. Fluconazole may be substituted for amphotericin B after clinical stability has been achieved. Again, susceptibility of the pathogen needs to be known prior to the treatment switch.

22.2.6 Candidal Cardiovascular Infection

Cardiovascular fungal infections are associated with a high rate of relapse and mortality. Removal of shunts, catheters, prosthetic devices, and valve replacement are an integral part of management and if not feasible, patients will need lifelong suppressive antifungal therapy. AMB-d (1 mg/kg/day), Fungisome (1–3 mg/kg/day) or, if available, liposomal AMB (3–5 mg/kg/day) for 2 weeks followed by a switch to fluconazole 400–800 mg/day until documented clearance of candidemia plus clinical, CSF, and radiological improvement may be reasonable.

Evidence for the use of isavuconazole as primary therapy for invasive candidiasis is lacking. Clinical studies do not show adequate comparative efficacy; hence, none of the guidelines have approved the use of isavuconazole for invasive candidiasis [44].

22.2.6.1 *Candida auris*: A Therapeutic Challenge

Since the first report of an ear canal infection with *C. auris* in 2009, this multi-drug-resistant pathogen has been reported from various centers around the world. A significant number of cases have been reported from India. Genotyping revealed that the Indian strains were clonally different from their counterparts in Japan and South Korea [45]. Four clades have been isolated from South Asia, South Africa, South America, and East Asia [46]. Most isolates are resistant to fluconazole and had variable susceptibilities to other azoles, polyenes, and echinocandins. Isolates that were initially identified as *C. haemulonii* were later confirmed to be *C. auris* by gene sequencing [47]. A report by Rudramurthy et al. that performed a subgroup analysis of all cases of candidemia (n = 1400) from 27 intensive care units in India showed that the incidence of *C. auris* was 5.3% and the majority of strains were clonal although hospitals were far apart, and resistance rates to fluconazole, amphotericin B, and caspofungin were 58.1%, 13.5%, and 9.5%, respectively [48]. Majority of cases were reported from public sector hospitals and a few trauma centers in northern parts of India. Major risk factors are a long stay in ICU, diabetes mellitus, malignancy, underlying respiratory illness, vascular surgery, medical interventions (central venous catheters, urinary catheters, post-operative drains, TPN), and prior antifungal exposure [49]. An outbreak of *C. auris* (50 cases) was reported from a cardiothoracic surgery hospital in London, further emphasizing the need for stringent infection control and preventive measures [50]. The overall crude mortality is

30–60%. Given the intrinsic resistance to fluconazole (MIC ≥32 μg/mL), *C. auris* infections remain a diagnostic and therapeutic challenge, with no consensus currently available for optimal treatment. Based on available data, resistance to fluconazole and voriconazole resistance are ~90% and ~50%, respectively. However, posaconazole (MIC 0.06–1 μg/mL) and isavuconazole (0.015–0.5 μg/mL) have shown excellent in vitro activity against *C. auris* and may be potential therapeutic options. Given the relatively low incidence of resistance (2–8%), echinocandins are the first-line therapy for *C. auris* infections. As echinocandins do not achieve optimal concentrations in urine, flucytosine (MIC 50 0.125–1 μg/mL) is preferred for management of urinary tract infections [51]. The global emergence of *C. auris* infections over the last few years has prompted the Center for Disease Control (CDC) to issue health alerts and publish guidelines on appropriate surveillance for prevention and management of these infections.

22.3 Epidemiology of Invasive Aspergillosis

Table 22.3 describes unique features/characteristics of invasive mold infections in the Indian setting [52, 53].

Table 22.3 Invasive mold infections in the Indian setting (aspergillosis, mucormycosis)

Likely factors contributing to increased frequency
1. Agricultural activities
• Poor protective equipment
• Contact with soil
• Exposure to high fungal spore burden
2. High frequency of trauma
• Eye/skin/soft tissue infection
3. Construction activities
• High exposure to fungal burden/poor protective equipment
4. Poor hygiene/suboptimal sanitary conditions
5. Hospital settings
• Suboptimal protection of compromised hosts
– No HEPA filters
– Open windows
• Poor hygienic conditions
6. High prevalence of poorly controlled diabetes mellitus
7. Liberal use of corticosteroids/antimicrobials—over-the-counter availability
Frequent features in India
1. Immunocompetent host: Not uncommon
2. Aspergillosis
• *A. flavus* most common
• Rhinosinusitis/endophthalmitis/CNS infections
3. Mucormycosis
• Linked to diabetes/trauma
• Renal mucormycosis—well described

In Western reports, *A. fumigatus* is the most common cause of invasive aspergillosis (IA) followed by *A. flavus, A. terreus, A. niger, A. ustus, and A. lentulus*. Several cancer centers have reported the emergence of *A. niger, A. flavus,* and *A. terreus* over recent years. Non-fumigatus Aspergillus species have a variable susceptibility pattern to the available antifungal agents. *Aspergillus flavus, A. ustus,* and *A. lentulus* are known to have higher MICs to voriconazole while *A. terreus* is intrinsically resistant to amphotericin B. Antifungal susceptibility of aspergillus is not performed in most clinical settings and until recently was not warranted in the routine management of invasive aspergillosis [1].

Clinical syndromes associated with aspergillosis in patients with preexisting lung disease include allergic pulmonary aspergillosis, chronic necrotizing aspergillosis, and aspergilloma. The most common forms reported in immunocompromised cancer patients are invasive pulmonary aspergillosis, cerebral aspergillosis, and disseminated infection.

A recent study reviewed invasive aspergillosis from 1970 to 2010 in developing countries including India. Authors report that suboptimal hospital practices, construction or renovation work in the vicinity, inappropriate use of steroids and broad-spectrum antibiotics, contaminated infusion fluids, and intravenous drug use were identified as important risk factors for IA. In addition to classical risk factors, liver failure, chronic obstructive pulmonary disease, diabetes, and tuberculosis have been identified as diseases associated with IA [53]. There is a geographic variation in the distribution of species, with *A. flavus* being reported as the predominant pathogen in South East Asia, the Middle East, and arid regions of Africa. A recent large-scale 1-year multicentric retrospective study assessed the incidence and clinical determinants of invasive mold infections in five countries (Thailand, Taiwan, Singapore, China, and India). Among patients without classic risk factors such as neutropenia and steroid use, diabetes and rheumatological diseases were frequently associated with IA. Aspergillosis (*A. fumigatus and A. flavus*) was the most common mold (71%), with a 90-day mortality rate of 32.9% [54]. Several studies are available regarding the incidence and prevalence of *Aspergillus* species from India. *A. flavus* is the second most common mold and is frequently associated with fungal rhinosinusitis, keratitis, and cerebral infections [55]. In a retrospective study performed over a 4-year period (2001–2004), Xess et al. reported that *A. flavus* (46.9%) was most frequently isolated from sinuses whereas *A. fumigatus* (37.7%) was the most common pathogen isolated from respiratory specimens followed by *A. niger* (15.1%) from nail samples [56]. Cases of invasive pulmonary aspergillosis have also been reported from patients with pulmonary tuberculosis [57]. Most Indian isolates of *A. fumigatus* remain susceptible to voriconazole, itraconazole, posaconazole, and echinocandins in vitro. However, azole resistance in *A. fumigatus*, as seen in the West, has been reported in India as well [58, 59].

Triazole resistance in *Aspergillus* is an increasing problem in both clinical and environmental isolates. Prevalence of resistance and its clinical impact in different countries are unclear. This phenomenon is well recognized in several European countries, likely related to widespread use of azole containing agricultural pesticides, and complicates diagnosis and treatment of aspergillosis. Patients with azole-resistant aspergillosis have a higher mortality compared to those with triazole susceptible infection. Recent ESCMID-ECMM-ERS aspergillus guideline recommends susceptibility testing in *A. fumigatus* and local resistance surveillance in regions of >10% azole resistance in aspergillus isolates. Moreover, many suggest that in regions where resistance rates exceed 10%, liposomal amphotericin B or a combination of triazole plus echinocandin should be considered as first-line therapy [60]. Based on scant resistance prevalence data, within Asia, it does not appear necessary to change current practice of management. However, regular local surveillance of resistance is prudent. Also, appropriate attention needs to be drawn to the inclusion of azoles in agricultural pesticides.

In comparison to the occurrence of IA in immunocompromised hosts in the western hemisphere, there are multiple Indian reports of chronic pulmonary aspergillosis [61, 62] and sino-orbital Aspergillosis in immunocompetent individuals. Reasons for the infections in immunocompetent host may be: (1) increased exposure with agriculture being a major factor in most rural and semi-urban areas, (2) environmental conditions resulting in several annual monsoons creating a favorable medium for fungal growth, (3) availability of systemic corticosteroids over the counter with widespread misuse by untrained health care professionals in rural and urban locations (4) intravenous drug use with products contaminated with fungal spores. Hence, the threshold for suspecting invasive mold infections needs to be much lower and needs to be strongly considered in the appropriate clinical setting regardless of the immune status of the patient.

22.4 Treatment of Invasive Aspergillosis

IDSA guideline recommends initiation of empiric therapy in patients at high risk with suggestive clinical and radiological findings [1]. Parenteral or oral voriconazole is generally preferred as empiric therapy. The latest addition to the anti-aspergillus armamentarium is isavuconazole. It was FDA (Food and Drug Administration) approved for treatment of invasive aspergillosis in 2015, based on compelling clinical efficacy established based on a randomized double-blind clinical comparative phase III trial (SECURE study), of patients who received either isavuconazole or voriconazole for invasive aspergillosis. ECIL 6 guidelines published in 2017 have included isavuconazole as first-line therapy for patients with IA, but not for salvage therapy. However, the IDSA guidelines have included isavuconazole as only alternative therapy in patients with invasive aspergillosis. It is recommended when drug interactions and/or toxicity preclude the use of voriconazole. It may also be considered in select clinical situations where broad empiric coverage for molds (including mucormycosis) is considered. Also, liposomal AMB may be used as alternative therapy, particularly in patients who are intolerant of or refractory to voriconazole. The recommendation for salvage therapy includes amphotericin B lipid complex (ABLC), posaconazole, itraconazole, or

Table 22.4 Treatment of Aspergillosis (IDSA, 2016—guidelines)

	Primary/alternative	Comment
Pulmonary[a]	Voriconazole; liposomal AmB or isavuconazole	No routine combination therapy
Endophthalmitis	IV/PO voriconazole + intravitreal AmB/voriconazole	Partial vitrectomy
Empiric/pre-emptive therapy	Liposomal AmB/voriconazole/ micafungin/caspofungin	
Prophylaxis	Posaconazole: Suspension/tablet/IV Altern: Vorizonazole/Itraconazole suspension/caspofungin/micafungin	
Other syndromes		
Aspergilloma	No surgery/ no drug Rx Alternative: Itraconazole/voriconazole	
Chronic Cavitary Pulmonary aspergillosis	Similar to invasive pulmonary aspergillosis	Consider long-term Rx; avoid surgery
Allergic syndromes		
Bronchopulmonary aspergillosis	Corticosteroids: Main Rx	Itraconazole Altern: Voriconazole/ posaconazole
Rhinosinusitis	Polypectomy/steroid washouts	If refractory, antifungal use

[a]Therapy similar in sinus/trachea-bronchial aspergillosis, CNS/cardiac/osteoarticular aspergillosis, cutaneous/peritoneal aspergillosis. Surgery in appropriate cases

micafungin/caspofungin. Guidelines do not support the use of combination therapy (antimold azole + echinocandin) for all patients with invasive aspergillosis. Duration of therapy is for 6–12 weeks or through the period of immunosuppression. Table 22.4 summarizes the IDSA recommendations for various syndromes of aspergillosis.

Most IDSA recommendations are applicable to the Asian setting. For chronic necrotizing aspergillosis, oral itraconazole may be suitable. As an alternative to voriconazole, for acute aspergillosis, AMB-d (1 mg/kg/day), or Fungisome (1–3 mg/kg/day) as initial therapy for 1–2 weeks followed by maintenance with oral itraconazole may be employed. With AMB-d use, close monitoring of electrolytes and renal function is important. Itraconazole has poor bio-availability and has not been examined as rigorously as voriconazole for the treatment of acute aspergillosis. Special situations include cardiac involvement where surgical removal of involved valves is the main stay of management followed by medical therapy with AMB-Dd (or Fungisome) for a minimum of 6 weeks, with subsequent lifelong suppression with itraconazole. Aspergillus endophthalmitis and keratitis may occur either as a result of direct contamination from agriculture-related activities, contaminated ophthalmic solutions, or due to poor sanitary conditions, and post-cataract surgery. Immediate vitreal aspiration with pars plana vitrectomy with parenteral and intravitreal AMB-Dd is indicated as a sight saving measure in these patients. High cost and limited availability may restrict the use of lipid form amphotericin B and the newer azole, isavuconazole.

22.5 Fungisome

The Indian preparation of liposomal amphotericin B, namely Fungisome TM, has demonstrated excellent efficacy, better tolerability and has two to four-fold lower MICs as compared to conventional AMB against aspergillus [63, 64]. In a post-marketing analysis, Fungisome demonstrated 74% complete response and 18% partial response, with significant cost savings. Recently, a multicentric, randomized, controlled clinical trial was conducted to compare low (1 mg/kg/day) vs. high dose (3 mg/kg/day) of Fungisome with conventional AMB (1 mg/kg/day) as empirical antifungal therapy for febrile neutropenia [65]. Although it was a small sample, Fungisome was equally effective but safer than conventional AMB, and low dose was as effective and well tolerated as the high dose. As Fungisome may be less expensive than the commercially available liposomal preparation of AMB, it may serve as an alternative therapy in the appropriate clinical setting. From the available literature, the product appears effective both in vitro and in vivo. More extensive clinical data against infections due to different fungi are urgently needed.

22.6 Treatment of Mucormycosis

Excellent reviews on mucormycosis in India have been published [66–70]. The emergence of mucormycosis in the USA and Europe has been noted in patients with hematological malignancies and transplant recipients, whereas cases in India are overwhelmingly associated with uncontrolled diabetes mellitus with or without ketoacidosis. The authors describe several unique features of mucormycosis from India including isolated renal mucormycosis in immunocompetent individuals. New risk factors such as renal failure and chronic liver disease have been reported [67]. The high incidence in India is likely related to the environmental factors such as the warm climate conducive for a high concentration of spores in the soil. A recent review of epidemiology of mucormycosis in India from 1960 to 2012, brought out some contrasting features of mucormycosis in India as compared to data from the USA or Europe. Most infections are rhino-cerebral (58%) followed by cutaneous involvement (14%) [68]. Another recent 10-year study from a teaching hospital in south India reported the emergence of *R. microsporus* (15.7%) and *Apophysomyces elegans* (10.8%) as important pathogens in addition to *R. arrhizus*. Paranasal sinuses (73.9%) followed by musculoskeletal system (15.2%) were frequently involved. *R. microsporus* was more common in patients with hematological conditions (25% vs 15.7%) and was less frequently a cause for sinusitis than *R. arrhizus* (27.58% vs 10.9%). The overall mortality was 30.97%. *Apophysomyces elegans* sensu lata typically produced skin and musculoskeletal disease in immunecompetent individuals, was secondary to trauma, and was associated with a lower mortality [70]. It is important to have a low threshold to include mucormycosis in the differential diagnosis of cutaneous, pulmonary, cerebral, or disseminated infections, particularly in those related to trauma.

The occurrence of renal mucormycosis in Indian patients with no underlying risk factors is unique. This entity carries a 50% mortality, route of entry is unknown, and has not been reported from other regions. Preferred treatment is nephrectomy along with IV AMB-d. Most frequent pathogens are *Rhizopus* species (*R. arrhizus*) followed by *Absidia*, *Rhizomucor*, and *Mucor*; there are emerging case reports of *Apophysomyces elegans* [68, 70] infections.

Isavuconazole was approved for treatment of mucormycosis in 2015, based on clinical efficacy established with data from the VITAL study, an open-label noncomparative study that comprised of a subgroup of 37 patients with proven or probable mucormycosis and results were evaluated by an independent data review committee. The 42-day all-cause mortality was 38% and a matched case control analysis with patient data from the Fungiscope Registry demonstrated comparable efficacy to amphotericin B [71]. With limited data, currently in the USA, the drug is more commonly used, not as primary therapy, but as step-down strategy once the acute infection is controlled with liposomal amphotericin B.

Guidelines for the management of mucormycosis are scant. The ECIL-6 (European Council on Infections in Leukemia) guidelines did not include isavuconazole for the treatment for mucormycosis, pointing out the scarcity of specific data in patients with leukemia [3]. Echinocandins and voriconazole have no reliable clinical activity against mucor infection. Oral posaconazole may be used in suspension or tablet form for salvage or step-down therapy.

The Italian guidelines suggest extensive debridement of all necrotic tissue, control of predisposing metabolic conditions, correction of neutropenia, reduction in immunosuppression, in conjunction with liposomal AMB at 5 mg/kg/day increased up to 12.5 mg/kg/day as tolerated, followed by a step-down to oral posaconazole. Conventional amphotericin B deoxycholate may be equally effective at 1–1.5 mg/kg/day, but its sustained use almost always will lead to unacceptably high nephrotoxicity. Fungisome may be an effective, less expensive and safer alternative, however more data are needed. In the Asian setting, a high index of suspicion needs to be maintained for early diagnosis. With cost considerations, amphotericin B deoxycholate is likely to remain as the main therapeutic agent for this infection.

22.7 Therapeutic Drug Monitoring

Ample data are published regarding serum level monitoring of itraconazole, voriconazole, and posaconazole. Clinical responses with isavuconazole occur across the observed range of MICs (minimum inhibitory concentration), thus monitoring serum levels is not currently recommended. Although data appear to support routine use of therapeutic drug monitoring of other triazoles to avoid toxicity and for optimal outcome, test for measuring drug levels is not readily available in most centers. For echinocandin or polyene use, measurements of serum levels are not recommended.

There are several treatment guidelines for the management of IFI that continue to be published from different regions of the world. Most offer evidence-based guidelines, learned from clinical trials, appropriate for a particular region. Such guidelines are immensely helpful in choosing appropriate therapy for a given patient in a given scenario. However, there are several factors that need to be considered prior to applying the recommendations from any guideline. Such factors include: (1) local epidemiology of the infection, (2) change in incidence of the infection over time, (3) etiologic pathogen and its susceptibility pattern, (4) specific risk factors in the host, (5) pharmacogenomics and drug toxicities, (6) patient care resources and financial limitations, and (7) availability of antifungal drugs. In the Indian setting, emergence of non-albicans Candida particularly *C. tropicalis, C. auris* and change in susceptibility to azoles among *C albicans* and non-albicans Candida are strikingly unique. As a soil fungus, not uncommonly, aspergillus infection is seen in the immunocompetent host setting, particularly with farm/agricultural environment. Also, a very high incidence of mucormycosis and unique presentations of infections due to aspergillus and mucor are noteworthy. Other critical factors to consider during the management of IFI include excessive empiric use of antimicrobial drugs with consequent emergence of multi-drug-resistant pathogens, poor quality control of drugs, and limited diagnostic capabilities for IFI.

References

1. Patterson TF, Thompson GR III, Denning DW, et al. Executive summary: practice guidelines for the diagnosis and management of aspergillosis: 2016 update by the Infectious Diseases Society of America. Clin Infect Dis. 2016;63:433–42.
2. Pappas PJ, Kauffman C, Andes DR, et al. Clinical practice guideline for the management of candidiasis: 2016 update by the Infectious Diseases Society of America. Clin Infect Dis. 2016;62:e1–e50.
3. Tissot F, Agrawal S, Pagano L, et al. ECIL-6 guidelines for the treatment of invasive candidiasis, aspergillosis and mucormycosis in leukemia and hematopoietic stem cell transplant patients. Haematologica. 2017:102433–44.
4. Schelenz S, Barnes RA, Barton RC, et al. British Society for Medical Mycology best practice recommendations for the diagnosis of serious fungal diseases. Lancet Infect Dis. 2015;15:461–74.
5. Bongomin F, Gago S, Oladele RO. Global and multi-national prevalence of fungal diseases—estimate precision. J Fungi. 2017;3(57):1–29.
6. Rotjanapan P, Chen YC, Chakrabarti A, et al. Epidemiology and clinical characteristics of invasive mould infections: a multicenter, retrospective analysis in five Asian countries. Med Mycol. 2018;56:186–96.
7. Ullmann AJ, Aguado JM, Arikan-Akdagli S, et al. Diagnosis and management of Aspergillus diseases: executive summary of the 2017 ESCMID ECMM-ERS guideline. Clin Microbiol Infect. 2018;24(Suppl 1):e1–e38.
8. Singh T, Kashyap AK, Ahluwalia G, et al. Epidemiology of fungal infections in critical care setting of a tertiary care teaching hospital in North India: a prospective surveillance study. J Clin Sci Res. 2014;3:14–25.
9. Slavin MA, Thursky KA, Worth LJ, et al. Introduction to the updated Australian and New Zealand consensus guidelines for the use of antifungal agents in the haematology/oncology setting, 2014. Intern Med J. 2014;44:1267–76.
10. Morrissey CO, Gilroy NM, Macesic N, et al. Consensus guidelines for the use of empiric and diagnostic-driven antifungal treatment strategies in haematological malignancy, 2014. Intern Med J. 2014;44:1298–314.

11. Fleming S, Yannakou CK, Haeusler GM, et al. Consensus guidelines for antifungal prophylaxis in haematological malignancy and haemopoietic stem cell transplantation, 2014. Intern Med J. 2014;44:1283–97.
12. Blyth CC, Gilroy NM, Guy SD, et al. Consensus guidelines for the treatment of invasive mould infections in haematological malignancy and haemopoietic stem cell transplantation, 2014. Intern Med J. 2014;44:1333–49.
13. Cornely OA, Arikan-Akdagli S, Dannaoui E, et al. European Society of Clinical Microbiology and Infectious Diseases Fungal Infection Study Group; European Confederation of Medical Mycology. ESCMID and ECMM joint clinical guidelines for the diagnosis and management of mucormycosis 2013. Clin Microbiol Infect. 2014;20 Suppl 3:5–26.
14. Girmenia C, Aversa F, Busca A, et al. Invasive Fungal Infections Cooperative Group of the European Organization for Research and Treatment of Cancer. A hematology consensus agreement on antifungal strategies for neutropenic patients with hematological malignancies and stem cell transplant recipients. Invasive Fungal Infections Cooperative Group of the European Organization for Research and Treatment of Cancer. Hematol Oncol. 2013;31:117–26.
15. Leroux S, Ullmann AJ. Management and diagnostic guidelines for fungal diseases in infectious diseases and clinical microbiology: critical appraisal. Clin Microbiol Infect. 2013;19:1115–21.
16. Chen SC, Sorrell TC, Chang CC, et al. Consensus guidelines for the treatment of yeast infections in the haematology, oncology and intensive care setting, 2014. Intern Med J. 2014;44:1315–32.
17. Ullmann AJ, Akova M, Herbrecht R, et al. ESCMID Fungal Infection Study Group. ESCMID guideline for the diagnosis and management of Candida diseases 2012: adults with haematological malignancies and after haematopoietic stem cell transplantation (HCT). Clin Microbiol Infect. 2012;18 Suppl 7:53–67.
18. Maertens J, Marchetti O, Herbrecht R, et al. Third European Conference on Infections in Leukemia. European guidelines for antifungal management in leukemia and hematopoietic stem cell transplant recipients: summary of the ECIL 3—2009 update. Bone Marrow Transplant. 2011;46:709–18.
19. Kullberg BJ, Verweij PE, Akova M, et al. European expert opinion on the management of invasive candidiasis in adults. Clin Microbiol Infect. 2011;17(Suppl 5):1–12.
20. Grossi PA, Gasperina DD, Barchiesi F, et al. Italian guidelines for diagnosis, prevention, and treatment of invasive fungal infections in solid organ transplant recipients. Transplant Proc. 2011;43:2463–71.
21. Prentice AG, Glasmacher A, Hobson RP, et al. Guidelines on the management of invasive fungal infection during therapy for haematological malignancy. British Committee for Standards in Haematology. March 2010. Electronic online version only. www.mycology.adelaide.edu.
22. Flückiger U, Marchetti O, Bille J, et al. Fungal Infection Network of Switzerland (FUNGINOS). Treatment options of invasive fungal infections in adults. Swiss Med Wkly. 2006;136:447–63.
23. Ruhnke M, Rickerts V, Cornely OA, et al. German Speaking Mycological Society, Paul-Ehrlich-Society for Chemotherapy. Diagnosis and therapy of Candida infections: joint recommendations of the German Speaking Mycological Society and the Paul-Ehrlich-Society for Chemotherapy. Mycoses. 2011;54:279–310.
24. Maertens JA, Raad II, Marr KA, et al. Isavuconazole versus voriconazole for primary treatment of invasive mould disease caused by Aspergillus and other filamentous fungi (SECURE): a phase 3, randomised-controlled, non-inferiority trial. Lancet. 2016;387:760–9.
25. Jenks JD, Salzer HJ, Prattes J, et al. Spotlight on isavuconazole in the treatment of invasive aspergillosis and mucormycosis: design, development, and place in therapy. Drug Des Devel Ther. 2018;30(12):1033–44.
26. Pfaller MA, Rhomberg PR, Wiederhold NP, et al. In vitro activity of isavuconazole against opportunistic fungal pathogens from two mycology reference laboratories. Antimicrob Agents Chemother. 2018;62:e01230–18.
27. Herbrecht R, Kuessner D, Pooley N, et al. Systematic review and network meta-analysis of clinical outcomes associated with isavuconazole versus relevant comparators for patients with invasive aspergillosis. Curr Med Res Opin. 2018;17:1–9.

28. Bagshaw E, Enoch DA, Blackney M, et al. Economic impact of treating invasive mold disease with isavuconazole compared with liposomal amphotericin B in the UK. Future Microbiol. 2018;13:1283–93.
29. Ledoux MP, Toussaint E, Denis J, et al. New pharmacological opportunities for the treatment of invasive mould diseases. J Antimicrob Chemother. 2017;72(Suppl 1):i48–58.
30. Groll AH, Townsend R, Desai A, et al. Drug-drug interactions between triazole antifungal agents used to treat invasive aspergillosis and immunosuppressants metabolized by cytochrome P450 3A4. Transpl Infect Dis. 2017;19:e12751.
31. Giri S, Kindo AJ. A review of *Candida* species causing blood stream infection. Indian Rev Med Microbiol. 2012;30:270–8.
32. Prasad RR, Shree V, Sagar S, et al. Prevalence and antifungal susceptibility of *Candida albicans* in Patna, India. Int J Curr Microbiol App Sci. 2016;5:957–61.
33. Falagas ME, Roussos N, Vardakas KZ. Relative frequency of albicans and the various non-albicans Candida spp among candidemia isolates from inpatients in various parts of the world: a systematic review. Int J Infect Dis. 2010;14:e954–66.
34. Chakrabarti A, Chatterjee SS, Rao KL, Zameer MM, Shivaprakash MR, Singhi S, Singh R, Varma SC. Recent experience with fungaemia: change in species distribution and azole resistance. Scand J Infect Dis. 2009;41:275–84.
35. Singla N, Gulati N, Kaistha N, et al. Candida colonization in urine samples of ICU patients: determination of etiology, antifungal susceptibility testing and evaluation of associated risk factors. Mycopathologia. 2012;174:149–55.
36. Jain M, Dogra V, Mishra B, et al. Candiduria in catheterized intensive care unit patients: emerging microbiological trends. Indian J Pathol Microbiol. 2011;54:552–5.
37. Chakrabarti A, Sood P, Rudramurthy SM, et al. Incidence, characteristics and outcome of ICU-acquired candidemia in India. Intensive Care Med. 2015;41:285–95.
38. Yesudhason BL, Mohanram K. Candida tropicalis as a predominant isolate from clinical specimens and its antifungal susceptibility pattern in a Tertiary Care Hospital in Southern India. J Clin Diagn Res. 2015;9:DC14–6.
39. Bhattacharjee P. Epidemiology and antifungal susceptibility of Candida species in a tertiary care hospital, Kolkata, India. Curr Med Mycol. 2016;2:20–7.
40. Rajalakshmi A, Shareek PS, Sureshkumar D, et al. Candidemia species distribution and emergence of Candida haemulonii complex isolates resistant to fluconazole in South India. J Contemp Clin Pract. 2018;4:47–52.
41. Sundaram C, Umabala P, Laxmi V, et al. Pathology of fungal infections in the central nervous system: 17 years' experience from Southern India. Histopathology. 2006;49:396–405.
42. Shankar SK, Mahadevan A, Sundaram C, Sarkar C, et al. Pathobiology of fungal infections of the central nervous system with special reference to Indian scenario. Neurol India. 2007;55:198–215.
43. Chakrabarti A, Shivaprakash MR, Singh R, Tarai B, et al. Fungal endophthalmitis: fourteen years' experience from a center in India. Retina. 2008;28:1400–7.
44. Kullberg BJ, Viscoli C, Pappas PG, et al. Treatment of candidemia and other invasive candida infections: the ACTIVE trial. Clin Infect Dis. 2018;68:1981–9. https://doi.org/10.1093/cid/ciy827.
45. Chowdhary A, Sharma C, Duggal S, et al. New clonal strain of Candida auris, Delhi, India. Emerg Infect Dis. 2013;19:1670–3.
46. Lockhart SR, Etienne KA, Vallabhaneni S, et al. Simultaneous emergence of multidrug-resistant *Candida auris* on 3 continents confirmed by whole-genome sequencing and epidemiological analyses. Clin Infect Dis. 2017;64:134–40.
47. Vallabhaneni S, Kallen A, Tsay S, et al. Investigation of the first seven reported cases of *Candida auris*, a globally emerging invasive, multidrug-resistant fungus-United States, May 2013-August 2016. MMWR Morb Mortal Wkly Rep. 2016;65:1234–7.
48. Rudramurthy SM, Chakrabarti A, Paul RA, et al. *Candida auris* candidaemia in Indian ICUs: analysis of risk factors. J Antimicrob Chemother. 2017;72:1794–801.

49. Mathur P, Hasan F, Singh PK, Malhotra R, Walia K, Chowdhary A. Five-year profile of candidaemia at an Indian trauma centre: high rates of *Candida auris* blood stream infections. Mycoses. 2018;61:674–80. https://doi.org/10.1111/myc.12790.
50. Schelenz S, Hagen F, Rhodes JL, et al. First hospital outbreak of the globally emerging *Candida auris* in a European hospital. Antimicrob Resist Infect Control. 2016;5: 2–7.
51. Chowdhary A, Sharma C, Meis JF. *Candida auris*: a rapidly emerging cause of hospital-acquired multidrug-resistant fungal infections globally. PLoS Pathog. 2017;13:e1006290.
52. Chakrabarti A, Singh R. The emerging epidemiology of mould infections in developing countries. Curr Opin Infect Dis. 2011;24:521–6.
53. Chakrabarti A, Chatterjee SS, Das A, et al. Invasive aspergillosis in developing countries. Med Mycol. 2011;49(Suppl 1):S35–47.
54. Rotjanapan P, Chen YC, Chakrabarti A, Li RY, Rudramurthy SM, Yu J, Kung HC, Watcharananan S, Tan AL, Saffari SE, Tan BH. Epidemiology and clinical characteristics of invasive mould infections: a multicenter, retrospective analysis in five Asian countries. Med Mycol. 2018;56(2):186–96.
55. Rudramurthy SM, de Valk HA, Chakrabarti A, et al. High resolution genotyping of clinical Aspergillus flavus isolates from India using microsatellites. PLoS One. 2011;6:e16086.
56. Xess I, Mohanty S, Jain N, Banerjee U. Prevalence of *Aspergillus* species in clinical samples isolated in an Indian tertiary care hospital. Indian J Med Sci. 2004;58:513–9.
57. Sivsankari S, Senthamarai S, Anitha C, et al. Prevalence of invasive aspergillosis among (PTB) patients in Kanchipuram, India. J Clin Diagn Res. 2014;8:22–3.
58. Chowdhary A, Kathuria S, Randhawa HS, et al. Isolation of multiple-triazole-resistant *Aspergillus fumigatus* strain carrying the TR/L98H mutations in the *cyp*51A gene in India. J Antimicrob Chemother. 2012;67:362–6.
59. Dabas Y, Xess I, Bakshi S, et al. Emergence of azole-resistant *Aspergillus fumigatus* from immunocompromised hosts in India. Antimicrob Agents Chemother. 2018;62: e02264–17.
60. Lestrade PPA, Meis JF, Melchers WJG, et al. Triazole resistance in *Aspergillus fumigatus*: recent insights and challenges for patient management. Clin Microbiol Infect. 2019;25(7):799–806. pii: S1198-743X(18)30780-8. https://doi.org/10.1016/j.cmi.2018.11.027.
61. Agarwal R, Denning DW, Chakrabarti A. Estimation of the burden of chronic and allergic pulmonary aspergillosis in India. PLoS One. 2014;9:e114745.
62. Maturu VN, Agarwal R. Itraconazole in chronic pulmonary aspergillosis: in whom, for how long, and at what dose? Lung India. 2015;32:309–12.
63. Sanath SS, Gogtay NJ, Kshirsagar NA. Post marketing study to assess the safety, tolerability and effectiveness of Fungisome: and Indian liposomal amphotericin B preparation. J Postgrad Med. 2005;51(Suppl 1):S58–63.
64. Rudramuthy SM, Jatana M, Singh R, et al. In *vitro* antifungal activity of Indian liposomal amphotericin B against clinical isolates of emerging species of yeast and moulds, and its comparison with amphotericin B deoxycholate, voriconazole, itraconazole and fluconazole. Mycoses. 2013;56:39–46.
65. Jadhav MP, Shinde VM, Chandrakala S, et al. A randomized comparative trial evaluating the safety and efficacy of liposomal amphotericin B (Fungisome) versus conventional amphotericin B in the empirical treatment of febrile neutropenia in India. Indian J Cancer. 2012;49: 107–13.
66. Bala K, Chander J, Handa U, et al. A prospective study of mucormycosis in North India: experience from a tertiary care hospital. Med Mycol. 2015;53:248–57.
67. Chakrabarti A, Singh R. Mucormycosis in India: unique features. Mycoses. 2014;57(Suppl 3):85–90.
68. Chakrabarti A, Dhaliwal M. Epidemiology of Mucormycosis in India. Curr Fungal Infect Rep. 2013;7:287–92.

69. Prakash H, Ghosh AK, Rudramurthy SM, et al. A prospective multicenter study on mucormycosis in India: epidemiology, diagnosis, and treatment. Med Mycol. 2019;57(4):395–402. https://doi.org/10.1093/mmy/myy060.
70. Manesh A, Rupali P, Sullivan MO, Raj PM, Rupa V, George B, Michael JS. Mucormycosis—a clinicoepidemiological review of cases over 10 years. Mycoses. 2019;62(4):391–8. https://doi.org/10.1111/myc.12897.
71. Marty FM, Ostrosky-Zeichner L, Cornely OA, et al. VITAL and FungiScope Mucormycosis Investigators. Isavuconazole treatment for mucormycosis: a single-arm open-label trial and case-control analysis. Lancet Infect Dis. 2016;16:828–37.

The manufacturer's authorised representative in the EU is Springer Nature Customer Service Centre GmbH, Europaplatz 3, 69115 Heidelberg, Germany. If you have any concerns regarding our products, please contact ProductSafety@springernature.com

Printed and bound by CPI Group (UK) Ltd, Croydon, CR0 4YY
24/07/2026
02175931-0006